ILLUSTRATED GUIDE
TO
GUIDE
HOMOEOPATHIC
TREATMENT

By

DR. HARBANS SINGH KHANEJA

B.Sc; R.M.P. (India) R.HOM (Canada)
Former Senior Vice President,
The Homoeopathic Medical Association
of India, Punjab State.

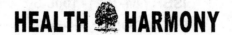

HEALTH 🌳 HARMONY

Published by :
Kuldeep Jain
For

HEALTH ⚕ HARMONY
an imprint of
B. Jain Publishers (P) Ltd.
1921, Street No. 10, Chuna Mandi,
Paharganj, New Delhi 110 055 (INDIA)
Phones : 3670430; 3670572; 3683200, 3683300
FAX : 011-3610471 & 3683400
Email : bjain@vsnl.com
Website : www.bjainindia.com

Printed in India by:
Unisons Techno Financial Consultants (P) Ltd.
522, FIE, Patpar Ganj, Delhi - 110 092

ISBN : 81-7021- 1006-6
BOOK CODE : BK-5450

PREFACE TO THE FIRST EDITION

The illustrated guide to homoeopathic treatment has been specially written for the benefit of the students of homoeopathy and laymen who want to treat their own diseases. Simple language and easy words have been used for easy understanding.

Illustrations are given where necessary. Diseases have been described for treatment in a non-boring way. This guide is useful as "Teacher's Notes" of practical homoeopathic therapeutics. Remedies have been arranged alphabetically for sake of convenience. That is not all. This book will also be found useful by the homoeopathic medical practitioners as being a short cut to the repertory of the homoeopathic materia medica and for easy selection of a remedy.

No definite and scientific guide is available for the selection of a potency. Some practitioners use high potencies with success and others use low potencies with satisfactory results. I use high potencies in chronic cases and low in acute and recent cases. I consider 30 C potency neither low nor high. Thus selection of a potency is a matter of one's own choice and experience. In this book where Q is mentioned against a remedy, it means mother tincture, where X is mentioned beside the potency, it means potency in decimal scale and where neither of these two are mentioned, it means potency in the centesimal scale and where no potency is mentioned, it means 30 in this scale.

It will be agreed that diseases like death, old age, etc. (about 10% in all) are not curable. Likewise all the diseases cannot be cured by oral medicines alone. Surgery is required in some cases like,fracture of bones,etc. I have given methods of surgery employed by surgeons in some cases because questions about it are generally asked by students as well as patients. Machines like X-rays, ultrasound scan or magnetic resonance imaging unit (M. R. I), etc. are used in surgical cases and also in some other cases. M. R. I. gives incredible snap shots of the body for detection of bone marrow illness, disorders of ligaments and cartilages and their injuries. It also detects tumors and nervous disorders.

Microscopic and other laboratory tests are useful in their own way like examination of stools for the presence and kind of worms,urine for presence of casts, etc. and blood for its disorders. Use of machines makes it easier for the homoeopath to treat the diseases and save the patient from surgery in several cases. It is very important that the cause of disease be known so that, the treatment can be directed at the source of the problem.

Our life depends upon the diet taken. Useful suggestions as to what can be taken and what should not be taken during ailments are given in each chapter. Medical science is a continuous process of study and research. Results of latest studies and research, as collected from various journals and news papers are incorporated to keep the homoeopaths abreast of the latest developments. I hope that this multipurpose book will be found useful by laymen, students, teachers of homoeopathy, homoeopathic medical practitioners, researchers and all those who love homoeopathy.

HARBANS SINGH KHANEJA

3134 MERRITT AVENUE,
MISSISSAUGA(ONTARIO),
CANADA L4T-IP3.

ACKNOWLEDGEMENTS

It is my pleasant duty to express my gratitude to thousands and thousands of different individuals who came to me for treatment since more than 50 years of my homoeopathic practice. They gave me all the practical knowledge and experience. My debt of gratitude also goes to several authors of homoeopathic books from whom I acquired the theoretical knowledge.

I remained as a president of the Homoeopathic Medical Association, Jalandhar (Punjab) and the senior vice president of its Punjab State Branch for several years. I continue to be a member of the National United Professional Association of Trained Homoeopaths in Canada. These two associations deserve my special thanks for enabling me to attend several homoeopathic conferences and seminars which added to my knowledge.

My thanks are also due to my wife Mrs. Harbans Kaur Khaneja who took off all the domestic worries from my shoulders during the years I remained busy writing this book. My thanks are also due to Dr. Jasleen Kaur Khaneja, D. H. M. S., Gold Medalist, for typing the book for me.

HARBANS SINGH KHANEJA

3134 MERRITT AVENUE,
MISSISSAUGA (ONTARIO),
CANADA L4T-IP3.

FOREWORD

It gives me pleasure to acknowledge that I read the pre-released copy of the "Illustrated Guide to Homoeopathic Treatment", by Dr. Harbans Singh Khaneja. The author has taken pains in compiling and arranging the guidelines for the homoeopathic treatment. He has given very valuable suggestions for taking selective foods during ailments. He has also given methods of surgery and has compared the conventional treatment with the homoeopathic treatment at places. He has suggested further fields of research for researchers. Naturally such a work cannot be very perfect and complete and reference to materia medica, etc. may become necessary in some cases. In my opinion this book is revolutionary and will prove useful for all the lovers of homoeopathy.

DR. FAROKH J. MASTER
Camp TORONTO M. D. (HOM)
Canada.

24th NOV, 98
Ratan Abad , Ground Floor,
Tukaram Javji Road,
In Bhatia Hospital Lane,
Bombay - 400 007,
India.

CONTENTS

■■

ABDOMEN

ABIES NIG. : Sensation of a lump at the cardiac end of stomach.

ACETICUM ACIDUM, AMMONIUM CARB., MEDORRHINUM, PODOPHYLLUM, STRAMONIUM : Feels relieved by lying on the abdomen.

AMBRA GRISEA : Sensation of weakness in the abdomen, in old people after passing a stool.

APOCYNUM CAN. 3X : Bloated due to dropsy. Has a very quick action. Reduces waist and weight within a month.

BACILLINIUM 200 : Once every 15 days, when abdomen is distended in thin, rickety children.

CALCAREA CARB. : Distention of abdomen in fat, scrofulous children. Increase of fat generally. Abdomen is sensitive to slightest touch and pressure. Patient cannot bear tight clothing around the waist.

CARBO VEG. : Distention of abdomen with contraction pain which extends to the chest. Cannot bear tight clothing around the waist and abdomen. Better passing wind.

CINA : Distention due to worms.

COLCHICUM AUTUM. : Abdomen bloated with gas. Cannot stretch legs.

CONIUM MAC. : Sensation of a lump about the liver region.

DIOSCOREA : Distention due to wind with pain in the belly.

HEDEOMA : Everything taken into the stomach causes pain.

KALIUM BICH. : Cutting pain in the abdomen, soon after eating.

KALIUM CARB. : Sensation of a lump in the pit of the stomach.

LYCOPODIUM : Distention of abdomen with or without constipation and due to flatulence.

LYCOPODIUM, RHUS TOX. : Abdomen is bloated immediately after a light meal.

MAGNESIUM PHOS. : Bloating of abdomen due to pain. Must pass flatus constantly.

PLUMBUM MET. : Sensation of abdomen being drawn to the spine by a string.

PODOPHYLLUM : Enlarged and hanging abdomen after giving birth to a baby.

SANICULA AQUA : Pot bellied children.

SELENIUM MET. : Sensation of pulsations in the abdomen after eating.

SEPIA : Pot bellied or distended abdomen in women, after giving birth to several children. Many brown spots on abdomen.

SILICEA	: Distention of abdomen in children generally with large heads and weak legs.
STAPHYSAGRIA	: Burning pains in the scar after abdominal operation.
SULPHUR	: Large abdomen of unmarried girls at puberty. Movements in the abdomen as if there is something alive in it.
TABACUM	: Wants abdomen uncovered.
THUJA OCC., CROCUS SAT.	: Hard distention with a feeling as if a living child or an animal were in the abdomen. Sense of fake pregnancy.
URANIUM NIT., KALIUM CARB., DOLICHOS	: Abdomen bloated with gas. Kali-c. has abdominal pain due to gas.

ABORTION (MISCARRIAGE)

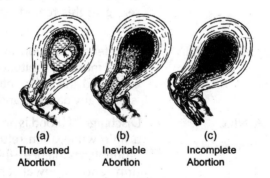

(a)	(b)	(c)
Threatened Abortion	Inevitable Abortion	Incomplete Abortion

ACONITUM NAP. 200	: If the abortion is threatened due to fear and excitement, repeat this remedy every 15 minutes.
ALETRIS FAR. Q	: Habitual tendency to abortion due to weakness and anemia.

APIS MEL.	: For abortion during 1st and 3rd months of the pregnancy.
ARNICA MONT.	: Threatened abortion due to an accident, shock and injury.
CAULOPHYLLUM 3X	: It is as helpful as Vib-p. in habitual abortions and when it is due to a weak uterus.
CHAMOMILLA	: If the abortion is threatened due to mental excitement.
CROCUS SAT.	: Threatened abortion during the first month of pregnancy.
CROTALUS H. 200	: If there is oozing of black blood which does not coagulate. Miscarriage during course of a septic disease or from other blood poisoning.
HELONIAS Q	: Use 5-10 drops 1/2 hourly if the abortion is threatened from over exertion or irritating emotions.
IPECACUANHA Q	: If there is a continuous flow of bright red blood, colic and nausea, give this remedy every 1/2 hour.
KALIUM CARB., SABINA	: Threatened abortion in the 2nd or 3rd month. Habitual abortion every 2nd and 3rd month. Blood is generally dark red and clotted.
PULSATILLA NIG.	: Discharge of blood is arrested for a little while, then returns with redoubled violence; this cessation and renewal are often repeated. Passes black blood with labor pains.
SEPIA 200	: Threatened abortion during 5-7 months of pregnancy.

SECALE COR.	: For abortion, more especially about the third month with copious flow of black, liquid blood.
SYPHILINUM	: Abortion due to syphilis.
THUJA OCC.	: It mends the tendency to abortion specially in women having a gonorrheal history in themselves or in their family.
THYROIDINUM	: It helps to avoid miscarriage and tendency to premature labor when the cause is not of a mechanical origin. It controls slow oozing from the uterus. Prevents threatened abortion when there is thyroid dysfunction.
TRILLIUM PEND. 3X, FICUS IND. Q	: Checks bleeding of abortion. Very effective remedies.
TUBERCULINUM	: Abortion due to tuberculosis.
VIBURNUM PRUN. Q, VIBURNUM OP. Q	: Their use helps to prevent habitual miscarriages. They also help to prevent abortion due to an accident or due to drugging.

ABORTION PRODUCING

Several countries have laws that make it illegal to cause an abortion in the healthy females. The following course can be tried only when the continuing of the pregnancy can cause damage to the health of the patient or to the baby when born and that also keeping in view the law of the land. It is risky to cause abortion after 12 weeks of pregnancy. It can cause complications.

1.   GOSSYPIUM Q + MACROTINUM Q - mixed in equal quantity and given in 40 drops a doze, thrice daily causes abortion within five days. If it does not occur in five days, wait for five more days before trying the second course. More than two courses are not advisable. Stop the treatment when the bleeding starts.

2.   CARICA PAPAYA Q induces abortion when locally applied to the mouth of the uterus.

NOTE : Both the treatments should be given simultaneously.

ABORTION, ILL EFFECTS OF

ARSENICUM ALB., NATRIUM MUR.	: Try either of the remedies when the patient has a feeling of a guilt having aborted.
CHINA OFF	: For weakness due to excessive bleeding.
KALIUM CARB.	: Removes weakness remaining after labor or miscarriage.
NUX VOM.	: Hemorrhage after abortion with sensation as if bowels wanted to move.
PULSATILLA NIG. Q	: It expedites expulsion of the fetus.
PYROGENIUM 200	: When there is fever and a danger of septicemia.
SABINA	: Pain in the lower back and genitals.
SEPIA	: Use it when the placenta has not been expelled or has been expelled partially.

THUJA OCC., PSORINUM : If there is a danger of illness after the miscarriage try either of the remedies according to the symptoms.

TRILLIUM PEND.Q : Give 5 drop doses every two hours if the bleeding prolongs in case of an induced abortion.

ABSCESS

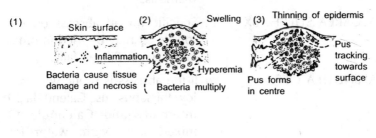

(1) Skin surface
Inflammation
Bacteria cause tissue damage and necrosis

(2) Swelling
Hyperemia
Bacteria multiply

(3) Thinning of epidermis
Pus tracking towards surface
Pus forms in centre

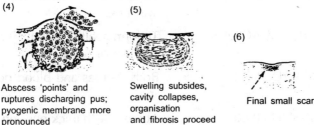

(4) Abscess 'points' and ruptures discharging pus; pyogenic membrane more pronounced

(5) Swelling subsides, cavity collapses, organisation and fibrosis proceed

(6) Final small scar

ANTHRACINUM IM : Carbuncles and boils with intense burning and high fever.

APIS MEL. : When there is swelling and pain is stinging and burning like the one produced by the sting of a honey bee. But there is no pus.

ARSENICUM ALB. : Unhealthy abscess which discharges offensive pus with burning. Restlessness and fever may be present.

BELLADONNA : Use it in the early stages when there is not much of swelling but there is redness and throbbing pain. Abscess and inflammation of the breast. The use of Belladonna will cure it. If Belladonna fails to cure, use Hep. after it.

CALCAREA CARB. 200 : Abscess in patients of tubercular diathesis.

CALCAREA SULPH. 6X : Specific for an abscess on the tonsils. It may be tried in other cases when Silicea fails.

CALENDULA OFF. : If the abscess is septic with yellow thick pus, use Calendula 30 internally and Calendula Q mixed with warm water for washing.

FLUORICUM ACIDUM : To form healthy granulation after the use of Silicea.

GUNPOWDER 3X : Boils, herpes and blood poisoning.

HEPAR SULPHURIS : Abscess with thick pus and great throbbing pain. When given in high potency (200 C) it will abort the pus and if given in low(3X) potency, will often open up the abscess. It is useful in the abscess near the ear. It is also useful in case of abscess in lungs. In 2X or 3X potency,it hastens suppuration and 1M or 10M potency checks suppuration.

MERCURIUS SOL. : If the pus has formed and the abscess is taking a septic form. The skin becomes bluish.

MYRISTICA SEB. : It often acts better and powerfully in the opening of abscess. It is known as a homoeopathic knife. Very effective for abscess at the end of fingers and phallenges.

PYROGENIUM IM : Recurring abscess, fever and septic conditions are cured by the use of this remedy.

RHUS TOX. : Abscess near the arm pit or the parotid gland. Pus is mixed with blood. It is useful for suppurating glands. Pus is thin, copious and corroding.

SILICEA : Ripens abscess and promotes suppuration. It helps to heal a boil which is of an obstinate nature.

STAPHYSAGRIA : Use it in the case of an abscess in the lumbar region.

SYMPHYTUM OFF. : After amputation of any part of the body or a limb, if an abscess is formed on the remaining part.

TARENTULA CUB. 200 : It is almost specific for an abscess in the armpit. One dose reduces the pain and either opens up the abscess when it is very ripe or aborts it. Hep. also acts likewise in such cases.

ABSENT MINDEDNESS
(SEE MEMORY)

ABUSIVENESS

ANACARDIUM ORI. : Tendency to use violent abusive language. The patient is generally mentally disturbed and wants to swear and curse. He uses abusive language during debates and discussions.

HYOSCYAMUS NIG. 200 : The patient is talkative and uses obscene and filthy language while talking. He will abuse if somebody engages him in arguments or when he suspects that somebody is doing mischief to him.

LILIUM TIG. : Constant inclination to weep and depressed; on being consoled uses abusive and obscene language for the person consoling him.

TUBERCULINUM 1M : The patient is cruel and destructive and desires to use foul language, curse and swear.

ACIDITY (HEARTBURN)

Heartburn is substernal (behind the chest bone) pain and burning sensation, usually associated with reflux of gastric juices into the oesophagus.

ACIDUM PHOS.

: Pyrosis with flatulence, diarrhea and debility. Thirst for cold milk. Craves juicy things.

ACIDUM SULPH.

: Chronic acidity. Burning in oesophagus. Nausea. If vomiting is very sour, even the teeth feel sour. Eructations are sour. Craves alcohol.

AMMONIUM CARB.

: Heartburn with pain in the pit of stomach. Nausea and waterbrash.

ARGENTUM NIT.

: Acidity and sour eructations in nervousness due to anticipation of coming events. Desire for sweets.

CALCAREA CARB.

: Acidity with pain in the chest and longing for cold drinks. Heartburn with loud belching. Great desire for eggs.

CAPSICUM

: Smarting in the stomach and oesophagus as if red pepper was sprayed there. Shuddering after each drink. Intense desire for stimulants.

CARBO VEG.

: Acidity after meals. Flatus is fetid. Much eructations, which relieve flatulence.

CONIUM MAC. 200

: Heartburn with nausea worse after going to bed and after few hours of taking meals. Amelioration from eating.

IRIS VERS.

: Hyperacidity. Sour and bitter belching, nausea and vomiting of bitter fluids, etc.

NATRIUM PHOS. 6X

: For an occasional acidity. Flatulence with sour risings. Spits mouthful of food. Specially suited to children.

NUX VOM.

: Acidity after about half an hour of taking food.

PULSATILLA NIG.

: Acidity after taking rich fatty food. There is no thirst or very little thirst.

ROBINIA

: Acidity worse at night. Vomiting. Acidity in children. Irritating eructations and frontal headache.

STRONTIUM BROM.

: It is an anti-fermentative and neutralizes excessive acidity. Nervous dyspepsia.

NOTE : To avoid acidity:
1. **Do not lie down soon after eating.**
2. **If overweight, lose weight.**
3. **Do not smoke or cut down smoking.**
4. **Avoid fatty and spicy foods, alcohol and foods containing caffeine.**
5. **In general, fruits and vegetables are alkali producing foods.**
6. **A cup full of cold milk without sugar taken during the attack,gives immediate but temporary relief.**

ACNE

(PIMPLES AND BLOTCHES i.e. PIMPLES WITH PUS)

Acne is one of the most common skin problem. It develops at puberty (teenage) when the sebaceous glands are most active. In the twenties, it gradually decreases, and is again seen, especially in women after the age of 28 (past-adolescent acne). It occurs in both girls and boys; in the latter, in a somewhat severer form.

ANTIMONIUM CRUD. : Pimples on the face and shoulders of fat persons with dry skin and indigestion.

ARSENICUM BROM. : Acne rosacea. Violet papules on nose; worse in spring weather. Pimples on face, nose, upper lip and chin of young girls.

ARSENICUM ALB. : Acne of the nose.

ASTERIAS RUB. : Red pimples on the sides of nose, chin and mouth. Pimples in the period between puberty and maturity.

BELLADONNA : Red pimples. May be burning and may be painful.

BERBERIS AQ. : Dry pimples. Blotches and pimples

BORAX 3X : Pimples on the nose and lips.

CALCAREA PHOS. 6X : Acne of anemic girls at puberty with menstrual troubles.

CALCAREA SULPH. : Pimples and pustules on the face and around the ears; discharging a yellowish secretion.

CALCAREA CARB.	:	Little pimples on the roots of the hair which bleed when scratched, in fat and flabby girls.
CALOTROPIS	:	It heals the ulcers and blotches from the skin and perfects the cure.
CAUSTICUM	:	Acne of the nose.
EUGENIA JAM.	:	Simple and indurated acne. Painful pimples. Blackhead pimples. Red pimples and rosy skin on the sides of the nose, chin and mouth. Useful for all ages.
FAGOPYRUM	:	Red and sore blotches here and there and also on the hairy parts. Itching worse by scratching.
GRAPHITES	:	Acne worse during and after periods, with a dry skin.
HEPAR SULPHURIS	:	Pimples which suppurate with white pus. May be as large as a pea.
HYDROCOTYLE A. 3X	:	Great dryness of the skin. Acne of red color on the face, nose and chin.
JUGLANS REG.	:	Blackhead and acne on the face. Red pustules.
KALIUM BROM.	:	Itchy pimples on the face, chest and shoulders. Blackheads, pustules with a depressed centre as if papular eruptions of smallpox with burning and pain. Acne may be associated with increased sexual urge, hormonal changes or puberty. It also helps removal of scars left after the cure of acne.

KALIUM MUR.	: Vesicular type of acne containing thick white contents.
KALIUM ARS.	: Acne; pustules worse during menses.
LEDUM PAL.	: Red pimples on the forehead and cheeks.
MAGNESIUM MUR.	: Pimples on face and forehead which appear before the start of menses and when the patient is constipated.
MEDORRHINUM 1M	: Blotches of red color on the face.
MERCURIUS SOL.	: Pimples. Vesicular and pustular eruptions along with the pimples. Skin is always moist with viscid sweat.
NATRIUM MUR. 200	: Pimples with oily skin. Earthy complexion.
OOPHORINUM 3X	: Acne rosacea and other skin disorders during climacteric.
PULSATILLA NIG.	: Pimples worse at puberty and at the start of menstruation especially in girls who are overweight and have delayed menses.
RADIUM BROM.	: Small pimples with itching, burning, swelling and redness. Great burning is the keynote for the use of this remedy. Acne rosacea, birth marks, moles and ulcers are influenced by its use.
SELENIUM MET.	: Black pimples and black corns.
SEPIA	: Pimples on the forehead near the root of hair.
SILICEA	: Rose colored blotches. Skin pale and waxy. Patient is chilly.

STREPTOCOCCINUM 200 : Chronic cases resisting treatment.

SULPHUR   : Acne in the orifice of the eye.

TARENTULA CUB.   : Septic, burning and painful red pimples.

THUJA OCC. 1M   : Blotches (i. e. pimples with pus) worse after scratching. An excellent remedy for acne on face. The skin is dry.

ACNE FACE LOTION

Take one gram (5 ml) each of BERBERIS AQUIFOLIUM Q, LEDUM PALUSTRE Q and ECHINACEA Q. Mix all the three with one ounce of glycerine and rub on the face which has previously been washed with soap and water and dried. It improves the complexion also. If desired, mustard oil can be used instead of glycerine. It is more useful as it contains Rhodallin which disolves scar tissue.

It is a very useful lotion and may obviate necessity for using any other medicine orally.

ADENOIDS

Hypertrophy of the adenoid tissue (pharyngeal tonsil) that normally exists in the nasopharynx of children.

AGRAPHIS NUTANS   : Child breathes through the mouth and has enlarged tonsils. Adenoids of the throat. Deafness. A good remedy for the disease.

BACILLINUM 200, TUBERCULINUM	: Weak children with history of TB in the family. Give a dose of either, weekly and start the treatment with this remedy.
BARYTA IOD. 3X	: Mentally retarded children and attacks of tonsillitis often.
BRAIN 3X (LERVEAU)	: An excellent remedy for sequel of surgical removal of adenoids.
CALCAREA CARB.	: Fat children, whose head perspires at night and who takes cold easily.
CALCAREA PHOS.	: Thin children with large tonsils. Chronic enlargement of adenoids.
STREPTOCOCCINUM	: For after effects of the removal of adenoids surgically.
SULPHUR	: Children who have a dread of bathing and are always hungry with nasal polyps.

AIDS
(ACQUIRED IMMUNO-DEFICIENCY SYNDROME)

No case with this label has ever come to me. It is possible that a patient not properly diagonised and who was unaware of the disease may have come to me. A homoeopath treats the diseases on its symptoms only. It is possible that such a patient may have been treated by me on its symptoms. Since the vital force of the patient is rendered deficient and the patient is unable to defend himself against diseases, the following medicines can prove useful taking into account the symptoms.

The following remedies may be used alongwith the indicated remedy of the disease of the patient:

CAMPHORA : The patient presents a picture of collapse. The body is icy cold. Strength appears sinking. Pulse is small and weak. Repeated drop doses of Camphora Q on a lump of sugar will strengthen the heart and raise his vital force. He will be able to fight the disease. The medicine can be repeated every 5 minutes till the condition of the patient improves.

CARBO VEG. : Vital force nearly exhausted. The disease has greatly depleted the patient. He cannot recover from it, and has cold copious sweat, cold breath,cold tongue and loss of voice. The patient appears to be in the last stages of life. In such cases, this remedy may save his life.

ECHINACEA Q : It is a great stimulant of the immune system. May be used with confidence in conditions of abnormal state of blood,blood poisoning and specific conditions. The patient has a tendency of malignancy in acute and sub-acute disorders. It increases the W. B. C. count and enhances the macrophage function which destroys foreign invaders in the body.

IODIUM : It arouses the defensive apparatus of the system by assembling the mononuclear leucocytes.

LAUROCERASUS Q : Lack of reaction in the chest, heart and lung affections.

LOBELIA PURP. : Overwhelming drowsiness as produced by the bite of a snake. Intense prostration. Cannot keep eyes open. Vital forces become very weak with a feeling of paralysis of the body, heart and lungs. Intense chill without shivering.

SILICEA 6X : It strengthens the vital and defensive forces. The patient is chilly and likes to keep the head covered. It cures deep seated diseases and as such may prove to be useful in the cure of Aids.

TUBERCULINUM 200 : Aids patient has low or no recuperative powers. He is always tired. Motion causes intense fatigue. Medicines, even well indicated, fail to improve the health of the patient. Tuberculinum acts in such cases.

AIR SICKNESS

ACONITUM NAP. : Person is afraid of travelling by air. A dose will remove his fear.

ARGENTUM NIT. : It removes fear of air raids.

ARNICA MONT. : It prevents mental and physical fatigue after a travel by air.

BELLADONNA : Give one dose as a preventive 20 minutes before travelling by air and one dose immediately before boarding the plane.

BORAX	: Use this when the stomach is upset or there is a fear when the plane descends to land. One or two doses of 30 potency will suffice.
PETROLEUM	: If inspite of the above treatment there is ringing and cracking in the ears or heaviness in the head or nausea or vomiting or heartburn on aviation, give one dose every 30 minutes till disappearance of the discomfort.

ALBUMINURIA

Albuminuria is the presence of protein in urine, chiefly albumin but also globulin; usually indicative of disease, but sometimes resulting from a temporary or trancient dysfunction.

ACIDUM PHOS.	: Presence of albumin during fever or after fever. Urine frequent, watery and milky.
APIS MEL.	: Presence of albumin in urine, either in pregnancy or in dropsy is cured by the use of this remedy. In dropsy, urine is scanty and there is swelling of the body.
CANTHARIS Q	: Urine is burning and is voided in drops. It contains albumin with infection of the kidney.
HELONIAS Q	: Albuminous and alkaline urine. Contains phosphates and is

profuse and clean. It is also useful in albuminuria of pregnancy.

MERCURIUS COR. : Albuminuria during the first few months of pregnancy.

MERCURIUS SOL. : Frequent urging. Burning in urethra on the start of urination.

PHOSPHORUS : Albuminuria in the later period of pregnancy or near the end of pregnancy at full term.

TEREBINTHINIAE Q : Albuminous urine with burning and drawing pain in urethra.

ALCOHOLISM

It may be noted that no help can be given to a patient who has no desire to leave such a habit. In such cases, hospitalisation is necessary to keep a strict watch over the patient so that he cannot consume alcohol. The following medicines may be tried in both the cases when the patient has a desire to abandon the habit or when the patient is admitted in the hospital and is under strict watch.

ACIDUM SULPH. Q : 5 drops a dose in water four times a day removes craving for wines and brandy. A dose may be given when the craving starts.

CHINA OFF. Q : It removes craving for alcohol in drunkards who wish to reform. Give10 drops in water twice a day.

PHOSPHORUS, QUERCUS : The use of this remedy takes away the craving for alcohol.

SEPIA, KALIUM BICH.	: Give alternately four times a day. It takes away longing for beer.
STERCULIA A. Q	: Its use lessens craving for liquors.
STRYCHNINUM NIT. 3X	: Removes craving for alcohol in any form, when used TDS for 3 weeks or earlier when the craving stops.
SULPHUR 200	: One dose per day in the morning if a person has great desire to drink alcohol all the time. Wants to drink from morning till evening or till awake.
SYPHILINUM 1M	: One dose a month to correct the hereditary tendency to alcoholism.

ALCOHOLISM, ILL-EFFECTS OF

ARSENICUM ALB.	: Helps in reducing the ill effects of excessive alcoholism.
CALCAREA ARS.	: Use it for all complaints remaining in drunkards who have now abstained themselves from drinking.
CARBONEUM SULPH.	: It is very useful in patients broken down by abuse of the alcohol. Impotency, sick headache, color blindness, etc. are cured by this remedy.
CARDUUS MAR.	: Liver troubles, liver pain, constipation alternating with diarrhea, caused by use of alcoholic drinks,

specially beer, are corrected by the use of this remedy.

CHIMAPHILA : Its use helps in the removal of renal and hepatic disorders in chronic alcoholics.

GELSEMIUM : This remedy is surely indicated when all the complaints of a patient are relieved by the use of alcoholic stimulants.

KALIUM BICH. : It cures nausea and vomiting after drinking beer. It is specifically useful for ladies. Nux-v. is more useful for men.

NUX VOM. 200 : It cures restlessness and giddiness after heavy drinking. It also cures vomiting after drinking.

PULSATILLA NIG., PETROLEUM : Use of either remedy cures vomiting immediately after drinking.

QUERCUS Q : Its use removes the bad effects of alcoholism.

RANUNCULUS BULB. : Cures, coma due to heavy drinking of alcohol and other bad effects of alcohol.

SECALE COR. : Insomnia due to the intake of alcohol.

ALLERGY

The main cause is the house dust mite, *Dermatophagoides pteronyssinus,* but allergy may develop to dust-containing animal or human hair (dandruff), cotton or other fibres.

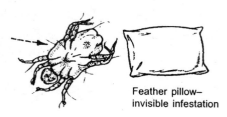

Feather pillow— invisible infestation

Allergy' is a condition when a person is susceptible to a substance which is harmless to a majority of people under similar conditions of environments, etc. For example, penicillin, one of a group of antibiotics, is borne by some people but it produces allergic conditions and toxic manifestations in others who are sensitive to it. This is a case with several other drugs and medicines - not homoeopathic. Such conditions can continue throughout the life, if not treated properly. One simpler method employed for determining allergy is the skin test. A scratch is made, usually on the arm, and the substance of which the allergy test is required, is applied upon it. If it produces irritation or some other symptoms, that person is allergic to that substance. More accurate methods are available in the clinical laboratories. Homoeopathic physician acting upon the law of "SIMILIA SIMILIBUS CURANTUR" or "let like's be treated by like's" will remove such an allergy by giving minute doses of the same allergen which is a causative factor. Iron cuts iron is the universal truth.

ACIDUM SULPH.	: Air pollen allergy.
AILANTHUS G.	: Smell of flowers causes asthma.
ALLIUM CEPA	: Allergic coryza with violent sneezing and worse in the "pollen season" i. e. August. Sensitive to the smell of flowers.
ANTIMONIUM CRUD.	: Cannot bear the heat of sun. The patient feels exhausted in warm weather. Gastric troubles increase.
ANTIPYRINUM 2X	: Allergic puffiness of eye lids, face, lips and sometimes penis.
APIS MEL. 200	: For skin allergy which is worse by heat and when there is puffiness with redness and burning. Allergic to heat.

ARALIA R., LYCOPERSICUM ESCU., POTHOS	:	Dust causes respiratory troubles and asthma.
ARGENTUM NIT.	:	Skin diseases due to any allergy. Skin withered and dried up.
ARSENICUM ALB.	:	For skin allergy worse by cold. Allergy to cold drinks.
ARUNDO, AMBROSIA, ARUM TRIPH.	:	Allergic watery coryza, sneezing, stuffed up feeling in the nose and asthma like attacks.
CARBO VEG., PULSATILLA NIG.	:	Allergic to poultry items, aspirin, salt and butter. Milk causes flatulence.
CHININUM ARS., NATRIUM MUR. 200	:	Allergic to eggs.
COCCULUS IND.	:	Heat of the sun produces rash and vertigo. Allergic to sun rays.
GELSEMIUM	:	General depression from the heat of sun.
HISTAMINUM 1M	:	Allergic to dust, smoke and perfumes. Allergic catarrh and coryza.
KALIUM BICH.	:	Allergic to beer and whisky.
LAC VACCINUM DEF., SEPIA, SULPHUR, TUBERCULINUM	:	Allergic to milk which disagrees.
LACHESIS 200	:	Allergic to vinegar, pickles and sour acidic foods.
MAGNESIUM CARB.	:	Allergic to milk.
NATRIUM CARB.	:	It removes allergy when the milk causes diarrhea.
NATRIUM MUR. 200	:	Allergic to bread, pickles and acidic foods.

NUX VOM.	: Allergic to coffee.
PETROLEUM	: Allergic to cabbage.
PSORINUM	: Allergic to wheat, which causes eczema.
PULSATILLA NIG.	: Allergic to orange juice which cases irritation of the skin. Allergic to pastry and rich ice cream mixed with fruits. Allergic to bakery foods.
RUMEX CRIS.	: Allergic to meat which causes eructations and itching.
SABADILLA	: Sensitiveness of all odours.
SACCHARUM OFF.	: Allergic to sugar.
SELENIUM MET.	: Allergic to lemonade.
SEPIA	: Allergic to fats and boiled milk, which cause diarrhea.
SULPHUR 200 or 6X	: Hair dyes produce eczema. Allergic reactions to antibiotics. Allergic to tomatoes, use of which turns face red and starts the cough.
TELLURIUM MET.	: Allergic to rice.
THUJA OCC.	: Onions cause coryza and ophthalmia.
THYROIDINUM 3X-6X	: Allergic urticaria. Allergy to lipstick.
ZINGIBER OFF.	: Allergic to melons.

ALOPECIA (BALDNESS)

Complete or partial baldness may occur naturally as a part of aging process. It may occur as effects of serious illness or it may be hereditary. It can occur also due to use of drugs. Following medicines are useful for the treatment:

ALUMEN 200, SELENIUM MET.	: For alopecia i. e. falling of hair of head, eye brows, eyelashes and other parts of the body.
ARSENICUM ALB.	: Alopecia due to use of metallic arsenic in forms other than potentised. Scalp itches intolerably. Circular patches of bare spots.
CALCAREA PHOS.	: Falling of hair in bunches.
FLUORICUM ACIDUM	: Alopecia of old age or of prematurely aged due to syphilis. Falling of hair in patches.
MANCINELLA 200	: For alopecia neurotica i. e. baldness after severe acute diseases or at the scar of a healed wound.
NATRIUM MUR.	: Falling of hair after delivery of a child and its nursing.
PIX LIQUIDA	: Alopecia due to the diseases of the scalp. Scalp itches intolerably and bleeds on scratching.
SANICULA AQUA 200, THUJA OCC. 200	: For alopecia furfuracea i. e. baldness which is chronic due to dandruff and lots of itching.
SELENIUM MET.	: It is useful in baldness of the whole head.
SEPIA	: Falling of hair in pregnancy.

SILICEA	: For premature alopecia i. e bald-ness, prematurely.
THALLIUM	: Alopecia after serious diseases. There is abnormal and excessive perspiration on the head. Total baldness.
TUBERCULINUM 200, THUJA OCC. 200	: Baldness in sharply defined cir-cumscribed patches i. e. alope-cia areata. Falling of hair due to dandruff.
VINCA MINOR	: Baldness is sharply defined, circumscribed patches which leave the scalp smooth and white or grey hair may grow on the bald spots like white wool. Hair may knit together.
WIESBADEN	: The hair grow rapidly and be-come darker by the use of this remedy. It also helps to cure the falling of hair.

NOTE: Onion slices rubbed on baldspots sometimes cures baldness.

ALZHEIMER'S DISEASE

It is a deteriotive mental state commonly known as presenile dementia occuring in the 40-60 years age group. Research has shown that it is developed due to excessive use of soluble aluminium which is generally found in widely used antacids and indigestion drugs and also cooking utensils. It has been found in greater amounts in the brains of people suffering from

Alzheimer's disease. Aluminium is partially blamed for this condition. According to the homoeopathic law "Alumina" is very useful for the treatment of this disease. If not treated early, this disease progressively destroys vital brain cells bringing changes in behaviour, difficulty in learning and remembering, impaired judgement, confusion, problems with speech, muscle co-ordination and restlessness. Disease requires constant supervision, care and proper use of the intelligently selected indicated remedy as mentioned in the chapter "SCHIZOPHRENIA".

If Alumina is indicated, there is straining at stools. Such patients are slow eaters and are seen rubbing their eyes often. Vitamin E-30C or 200C sometimes prove to be antidotal to aluminum. The following symptoms point towards this disease and study of the patient with reference to them will narrow the circle for choice of the indicated remedy.

1. Extremely suspicious, withdrawn and fearful.

2. Rapid swing in mood - weeping to laughter or anger.

3. Puts the things in wrong places like a watch in the sugar bowl or an iron in the fridge.

4. He/She may wear warm clothes in summer and summer clothes in winter.

5. He may get lost in his own street. He has no regard for time and place.

6. Loss of memory. Forgets the names of familiar persons. Forgets that the carrots were left for cooking on the stove until they are burned. Cannot find appropriate words at the right occassion.

AMENORRHEA
(ABSENCE AND SUPPRESSION OF MENSES)

Amenorrhea is absence or abnormal cessation of the menses. It may be primary or secondary (due to some other reasons like lactation, emotional, dietary, exercise induced, etc.).

ACONITUM NAP., PLATINUM MET.	: Menses suppressed in plethoric girls. Plat. acts very promptly.
ACONITUM NAP.	: Menstruation stopped suddenly due to a great emotional shock, stress or from exposure to dry windy cold weather.
APIS MEL.	: Menses suppressed with head symptoms or due to a tumor in the ovaries. It acts very well specially in young girls when it appears that the menses are about to start but do not.
APOCYNUM CAN.	: Absence of menses in tropical conditions. Women become weak and nervous due to non appearance of menses.
ARGENTUM NIT.	: A mere spot of blood instead of regular menses.
ARISTOLOCHIA CLEM. 200	: Young women at the helm of their youth lose their menses after the hormonal treatment. It combines the properties of Sepia and Pulsatilla nig.
CALCAREA CARB.	: Menses suppressed in fat girls.
CAUSTICUM, CYCLAMEN	: Menses during day time only, ceases at night.

CIMICIFUGA 3X	: Menses absent or scanty due to hormonal imbalance.
DAMIANA Q	: Aids the establishment of normal menstrual flow in young girls.
DULCAMARA	: Suppression of menses from cold or dampness. Before appearance of menses, a rash appears on the skin or sexual excitement.
EUPHRASIA	: Menses last for one hour only.
GOSSYPIUM Q	: Menses suppressed due to uterine troubles. Sensation that the flow is about to start but it does not. It is a powerful remedy and brings about menses in most cases.
GRAPHITES	: Menses are suppressed, delayed or scanty. This is usually accompanied by constipation with ball like stools.
IGNATIA AMARA	: Suppressed menses in patients with very changeable moods-crying and laughing at unexpected times or hysterical patients.
KALIUM CARB.	: Menses delayed in young girls. Difficult first menses.
LYCOPODIUM	: Young girls with non development of breasts and with absence of menses. This remedy will develop the breast and make the course appear.
MACROTINUM 2X	: 5 drops of it in a little water given every two hours at the time when the flow was due, but

failed to come on, makes the menses appear.

ONOSMODIUM : Feels as if menses would appear but it does not. There is severe intense pain and aching in the breasts.

PHOSPHORUS : Amenorrhea. Bleeding from nose, breasts or eyes instead of menses. Weeps before menses. Corrosive leucorrhea instead of menses.

PINUS LAMBERTIANA Q : Menses suppressed or delayed. Give in 15 drop doses, thrice or four times daily.

PITUITRINUM 3X : When menses fail to appear at puberty and when the breasts are defective in their development.

PULSATILLA NIG. Q : Stoppage of menses due to any cause.

SABADILLA : Menses too late. Menses come and stop and comes again by fits and starts, due to the congestion of the uterus and anemia. Worse cold and cold drinks and better warm food and warm drinks.

SABINA Q : Young girls having no menses for months together. One breast is smaller than the other.

SARACA INDICA Q : Delayed or irregular menses. Headache due to the suppression of menses. Menstrual discharge is scanty, pale, watery, foul smelling and blackish. Amenorrhea at puberty with pain in the head.

SENECIO AUR. : Menses retarded and suppressed due to functional disorders in young girls with backache.

SEPIA : When menses do not start after the mother has ceased breast feeding the child. The women feels troubled mentally. Sepia not only starts the menses but also cures all symptoms due to the suppression of menses.

SULPHUR : Menses too late, scanty and difficult. Blood thick, black, acrid and makes the parts sore. Menses preceded by headache.

THYROIDINUM 3X : When the menses are suppressed due to the over activity of pituitary or thyroid gland.

TUBERCULINUM 200 : Use it when various indicated remedies fail.

AMOEBIASIS
(AMOEBIC DYSENTERY)

This disease is generally characterised by dysentery, diarrhea, weakness and prostration. Nausea, vomiting and pain may be present. In chronic cases, ulceration of the colon occurs. The microscopic examination of the stool shows presence of a single cell pratozoa, Entamoeba hystolytica or Giardiasis lamblia.

ALOE SOC. : A lot of mucus with the stools. Copious flatus and pain in the rectum after the stool.

CALCAREA IOD. 3X   : Some practitioners recommend it for the disease.

EMETINUM 1X   : It is specific for the disease. Give in drop doses, four times a day.

SYMPHYTUM OFF. 1M   : Give one dose fortnightly when ulceration of the large intestines is present.

THUJA OCC. Q   : It is an excellent remedy for this disease and the treatment should be started with it. No other remedy must be given for the next 24 hours.

MERCURIUS COR.   : Constant cutting pains in the abdomen and intolerable, almost ineffectual pressing, straining and tenesmus; only frequent, scanty discharges of bloody slime, day and night.

ANEMIA

ACIDUM PHOS.   : Anemia due to grief or loss of seminal fluids.

ARGENTUM NIT.   : Anemia due to excessive vomiting and indigestion.

ARSENICUM ALB.   : Anemia due to malaria. There is lot of prostration and anxiety. The patient drinks often but little at a time.

CALCAREA ARS.   : By its use, the hemoglobin and red blood corpuscles increase in a short time.

CALCAREA PHOS. 6X : Anemia of children, who are pale but flabby and suffer from tonsillitis.

CALOTROPIS Q : Primary anemia of syphilitics. Heat in the stomach is a good guiding symptom for the use of this remedy.

CEANOTHUS A. Q : Anemia due to the dysfunction of liver and spleen. Violent dyspnea. Bronchitis with profound secretion.

CHINA OFF. 1X, CALCAREA CARB. : If anemia is caused by loss of blood or vital fluids.

FERRUM PHOS. 1X, FERRUM PROTOXALATUM 1X : This may be given once daily for a week if the anemia is due to lack of iron. It will cause a rapid increase of hemoglobin. If it does no good, stop its administration and if improvement is noticed continue it, till cured.

IRIDIUM MET. : Anemia after exhausting diseases or due to old age or in children growing too fast. It increases red blood corpuscles.

KALIUM CARB. : Blood lacks red blood corpuscles. The skin is milky white or watery with great debility. Young ladies at the time of puberty have menstrual troubles on account of great weakness. There is bloating of face, eyelids and backache in the lower back. If such conditions occur during menopause, specially the bloating, this remedy is again indicated. This remedy has a profound influence over blood making.

LECITHINUM 1X to 3X : It has a favourable influence upon the nutritive conditions of blood. Increases the number of red blood corpuscles and amount of hemoglobin. Loss of flesh and general breakdown may be noticed.

NATRIUM CACODYL. 1X : It increases the number of red blood corpuscles to double. Give four doses a day.

NATRIUM MUR. : The patient is constipated. The face is pale and there is palpitation. It is also useful for anemia after malaria.

NUX VOM. : Anemia due to indigestion, especially in persons of sedentary habits or given to high living or debauchary.

OSTRYA VIRGINICA : It is of great value in anemia from malaria.

PETROLEUM : When anemia is accompanied with fever and the patient vomits the food taken.

PHOSPHORUS : Anemia due to kidney diseases and when there is puffiness all over the body.

PULSATILLA NIG. : Patients who were heavily and irrelevantly drugged by medication and tonics or due to accidental stoppage of menses.

SILICEA 6X : Anemia of infants with tendency to rickets.

STROPHANTHUS HISP. Q : Anemia with palpitations and breathlessness. It tones up the heart and is safer for the aged. Dyspnea specially on ascending. Lungs congested.

STRYCHNINUM PHOS. 3X : An excellent remedy for anemia of the spinal cord. Aching, burning and weakness of the spine is present. Tenderness in the mid dorsal region on pressure.

TEUCRIUM MAR. 10M or CM : One dose fortnightly will cure anemia which is due to pin worms. It will also eradicate worms.

NOTE 1 : 1 : Patients suffering iron deficiency anemia can also increase the amount of iron in the hemoglobin by use of cast-iron cooking vessels. The following foods top in iron content:

a. **Meat, poulty, fish and eggs.**

b. **Whole grains, dried fruits (like apricots, prunes and raisins), dark green leafy vegetables, beans, peas, lentils, nuts and jaggery.**

NOTE 2 : Coffee and tea with meals interferes in the absorption of iron by the body.

ANGER
(ANNOYANCE)

ANTIMONIUM CRUD. : Cannot bear to be touched or looked at. When done so, feels angry.

ARNICA MONT. : Anger following fright.

ARSENICUM ALB. : Anger caused by noise or light.

ARUM TRIPH. : Trembling when angry. Must

quarrel with somebody or beat and hit children to give vent to his feelings.

CALCAREA ARS.	:	Anxiety with anger.
CALCAREA CARB.	:	Anger after coition.
CEREUS SERP.	:	Wild anger. Low morals. Tendency to swear.
CHAMOMILLA	:	Anger of children who are irritable. They will want this or that and refuse and throw it away when offered. Anger almost furious. Anger results in diarrhea. Perspires when angry.
COLOCYNTHIS	:	Abdominal pain after anger. Great indignation and other ill effects of anger.
CONIUM MAC.	:	Trifling matters cause annoyance.
CROCUS SAT.	:	Anger with violence followed by repentance, laughs a lot, involuntarily.
IGNATIA AMARA	:	Unbearable anger. Headache following anger.
LYCOPODIUM	:	Angry due to a feeling of insecurity and lack of self confidence. Coward with fear of future events.
MERCURIUS SOL.	:	Sudden anger with an impulse to do violence.
NATRIUM MUR.	:	Ill effects from anger with fear.
NUX VOM.	:	Violent temper. Cannot bear contradiction. Generally irritable and angry. Anger from loud noises which are painful. The anger

may lead to indigestion. Very impatient and difficult to live with.

NUX VOM., AURUM MET.	: Anger from least contradiction and disagreement.
PHOSPHORUS	: It is specially indicated in children who have a wild temper. Always fighting with other children and ever with mother and teachers.
STAPHYSAGRIA	: Ill effects of anger and insults. Colic after anger. Suppressed anger and indignation, which results in uncontrollable outbreaks of anger.
STRAMONIUM	: Anger almost furious.
TARENTULA HIS.	: Anger which often results in violence. Anger from contradictions.
TUBERCULINUM	: Children always angry, become violent on trifles. People who never smile and have always an angry look.

ANGINA PECTORIS
(SEE HEART ALSO)

Angina pectoris is a severe constricting pain in the chest, often radiating from the precordium (heart) to a shoulder (usually left) and down the arm.

British researches team of Cambridge University, scientists headed by Prof. Morris Brown said that vitamin E cuts heart attack risk by 75%. Vitamin E occurs naturally in foods such as vegetable oils, nuts, butter, leafy vegetables and whole grains. Daily average intake of vitamin E is recommended to be 15 to 30 international units.

ACONITUM NAP.   : Sudden attack of angina with acute pain in the region of heart, arm and left shoulder. Palpitation, pulse full, hard and bouding. Restlessness, constant pressure in the chest obstructing smooth breathing. Cough may be present. It should be given immediately at the onset of the feeling of pain when there is a previous history of the disease in the patient.

AMMONIUM CARB. 30   : Danger of heart failure of heart due to a prolonged illness. Give a dose every half hour.

AMYLENUM NIT. Q   : A little cotton drenched in it may be placed near the nostril of the patient for inhaling. It gives immediate relief after which the indicated remedy can be used.

ARGENTUM NIT.   : It is best applicable when the heart attack occurs after taking meals. Angina pain is worse at night.

ARSENICUM IOD. 3X   : If this remedy is indicated, give one dose at night and one dose in the morning immediately after the food.

BRYONIA ALBA Q   : If the pain persists and is worse by motion use this remedy.

CACTUS Q   : Acute pain, suffocation and contraction in heart region. 10-15 drops every 15 minutes.

CIMICIFUGA : Pain in the heart region and the left arm. Heart action ceases suddenly and there is an impending suffocation.

CRATAEGUS OXY. Q : Pain in the region of heart and under the left collar bone. Cardiac cough. Pulse accelerated, irregular and feeble. Valvular murmurs, blueness of the fingers and the toes. Sustains heart in infectious diseases.

CUPRUM ACET. : It may be given thrice daily. It may prove to be of great value.

DIGITALIS : Angina pectoris with a feeling as if the heart would cease working. Pulse is slow and the patient is worse by movement.

GLONOINUM 30 : Violent beating of the heart as if it will burst open. Strenous breathing. Pains radiate in all directions, down the left arm with weakness.

KALMIA LAT. : Weak, slow pulse. Palpitation; worse leaning forward. Sharp pains take away the breath. Shooting through chest above the heart into shoulder blades. Heart's action tumultuous, rapid and visible.

LACHESIS 30 : Shooting pain of the heart and arteries on the left portion of the chest and left arm.

LATRODECTUS MAC. 6X : There may be restlessness, depression and pain after the attack is over. There may be still pain in the chest muscles, left shoulder, back and neck. Pain may extend to abdomen. This remedy is almost specific in curing this dreaded disease. Continue its use after the attack till all the symptoms disappear. Pains radiate from the chest to left arm and fingers.

LILIUM TIG. : Angina pectoris with pain in the right arm. Suffocation, pulsations all over the body.

MAGNESIUM PHOS. 12X : Use it for nervous spasmodic palpitation, constrictive pains around the heart. It relieves pain and calms the patient. Give it with hot water or dry on the tongue and repeat often, every fifteen minutes. Before its use, relief may be obtained by inhaling Amylenum nitrosum Q.

NAJA TRI. : Heart cases without clear cut symptoms. A dose every half an hour - two or three doses will relieve speedily, if the remedy is useful. After 3 doses look for another remedy which is indicated. Special symptoms for the use of this remedy is a feeling of weight on the heart. Angina pains extend to the neck, left shoulder and left arm. Fear and anxiety is present. There may be pain in the forehead and temples.

PITUITRINUM 3X : In heart attacks of old people, where sometimes it becomes almost impossible to select a well indicated remedy. It has a specific action on anginal attack due to coronary trouble from chronic uremic conditions as well as in allergic subjects where it relieves greatly.

SECALE COR. : Angina pectoris is caused by spasms or contractions of the coronary artery which supplies the heart muscles. This medicine lessens the contractions and softens the attacks.

SPIGELIA : Pressure, oppression, darting shooting and stabbing pains in the chest and down the left arm. Breathlessness. It is specially indicated in smokers and drunkards.

STROPHANTHUS HISP. Q : Angina due to weakness of the heart. 10 drops three hourly or earlier, if required.

TERMINALIA ARJUNA Q : Angina pectoris, weakness of the heart with palpitation.

VERATRUM ALB. : Heart cases of tobacco chewers. There is palpitation and anxiety and rapid audible respiration. Pulse is feeble and irregular. There is a feeling of extreme coldness. It presents a picture of collapse with blueness of the face. Cold perspiration on the forehead is a good indication for the use of this remedy.

VIBURNUM OP. Q	:	Angina with cramps in the heart. 5-10 drops, 1/2 hourly.
DIET	:	**Special attention should be paid to the diet. Spicy, fried and fatty foods should be avoided. Only vegetarian food should be taken.**

ANKLES

AMMONIUM CARB.	:	Tearing in the bones of ankles and feet.
APIS MEL.	:	Simple swelling of ankles.
ARNICA MONT.	:	It cures sprains, swelling with black and blue appearance of the skin in a short time.
BELLIS P.	:	It is an excellent remedy for sprains of all joints.
CALCAREA PHOS.	:	Generally weak ankles. Also good for weak ankles of children and in almost all the other cases.
CAUSTICUM	:	Weak ankles. Walking causes suffering.
CROCUS SAT.	:	Pain in the ankles.
LEDUM PAL.	:	Easy spraining of the ankle.
MANGANUM ACET.	:	Growing pains and weak ankles.
MIMOSA P.	:	Swelling of ankles and legs.
NATRIUM CARB.	:	Easy dislocation and spraining of ankles. Ankles are very weak. Old sprains are cured by the use of this remedy.

NATRIUM MUR., SILICEA : Weak ankles, gives difficulty in walking. It is specially indicated in children who are late in learning to walk.

PROPYLAMINUM Q : Pain in ankles, unable to stand. Use 10-15 drops in a glass of water. A teaspoonful every 2 hours.

PSORINUM : Ulcer of ankles and lower legs.

RUTA G. : Aching pains in ankles with restlessness.

STRONTIUM CARB. : Sprain of ankles which is chronic and when there is swelling.

ANNUAL COMPLAINTS

ARSENICUM ALBUM and NAJA TRIPUDIANS may be compared in respect of complaints and diseases which occur annually.

CARBO VEGETABILIS, LACHESIS, SULPHUR and THUJA OCCIDENTALIS also have complaints that recur annually. URTICA URENS has complaints at the same time every year.

ANTIBIOTICS, ILL-EFFECTS OF

Antibiotics are a variety of drugs prepared both from natural and synthetic substances to destroy micro-organisms infecting the bodies of humans, animals, birds and plants, producing diseases. These are most misused and overused drugs of modern allopathic practice. More or less every antibiotic drug has side effects because their use disturbs the normal function of the organs of the body and the composition of the blood. The patient may develop disturbances in digestion, discomfort, unsteadiness, diarrhea, sore throat, aphthae, fever, etc. The following medicines may be prescribed to remove the ill-effects of antibiotics. The use of antibiotics should be stopped when any ill effect is noticed.

ACIDUM PHOS. : For general debility after use of antibiotics.

ANTIMONIUM TART. : When there is rattling of mucus but little comes up on coughing.

BORAX : For thrush of tongue and mouth or vagina.

BRYONIA ALBA : Bronchitis with lot of thirst. The patient drinks often and in large quantities. Cough is worse in a warm room and the chest is sore. Give every three hours.

IPECACUANHA : For constant nausea.

NITRICUM ACIDUM : Diarrhea is a very common side effect and it is cured by this remedy.

PULSATILLA NIG. : Persistant catarrh of the throat and nose.

SULPHUR 200 : One dose, usually to overcome the, so called "drug rash".

THUJA OCC. 200 : It has a specific antibacterial action.

DIET : **In all such cases, yogurt, garlic capsules and juices are the best diets.**

ANTIDOTES

Antidote is an agent that neutralizes a poison or counteracts its effects.

AGARICUS MUS.	: Antidotes effects of alcohol.
ALUMEN	: Antidotes lead poisoning.
ARSENICUM ALB.	: Antidotes pencillin and carbolic acid.
CARBO VEG.	: Antidotes fumes of gases.
CHAMOMILLA	: Antidotes the bad effects of excessive coffee drinking.
FLUORICUM ACIDUM	: Antidote to radiation.
GRAPHITES	: Antidotes skin troubles from arsenic poisoning.
INSULINUM 200	: Antidote to insulin.
IPECACUANHA	: Antidotes the bad effects of quinine and opium poisoning.
LEDUM PAL.	: Antidotes the poisons of animals and insects.
NITRICUM ACIDUM	: Antidotes the effects of antibiotics specially mycins which have caused diarrhea.
NUX VOM. 200	: Antidotes stimulants like wine, whisky, tea and coffee.
PHOSPHORUS, AMMONIUM CARB.	: Antidotes effects of chloroform or other anesthetic drugs.
PULSATILLA NIG.	: It is a better antidote to whisky than even Nux-v.
THUJA OCC.	: Antidotes tea and vaccination.
TUBERCULINUM, SULPHUR 200	: Antidotes bad effects of hair dyes.

ANTISEPTIC

Antiseptic is an agent or substance capable of prevention of infection by inhibiting the growth of infectious agents.

CALENDULA OFF. Q : It is a great homoeopathic antiseptic and a remarkable healing agent. It promotes rapid healing of open wounds. Use internally and externally. Lotion for external use is prepared with one part of Calendula Q mixed with six parts of hot water.

CINNAMOMUM Q : Lotion prepared with 3-4 drops in about 2 litres of hot water is used as an antiseptic agent in washing of wounds and even cancer parts when the skin is intact. It is also used for hemorrhage after child birth when an offensive odour is present.

MYRISTICA SEB. : It has a great antiseptic power for inflammation and suppuration of the covering membranes of the bones, wounds, fistula, abscess, carbuncles and boils. Hastens suppuration and shortens its duration. Acts more powerfully than Silicea and Hepar sulphuris.

ECHINACEA Q : Old ulcers. Irritations from insect bites and poisonous plants. Recurring boils. Apply locally, as a cleaning and antiseptic wash.

ANUS

ALOE SOC.	: Itching and burning of anus. Patient is always scratching the anus and feels pleasure in boring the finger in the anus. The itching compels him to sodomy and anal intercourse.
ANACARDIUM ORI., ANTIMONIUM CRUD.	: Constant oozing of moisture from the anus or constant oozing of mucus from it. Hard lumps with watery discharge.
CALCAREA SULPH.	: Painful abscess around anus and fistula of the anus.
IGNATIA AMARA	: Violent itching and crawling in the anus and in the rectum.
MEDORRHINUM 1M	: Intense itching of the anus worse while thinking of it. Oozing of foul moisture from the anus.
NITRICUM ACIDUM	: Anal fissure. Sharp cuttiing pain during and after stools. Constipation may be present.
RATANHIA PERU.	: Fissure burning like fire. Stool after lot of straining.
SEPIA	: Almost constant oozing from anus.
SULPHUR	: Itching and redness of the anus in children. Diaper rash.

ANXIETY

Anxiety is an apprehension of danger and dread accompanied by restlessness, tension and dyspnea unattached to a clearly identifiable stimulus.

ACONITUM NAP.   : Acute anxiety with agonising terrors and fear of death. Frequent palpitations. The patient is inconsolable and restless.

ANACARDIUM ORI.   : Anxiety vanishes on eating.

ARGENTUM NIT.   : Anticipatory anxiety with diarrhea. Hurried, irritable, nervous and lacking in self confidence.

ARSENICUM ALB.   : Intense anxiety with great restlessness. Fears something terrible will happen. He is worse during night and after midnight. Very chilly, exact and fault finding. He is meticulously tidy.

BORAX   : Anxiety leading to nausea with fear of downward motion. He is worse until 11 P.M.

BRYONIA ALBA   : Anxious about business even though seriously ill.

CALCAREA CARB.   : The patient thinks that he has done something wrong. He feels uneasy and anxious with palpitations. Fears loss of reason. Desperate of life. Fears insanity. Bores others by repeatedly describing his ailments.

CARBO VEG.   : Anxiety is worse felt lying in the bed with eyes closed.

CAUSTICUM	: Anxiety worse in the evening due to apprehension.
GELSEMIUM	: Anxiety due to fright, fear, emotions, exciting news or forthcoming examination and interview.
IGNATIA AMARA	: Anxiety due to any grief.
LACHESIS	: Nocturnal attacks of anxiety. Cramps in legs from fear.
LYCOPODIUM	: Anxiety with lack of confidence. The patient is unable to sleep due to the happenings during the day. Anxiety about forthcoming events.
MANGANUM ACET.	: Anxiety worse while lying still. Sad music decreases the anxiety.
NATRIUM MUR.	: Anxious about everything, even has anxious dreams.
PHOSPHORUS	: Very restless patients who are sensitive. They need security and constant reassurance. Anxious, restless and nervous due to the fear of darkness, thunder, alone or dying.
PULSATILLA NIG.	: Anxiety after bad news or an emotional upset. The patient is weepy, touchy and needs company.
SULPHUR	: Anxiety is worse felt in the morning with profuse sweating and fainting spells.
SEPIA	: Anxious towards evening: Dreads to be alone. Indifferent to those loved best.

APHTHAE

ACIDUM MUR.   : Foul smell from the mouth with soreness of the teeth and gums.

ACIDUM SULPH.   : Gums bleed easily. Pyorrhea. Tongue swollen. Excessive salivation.

ARSENICUM ALB.   : Burning blisters. Sips water frequently.

BORAX   : Painful whitish blisters in the mouth which bleed easily. Fungus like growths in the mouth.

HYDRASTIS CAN.   : Aphthae and ulceration of the membrane of mouth. Tongue is yellowish in color and there is constipation.

LACHESIS   : Severe form of aphthae. Swollen gums with burning. Gums spongy and bleed easily.

MERCURIUS SOL.   : Painful blisters with foul smell from the mouth. Saliva increased.

NITRICUM ACIDUM   : Painful blisters with offensive and acrid saliva.

THUJA OCC. 1M   : White blisters on the sides close to the root of the tongue. Painful and sore. This remedy has a specific antibacterial action and destroys the fungus growths.

APOPLEXY
(SEE BRAIN HEMORRHAGE)

APPENDICITIS

Appendicitis is an inflammation of the vermiform appendix.

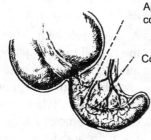

Appendix swollen and congested

Congestion of vessels

BAPTISIA TINC. CM	: One dose given in the acute form of the disease may abort the need for surgery.
BELLADONNA 200	: In the early stages of acute appendicitis when the patient tosses about restlessly, he has headache and fever without perspiration. It can be repeated frequently.
BRYONIA ALBA 10M	: In acute appendicitis, when the pains are worse from movements and better by lying on the painful side.
DIOSCOREA Q	: 15 drops in hot water fades the pains of appendicitis.
ECHINACEA 3X, PYROGENIUM 3X	: Any of these two remedies may be used in septic conditions of appendicitis.
IRIS TENAX 2X	: It is very near specific for appendicitis and can be used when no special indications for other remedies are present.

LACHESIS	:	Pain of appendicitis or any pain, which is aggravated from the lightest touch even with a feather.
LYCOPODIUM	:	Can be given on the outset of the disease provided indications for its use are present.
NATRIUM SULPH.	:	Acute attack with acute pains in the caecal region. Jaundice usually accompanies inflammation and abscess of the appendix and fever. Cases where the appendix was removed surgically but the pain and fever persisted.
PSORINUM 200	:	Give it after an acute attack is over to prevent return of the disease.
RHUS TOX.	:	It is a homoeopathic knife in case of appendicitis.

NOTE: Cases of appendicitis during pregnancy should be immediately referred to the hospital for surgery. Any waste of time can cause abortion or even death. Abdominal pain that has continued without intermission for several hours specially if associated with vomitting and restlessness can be due to acute appendicitis.

APPETITE (LOST)

ALFALFA Q, GENTIANA LUTEA Q	:	A mixture of both in equal quantity and a ten drops dose is a good appetiser.
ANTIMONIUM CRUD.	:	Loss of appetite. Desire for pickles and acidic things. Eructa-

		tions taste of ingesta. Tongue thickly coated white.
AURUM ARS.	:	It causes rapid increase of appetite specially in anemia and chlorosis.
CALCAREA CARB.	:	Aversion to meat. This remedy will remove it.
CHINA OFF.	:	Hungry without an appetite.
FERRUM PHOS.	:	Aversion to meat and milk. Sour eructations.
GENTIANA LUTEA Q	:	Simple loss of appetite. Acts as a tonic and increases appetite. Loss of appetite after illness. Give five drops before each meal.
IGNATIA AMARA 30	:	Complete loss of appetite for all foods, drinks and tobacco. He has no bad taste for these things.
LECITHINUM 3X	:	Loss of appetite with craving for wine and coffee.
NUX VOM. 200	:	Bitter taste, tongue coated yellow at the back with loss of appetite.
RHUS TOX.	:	Loss of appetite for everything, except milk, which he craves.
SANGUINARIA CAN.	:	Craves toffees, gol gappas, ice cream and things of that sort but does not take bread.
THUJA OCC. 200	:	Complete loss of appetite. Dislike for fresh meat, potatoes and onions. Rancid eructations after fat food.

APPETITE (INCREASED)

COLOCYNTHIS	: Canine hunger. Acidic eructations after eating.
CINA	: Gets hungry soon after eating. Hunger causes digging and gnawing in the stomach. A hunger remedy for children.
FERRUM MET., CHINA OFF.	: Canine hunger alternating with complete loss of appetite. Regurgitation of food and eructations after eating. Wants bread and butter but meat, beer and tea disagree.
GAULTHERIA Q	: Uncontrollable appetite, despite eating, causes sickness in the stomach and pain.
IODIUM	: Anxious and worried if he does not eat. Faints if kept hungry for a few hours. Eats often and much but still loses flesh. All symptoms are relieved by eating.
LYCOPODIUM	: Wakes at night feeling hungry-partiularly, a child. The patient starts eating being hungry,but is full after only a few mouthfuls.
NATRIUM MUR. 200	: Feels nice after eating but soon after he feels sleepy and tired.
PETROLEUM	: Hungry immediately after stool.
PHOSPHORUS	: Hunger soon after eating. Sour taste. Belching large quantities of wind after eating.

PSORINUM 200	: Very hungry always. Must have something to eat in the middle of night.
RHUS TOX.	: Canine hunger without appetite.
SULPHUR	: Complete loss or excessive appetite. Very weak and faint at about 11A.M. must have something to eat.

ARMPIT (AXILLAE)

BARYTA CARB.	: Inflammation of the axillary glands.
HEPAR SULPHURIS	: Painful abscess with other symptoms of the medicine.
JUGLANS REG.	: Itching red pustules or pain with or without swelling.
KALIUM CARB.	: Excessive perspiration under the armpits. Parts of the undergarment or shirt under the armpit is always wet.
NITRICUM ACIDUM	: For offensive perspiration under the armpits.
TARENTULA CUB.	: A near specific for painful abscess under the armpit.

ARROGANCE

LYCOPODIUM	: Headstrong and haughty when ill.

PLATINUM MET.   : Very proud and has a contempt
                            for others.

ARTERIES

ADRENALINUM 30   : It contracts arteries.

CACTUS Q.   : Thickening of the coats of the
                            arteries.

CALCAREA CARB.   : Inflammation of the arteries.

CRATAEGUS OXY.   : Hardness of the arteries. It has a
                            solvent power upon the crusta-
                            ceous and calcareous deposits in
                            the arteries.

SUMBULUS   : A remedy for sclerosed arteries.

THIOSINAMINUM   : Hardening of the arteries.

THYROIDINUM 3X   : The use of this remedy dialates
                            arteries.

ARTHRITIS - GOUT
(JOINT PAINS)

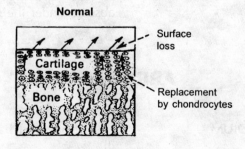

At site of pressure

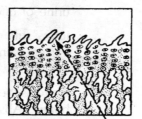

Early

Flaking and fibrillation
of surface

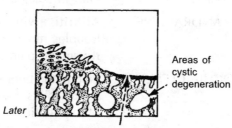

Areas of
cystic
degeneration

Later

Loss of cartilage; exposure of bone.

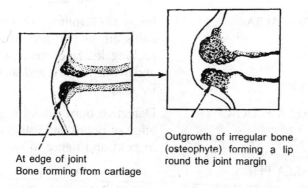

At edge of joint
Bone forming from cartiage

Outgrowth of irregular bone
(osteophyte) forming a lip
round the joint margin

APIS MEL. : Acute arthritis. The affected part is red, shiny and swollen. There is great tenderness to touch; better by applying cold water.

BENZOICUM ACIDUM : Pain and swelling in knees. Gout starting in right great toe with urine of offensive odor.

CAUSTICUM : Joints stiff; toes or fingers contracted; pains relieved by warmth of bed.

ACIDUM FLUOR. : Corrects the abnormal growth of bones. Absorbs nodes and softens bones. Painful parts are red in color.

ACIDUM TART. : Pain in soles and heels.

ARBUTUS ANDRACHNE : Arthritis with eczema. Skin troubles move to joints causing rheumatic pains.

ARISTOLOCHIA CLEM. : Pain in the bones of the ball and socket joints. Pain in heels, back of extremities.

BERBERIS VULG. 3X : Four doses do away the swelling and the pain. Pain in joints with urinary disturbances.

BRYONIA ALBA : Joints are swollen, hot and red. Pains are tearing and worse by rubbing, least movement, warmth and in the morning and are better by rest.

CALCAREA FLUOR. : Defective bony growths. Ulceration of bones and fistula worse in cold and better in warmth.

CALCAREA PHOS. : Arthritis of the neck and shoulders with weakness and softness of bones.

CAULOPHYLLUM 3X : Cutting pains in joints specially in the finger joints while closing the fist.

CHAMOMILLA : Arthritis with sensation of pain far more in excess than the actual pain. There is numbness with pain which is worse during night.

COLCHICUM AUTUM. 3X : Swelling and pain of finger joints and knees. A useful remedy for post traumatic arthritis of small joints following surgery or fracture.

ELATERIUM : Sharp pains in fingers, thumbs, knees, and the hollow of sole. Pains extend downwards. Arthritic nodules. Gouty pains in the great toe and hip joints.

FORMICA RUFA 6X : Arthritis which is not due to an injury. Start with 3 doses a day and gradually reduce it in comparison with the cure.

GAULTHERIA OIL : In 10-20 drops a dose arrest the pains of arthritis.

NATRIUM PHOS. : Gout of the elbow.

PICRICUM ACIDUM : Arthritis deformans. Pins and needles sensation in the extremities.

PULSATILLA NIG. : Gout of the knees. Boring pains in heels towards evening.

RADIUM BROM. : Chronic rheumatic arthritis. Severe pain in all the limbs and joints. Knees and ankles are specially affected. Severe pain in shoulders, arms, hands, fingers, toes, calves, etc. Better open air and continuous motion.

RHAMNUS CAL. : A positive remedy for muscular pains and rheumatism, worse in the evening.

RHUS TOX.	:	Attacks of gout and rheumatism become worse during winters, rain and dampness. Restlessness, stiffness and tearing pains are worse while at rest. Lumbago. Pains better by motion.
SALICYLICUM ACIDUM	:	Rheumatism of the knee and the elbow joints with great redness and high fever.
SANGUINARIA CAN.	:	Rheumatoid arthritis of shoulder joints.
STICTA PULM.	:	Rheumatism of the right shoulder blade, joint, wrist, ankles or knee joint.
SULPHUR	:	Rheumatic pain in the left shoulder and other gouty symptoms accompanied by itching of the skin. Pains are worse at rest or standing, warmth of the bed and washing. Better in dry and warm weather. Stiffness of knees and ankles.
SYMPHYTUM OFF. 1M, RUTA G. Q	:	Joint pains are due to an injury or fracture- simple or compound.
THUJA OCC.	:	Arthritis due to gonorrhea. Cracking in joints.
TRIMETHYLAMINUM	:	Pain in wrists and ankles with fever.
TUBERCULINUM 1M	:	Acute inflammatory arthritis of joints; worse by motion, standing, dampness, early morning, after sleep. Better in open air.

NOTE: Rheumatoid arthritis affects the   joint lining and synovial tissue all over the body and osteoarthritis affects the bone tissue of joints because of wear and tear of aging and gradual destruction of irreplacable cartilage inside the joints.

ASCITES
(SEE DROPSY)

ASTHMA

● **When asthma strikes**
Asthma occurs when the linings of the lungs' bronchial airways become inflamed or swollen, usually due to allergies, airways carry oxygen to the blood, and the length and severity of an attack can be fatal. Because the drugs that treat attacks increase oxygen levels in the blood, helping muscles to work harder and longer, many are banned for Olympic competitors.

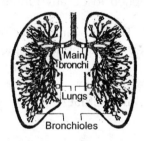

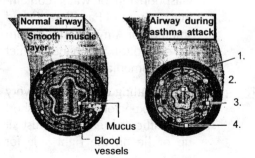

● **Impact on airways**
There are four main ways an asthma attack results in blocked airways:
1. Mucus secretion increases.
2. Smooth muscle contracts.
3. Blood vessels widen in allergic reactions.
4. Swelling and inflammation.

In serious asthmatic attacks, physicians of the old system of medicine utilise steroids. These are no doubt,great as they reduce the life threatening symptoms of asthma. Despite their essential value,however,steroids do not cure the disease and the side effects from their long term use are so serious that even the American Academy of Allergy does not condone their use except in life threatening situations. Inhalers are useful when used correctly for less severe symptoms of asthma as they have less severe side effects generally. Inhalers dry the lung secretions making it difficult for the asthmatics to clear their chest and throat from mucus and clog their breathing passages. This is why homoeopathic medicines are more trustworthy and workable under such circumstances. Most commonly a single medicine is not enough to effect cure and a series of medicines over a period of several months or years are needed. The homoeopathic physician should himself bear this in mind and tell the patient accordingly. The medicines should be changed only when it has stopped to do any further good.

The following medicines are generally indicated and may be used according to symptoms.

AMBRA GRISEA	: Asthma on attempting coition. Asthma accompanied by cardiac symptoms.
AMYLENUM NIT. Q, PASSIFLORA Q	: During the attack of asthma a teaspoon full of water containing 10 drops of Passiflora Q and smelling of Amylenum nitrosum Q on cotton or handkerchief gives immediate relief.
ANTIMONIUM TART.	: Great rattling of mucus but very little is expectorated. Rapid, short and difficult breathing. Must sit up or lie on the right side for relief.
ARSENICUM ALB.	: Asthma worse midnight. Unable to lie down, fears suffocation.

Burning in the chest. Expectoration is scanty and frothy. Wheezing respiration. For treatment give 30 potency and during attack give 200 potency in alteration with Blatta orientalis 200. It offers great relief.

ARUM TRIPH. : Allergic asthma.

ASPIDOSPERMA Q : The tonic for lungs. Removes temporary obstruction of the oxidation of blood by stimulating respiratory centres. Give a few drops doses till the feeling "want of breath" is over. It is very useful in cardiac asthma.

BLATTA ORIENT. : It is an excellent remedy for asthma. In acute cases acts better in lower potencies - mother tincture to 3X. But in chronic cases it needs higher potencies 200 to 1000. Patient gets worse in the rainy weather. Cough with much pus like mucus. When improvement is noticed, discontinue the medicine.

BROMIUM : Asthma with dry, spasmodic, wheezing and rattling cough. Inspiration very difficult. Feels better near rivers and sea and worse in dry climate.

CANNABIS IND. : Humid asthma. Chest oppressed with deep, laboured breathing.

CARBO VEG. : Asthma in old people. Cough spasmodic with gagging and vomiting of mucus. Bluish face. Offensive expectoration. Asthma due to ill treated and neglected pneumonia. Asthma from abdominal orientation, with marked flatulence. Asthma of old or debilitated people.

CASSIA SOPHERA : Dyspnea worse during winter, change of weather, inhaling of dust, cold drinks and exertion. Cough hurts the chest and there is hoarseness.

CINA 200 : Asthma of children with history of worms.

CUPRUM MET. : A real asthma, cough has a gurgling sound and is relieved by drinking cold water. Suffocative attacks worse 3 A.M. and cold weather. Vomiting after the attacks.

GRINDELIA ROB. Q : Suffocation by lying in bed. An effective remedy for wheezing and oppression of breathing. Mucus is foamy and difficult to detach. Cannot breath when lying down. Must sit up to breathe.

HYDROCYANICUM ACIDUM : Recent and uncomplicated asthma. Noisy breathing. Dry cough, with contraction of the throat.

IPECACUANHA : Violent, wheezing cough. Chest seems full of phlegm but does not come out on coughing. Very useful in children. Child becomes stiff and blue in the face. Given in alteration with Nat-s. in 30 potency, often cures asthma in children. During the attack Ip.

1X in alteration with Acon. 1X has proved to be a great palliative. Nausea may or may not be present. Attacks which occur yearly are also cured by the use of this remedy.

KALIUM CARB.

: Asthma from 3 to 5 A.M. Dry hard cough with pain in the chest. Expectoration is scanty, tenacious and offensive. Wheezing better in warm climate.

LACHESIS

: Asthma worse after sleep. The patient sleeps into aggravation and worse after taking pickles and other sour things.

LINUM USITAT.

: It is used in asthma with eczema and skin diseases and difficulties in urinary passages.

LUETICUM 1000

: Chronic asthma in summer. Wheezing and rattling. Cough dry, hard and (Syphilinum) worse at night. Wind pipe sensitive to touch.

LYCOPERSICUM ESCU.

: Asthma on breathing the least dust with frequent urination.

MEDORRHINUM

: Much oppressed breathing. Hoarseness. Pain and soreness through chest and mammae. Incessant, dry cough at night. Asthma better by lying in knee-elbow position.

NAJA TRI.

: The patient grasps the neck during attack. Intense sneezing. Patient cannot lie down. Choking. Sticky mucus.

NATRIUM ARS.	: Asthma of children beyond the age of 7 years and before puberty.
NATRIUM MUR.	: Asthma at sea shore with tears in the eyes during attack. Shortness of breath especially on going upstairs.
NATRIUM SULPH.	: Asthma of children. Dyspnea. Springs up in bed as cough hurts and holds the chest with both hands. Rattling cough worse at 4 and 5 A.M.
	Expectoration is greenish. Every fresh cold brings fresh attack. Chronic asthma worse in damp or rainy weather, from living in basements or cellars.
NUX VOM.	: Attacks occur only in the morning frequently induced by the disorder of the stomach. Scraping in the throat. Asthma with fullness of stomach in the morning or after eating. Shallow respiration and oppressed breathing.
POTHOS	: Asthmatic complaints worse inhaling the least dust. Asthma relieved after passing the stool.
PSORINUM 200	: Asthma with a peculiar symptom of relief by lying on the back with arms spread apart.
SENEGA Q	: In old people,who are asthmatic and have to sit up in the bed. Dyspnea. Great accumulation of mucus with much rattling and wheezing. Give 7 to 10 drops in

a teaspoon full of water, every hour till relieved. Talking hurts and cough often ends in a sneeze. Difficult raising of tough, profuse mucus, in the aged.

SUCCINICUM ACIDUM 3X : Asthma of hysterical persons and due to the inflammation of the respiratory tract with pain in the chest.

SULPHUR : Dyspnea, worse midnight and early morning. Wants windows open and craves open and fresh air.

SUMBULUS : Cardiac asthma. Loses breath on any exertion.

THUJA OCC. 200 : Asthma of children. Give one dose, a week. On that day no other medicine is to be taken. On other days give Nat-s. 30 and Ip. 30, in alternation. This course often cures asthma of children. If given occasionally prevents recurrence and bronchitis.

THYMUS Q : A useful remedy for respiratory infections in children. Dry, nervous asthma with severe spasms, but only a little sputum is expectorated.

TUBERCULINUM 1000 : Hard, hacking cough with profuse sweating and loss of weight. Rales all over the chest. Deposits begin on the apex of lungs. This medicine should be used intercurrently. One dose a day and then wait for the symptoms to develop indicatively for the medicines to be prescribed. Syphilinum often follows well advantageously producing a reaction.

VALERIANA Q : Choking on falling asleep. Nervous and spasmodic asthma.

AVERSION

ABIES CAN. : Aversion to pickles.

ACONIUM NAP. : Aversion to music. Music makes her sad.

AMBRA GRISEA : Aversion to smiling faces.

AMMONIUM CARB. : Aversion to water, cannot bear to touch it.

AMMONIUM MUR. : Aversion to some particular person.

ANTIMONIUM TART. : Aversion to milk as it causes nausea. Aversion to apples.

ARGENTUM MET., LACHESIS : Aversion to work in melancholia.

ARSENICUM ALB. : Aversion to cold drinks.

BARYTA CARB. : Aversion to bananas and plums.

CADMIUM SULPH. : Aversion to do any thing mental or physical.

CALCAREA CARB. : Aversion to water and washing as it aggravates ailments. It is very helpful when taking cold

	while bathing specially in rivers or pools. Aversion to coffee.
CARBO VEG.	: Aversion to cabbage and brandy.
CINA	: Aversion to butter, milk but craving for sweets.
CONIUM MAC.	: Aversion to work but attraction towards playing. During pregnancy aversion to friends.
CYCLAMEN	: Aversion to bread, butter and beer.
FERRUM MET.	: Aversion to eggs.
FLUORICUM ACIDUM	: Aversion to parents and wife.
GLONOINUM	: Aversion to husband.
GRAPHITES	: Aversion to music which makes her weep. Decided aversion to coitus. Aversion to fish and hot drinks.
HYDROPHOBINUM	: Aversion to water and dazzling light and they bring about convulsion.
IGNATIA AMARA	: Aversion to amusement and extreme aversion to tobacco smoke.
KALIUM BICH., CALCAREA CARB.	: Aversion to meat.
LAC VACCINUM DEF.	: Aversion to milk and every body.
LYCOPODIUM	: Aversion to coffee and meat.
MAGNESIUM CARB.	: Aversion to vegetables generally.
MERCURIUS SOL.	: Aversion to beef and brandy.
NATRIUM CARB.	: Aversion to milk which causes diarrhea and wind. Inability to

work due to over study. Aversion to honey also.

NATRIUM MUR.	: Aversion to bread, butter, hot food, rich food and melons.
NUX VOM.	: Aversion to beer.
PICRICUM ACIDUM	: Aversion to marriage and the very talks of marriage.
PLATINUM MET.	: Aversion to family members. irresistable impulse to kill. Aversion to wise people and advice because of his arrogance and pride. Aversion to her own children. Aversion to women in homosexuals.
PLUMBUM MET.	: Aversion to work with chronic constipation.
PULSATILLA NIG.	: Aversion to women, coition and marriage.
RADIUM BROM.	: Aversion to ice-cream.
RAPHANUS	: Aversion in women to men.
SABADILLA	: Aversion to cold water, onions, garlic and wine.
SEPIA	: Aversion to family members. Indifferent to those loved best. Aversion to occupation and opposite sex. Aversion to coition.
SILICEA	: Aversion to mother's milk as it causes vomiting. Aversion to pastry and melons.
STRAMONIUM	: Aversion to water as the very sight of water or anything glittering brings on spasms.
SULPHUR	: Aversion to being washed.

BACKACHE · LUMBAGO

Lumbago is pain in the mid and lower back.

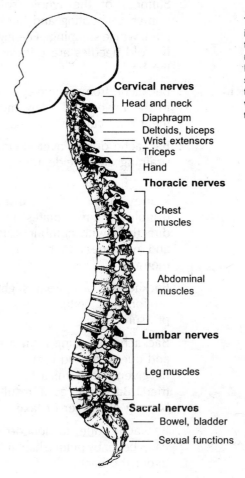

The spinal cord is a vital part of the central nervous system. Different sections control the functions of various parts of the body.

Cervical nerves
Head and neck
Diaphragm
Deltoids, biceps
Wrist extensors
Triceps
Hand
Thoracic nerves

Chest muscles

Abdominal muscles

Lumbar nerves

Leg muscles

Sacral nerves
Bowel, bladder
Sexual functions

ACETICUM ACIDUM : Pain in the back relieved only by lying on abdomen.

ACONITUM NAP. : Sudden backache on exposure to cold dry winds. Stiffness and shooting pain in lower back.

AESCULUS HIP.	: Backache in the lower region due to constipation and piles. Patient feels better by standing. Backache due to hard work.
AGARICUS MUS.	: Stiffness of the whole spine. Immense shooting and burning pain, worse stooping. Feeling as if cold needles are pricking in the back.
ANTIMONIUM TART.	: Backache from fatigue specially in the lower back. Any movement may cause vomiting.
ARNICA MONT.	: Backache due to over exertion, straining and accident.
BERBERIS VULG.	: Backache due to stones in the kidney and due to urinary troubles. Pain radiates in all directions with numbness. Pain and numbness in back during menses.
BRYONIA ALBA	: Backache worse from slightest motion and better by rest and pressure.
CALCAREA CARB.	: Backache on rising from a seat and due to an old hurt. It may be given after Arnica has been tried. Backache as a result of bathing in a river or lake.
CALCAREA PHOS., NATRIUM MUR. 6X	: Backache due to leucorrhea. Pains better by putting hard things under the back.
CANNABIS IND.	: Backache after sexual intercourse.
CHINA OFF.	: Backache extending to the hollow of the knee. Worse morning and sitting. Better standing.

CIMICIFUGA : Rheumatic pains in the lumbar and sacral region extending to the thighs. Pain in the scapulae and right shoulder. Restlessness and sleeplessness.

CAUSTICUM : Pain in back during menses. Pressing, cramp like pain in small of back and renal region while sitting, better after rising.

COLOCYNTHIS : Pain in the back, buttocks and thighs. Severe burning pain along the sacrum.

CONIUM MAC. : Backache from coition.

DULCAMARA, NATRIUM SULPH. : Backache due to living in damp houses and in dwellers of basements.

EUPATORIUM PERF. : Backache due to pain in the bones of the spine.

GNAPHALIUM : Chronic rheumatic character of the muscles of the back and neck. Worse continued motion, better resting specially on the back. This remedy is indicated in severe chronic backache. It is specially useful when the pain is associated with numbness.

HYPERICUM PERF. : Backache due to injuries to the nerves. Violent pain and inability to walk or stoop after a fall on coccyx.

KALIUM CARB. : Backache in the lower part of the back and in pregnant women. Pain is constant, back and the legs gives out. The patient has to sit.

KALMIA LAT.	: Backache with numbness. Pain extends to the scapulae. Pains are descending.
LACHESIS	: Pain in coccyx and sacrum, especially on rising from a sitting position.
MAGNESIUM PHOS.	: Pains better by heat and pressure and worse in cold.
MEDORRHINUM 200	: Backache from neck to sacrum.
NATRIUM MUR.	: Backache better by hard pressure. The patient walks with hands around his hips and back.
NUX VOM.	: Backache in the bed on lying. Must sit up or turn side. Pain is located in the lumbar region. Hemorrhoids may be present. Backache in chilly and constipated patients, who lead a sedentary life.
OVA TOSTA 3X	: Backache with leucorrhea. A feeling as if the spine was broken and wired or tied together with a string.
PHYTOLACCA DEC.	: Pains in the lumbar region. Backache especially in the morning, on rising.
PULSATILLA NIG.,	: Backache during menstruation.
CIMICIFUGA, RHUS TOX.	: Backache resulting from an old hurt. Backache due to sprain, exposure to cold weather, sleeping with damp clothes or damp ground or getting wet in rains or taking bath when perspiring or over lifting. Worse rising from a seat and better by movement.

SEPIA	: Backache better by belching. Chilly patients. Relief by hand pressure.
STAPHYSAGRIA	: Backache worse in the morning after rising and after sexual excesses or on indignation.
SULPHUR	: Pain between shoulders. Stiffness of the nape of the neck. Backache after physical exertion, cannot straighten up immediately after exertion. Backache worse on standing.
	Severe pain in the lower back and coccyx. Cannot walk erect. Pain worse night and cold.
SYMPHYTUM OFF.	: Backache due to excessive indulgence in sex.
THUJA OCC.	: Drawing pain in small of back after prolonged sitting.

BACKWARD CHILDREN
(DWARFISHNESS)

AETHUSA CYN.	: Confused children with impaired memory. Dull in studies.
AGARICUS MUS.	: Child has a weak memory due to slow development of brain. Late learning to walk and talk.
BARYTA CARB.	: Shy children who do not develop properly. Low intelligence due to slow development of brain. Cannot concentrate.
BARYTA MUR.	: Patient walks about with mouth open and appears stupid.

CALCAREA CARB.	: Child does not grow properly. Has a big head and a big belly. Profuse perspiration on the head, wets the pillow. They are slow to understand and slow in learning to walk. Tendency to obstinacy.
CALCAREA PHOS.	: Pale, sickly or lean children who do not grow properly. They are late in learning to walk.
NATRIUM MUR.	: Child is late in learning to talk.
STRAMONIUM	: Restless and angry children. Always crying. Cat nap sleep. Easily frightened. Look and behave stupidly.
SYPHILINUM 1M	: A dose can be given every month with a gap of 15 days after taking Tuberculinum.
TUBERCULINUM 1M	: Retarded development of a child. The treatment should be started with this remedy and it should be repeated each month.

BALDNESS
(SEE ALOPECIA)

BATHING FEAR

HYDROPHOBINUM	: The person is terribly afraid of water, specially running water.

and as such does not like to take a bath, specially in a lake or in a river.

SULPHUR : A person wants to remain dirty. He has no inclination to look smart and clean and hence hates to be washed or bathed.

BEARD

SPHINGURUS MAR. : Hair fall out from the beard. Women's face in grown up men without a beard.

ARSENICUM IOD. : Eczema of the beard.

HEPAR SULPHURIS 6 : Pustular eruptions on beard.

BED SORES

ARNICA MONT. : Generally indicated in bed sores when a patient is confined to a bed for a long time and feels bruised all over before ulceration.

BAPTISIA TINC. : Bed sores specially during typhoid fever.

NOTE : Bed sores develop on account of lying in one position for a long time such as is necessary in orthopedic or similar problems. Precaution is easier than cure. The patient should be sponged daily with luke warm water and any talcum powder be sprinkled on him after this. If ulcers have developed, Calendula Q - a few drops may be added to water used for sponging.

BED WETTING
(SEE   ENURESIS)

NOTE: No liquid diet should be given to a patient suffering from enuresis before one hour of bed time. In children, parents should take the trouble of getting up before the time when the children wet the bed and make them urinate in the urinal. Ten days of this trouble usually breaks this habit. The child should never be rebuked for this bad habit.

BEE STINGS

Apply URTICA URENS Q or LEDUM PALUSTRE Q at the site of the sting. It will remove burning, pain and swelling within a short time.

BELCHING
(SEE ERUCTATIONS)

BEREAVEMENT

It is an acute state of intense psychological sadness and suffering experienced after the tragic loss of a loved one or some priceless possession.

ARNICA MONT.	: Shock on account of sudden death of a loved one. Sits with head between the knees and does not desire to be spoken to and to be left alone.
ACONITUM NAP.	: Grief on account of a sudden loss of a friend or a relative. Extreme restlessness and fear of death.
IGNATIA AMARA	: Consequences of suppression of grief. Hysterical mood. Laughing at one time, sighing or crying at another time. She is relieved by passing urine or eating something.
STAPHYSAGRIA	: Chronic grief due to indignation, humiliation and insults.

BILIOUS ATTACK

ARSENICUM ALB.	: Diarrhea due to bilious attack.
BERBERIS AQ. Q	: Attack of biliousness. Nausea and vomiting of bile. Bitter taste.
CHAMOMILLA	: Diarrhea due to biliousness. Stools slimy green.
CHELIDONIUM	: Bilious attacks relieved by eating.
CHINA OFF. 1X	: Complete suppression of bile. This causes pale stools and yellowish tinge of skin. Four doses of 2 drops each in a day.
IRIS VERS.	: Attacks of nausea, vomiting, diarrhea and severe headache.

MANGANUM SULPH.	: Excess of bile.
MERCURIUS SOL.	: Dysentery due to biliousness.
NUX VOM.	: Biliousness after over indulging in alcohol.
PULSATILLA NIG.	: Bilious attack after eating fried and rich foods. Vomiting of bile.

BIRTH CONTROL

NATRIUM MUR. 200	: Three doses - one each day, on the first, second and the third, after cessation of menses; acts as an oral contraceptive and makes pregnancy unlikely for one month.
PULSATILLA NIG. 200	: Three doses - one each day, for three days before starting of menstruation; also gives protection against pregnancy for the next month.

NOTE: In females, every month during the menstrual cycle, an ovum is released from the ovary into the fallopian tube where it can be fertilized by the male sperm and then it travels to the uterus. If the egg is not fertilized, each months menstruation occurs and the lining of the uterus is shed through the vagina. If the egg is fertilized, it results in pregnancy. The best way to avoid pregnancy is to avoid the combination of ovum and sperm. This can be done by man by using a condom during intercourse and by the women by using a cervical cap which blocks the entry of sperms into the cervical canal. Surgical and some other oral methods are also available.

BITES
(SEE ALSO STINGS)

ACETICUM ACIDUM : Bad effects from stings and bites are cured by the use of this remedy.

APIS MEL. : Bites by bees.

ARNICA MONT. Q : Apply externally for wasp stings and give Cantharis 200 orally.

CEDRON Q : Bites of serpents and poisonous insects are antidoted by this remedy.

CISTUS CAN. : For bites of mad dogs and other mad animals. Locally as a wash to arrest fetid discharge.

ECHINACEA Q : A general but a good remedy for stings and even bites of venomous animals like snake.

EUPHORBIA PROSTATA Q : It is said to be an infallible remedy for bites of snakes, specially rattle snakes. Dose, 15 drops every 10 minutes.

GUACO : For stings of scorpions. Apply Drona Q (an Indian remedy) locally.

GOLONDRINA Q : An antidote to the snake poison. Its use renders the body immune to the influence of snake venom. May be used as a preventive at places where incidents of poisonous snake bites are common.

HYPERICUM PERF. 3X : Bites of bugs. There is burning at the site of bite.

INDIGO TINC.	:	Pure powder of remedy placed on the wound caused by bites of snakes and spiders cures the effects of poison.
LACHESIS 200	:	For bites of dogs which are not mad. Also for bites of leeches.
LEDUM PAL. Q or 200	:	For bites of all animals, rats, cats, dogs, scorpions, etc. Apply Q locally and give 200 orally. It acts as an anti-tetanus remedy.
LYSSINUM 200	:	Dog bites.
PULEX IRRITANS	:	Flea bites and bites of dust mite. There is prickly itching of the skin.
STAPHYSAGRIA	:	Bites of mosquitoes.
URTICA URENS Q	:	A very good remedy for bee stings. Use orally in drops and apply externally at the site of bite.

BITING

AMMONIUM BROM.	:	Irritable feeling under the finger nails. Relieved only by biting them.
ARUM TRIPH.	:	Biting of lips and biting of fingers and nails.
CAUSTICUM	:	Biting of cheeks or tongue while eating.
IGNATIA AMARA	:	Biting inside of cheeks while eating or biting of tongue while eating.

PHYTOLA CA DEC.   : Irresitible desire to bite gums
                           and teeth together.

BLADDER
(SEE ALSO CYSTITIS)

ARSENICUM ALB.   : Burning pain in the urethra on
                           urination, with unquenchable
                           thirst for cold water.

BERBERIS VULG. Q   : Burning and cutting pains in the
                           urethra when not urinating.
                           Sensation as if some urine
                           remained after urination. Pain in
                           thighs and loins on urinating,
                           specially in women.

CALCAREA REN. 30,   : Stone in the bladder with sharp
HYDRANGEA Q   pains in the loins.

CANTHARIS   : Intolerable urging and tenseness.
                           Nephrites with burning in the
                           urethra while passing urine.
                           Urine is passed drop by drop.

CAUSTICUM   : Paralysis of the bladder resulting
                           in dribbling of urine and invol-
                           untary spurting of urine on sneez-
                           ing and coughing. Involuntary
                           urination during first sleep at
                           night or from excitement.

CONIUM MAC. 200   : Much difficulty in passing urine
                           due to inflammation of the
                           bladder.

OPIUM   : Bladder weak, no expulsion
                           power.

PYRUS AMERICANA	:	Prolapse of bladder.
TARAXACUM Q	:	Cancer of bladder.
TEREBINTHINIAEQ	:	Burning pain on urinating. Urine is passed drop by drop. Strangury with bloody urine. Urethritis with painful erections. In women there is intense burning in the uterine region.

BLEEDING

ACETICUM ACIDUM	:	Bleeding from mucous membranes.
CALENDULA OFF. Q	:	A very good healing and antiseptic agent; checks bleeding of wounds and bleeding after tooth extraction. Use externally or internally.
FERRUM PHOS. 3X	:	Bleeding of bright red blood from any outlet of the body.
FICUS IND. Q	:	It possesses great anti-hemorrhagic properties, more than Fic-r. Blood should be pure red.
FICUS REL. Q	:	Bleeding of any kind. It will arrest hemorrhage from any part of the 'body.
HAMAMELIS Q	:	Bleeding from veins. Give internally and apply externally.
LACHESIS	:	Bleeding from any part, when the blood is blue, black or dark.

If there is a continuous bleeding due to a sexually transmitted disease.

MILLEFOLIUM Q,
HAMAMELIS Q,
FICUS IND. Q

: Small wounds bleed profusely and for a long time because the blood does not coagulate easily and early. All the three can be mixed together in equal parts. 10 drops a dose.

TRILLIUM PEND. Q

: Checks bleeding after tooth extraction and operation (surgical). Use externally and internally.

BLEMISHES

Blemish is a small circumscribed alteration of the skin.

CIMICIFUGA

: Blemishes on the face of a young woman. There are stains and defective skin color of the face.

CAULOPHYLLUM 3X

: Discoloration of the facial skin on account of troubles of menstruation and uterine disorders.

LYCOPODIUM

: Freckles, nitching liver spots; yellow gray complexion.

SEPIA

: Yellow spots on face. Bluishness in married woman having menstrual and uterine disorders.

BLEPHARITIS
(INFLAMMATION OF EYES OR EYELIDS)

CHRYSAROBINUM : Eruptions and itching of the eyelids. Lids are red and covered with dandruff like scales.

HEPAR SULPHURIS : Throbbing pain in the lids and their inflammation. This will be used in the beginning of the treatment. Petroleum in the middle of the treatment and Chrysarobinum should be tried last of all.

PETROLEUM : Loss of eye lashes. Lot of itching in the eye lashes. Margins of the lids are swollen and red.

BLINDNESS

Blindness is loss of vision. It may be congenital (from birth) or acquired (due to some eye disease etc.)

Blindness from birth, blindness from small pox, eruptions in the eyes and blindness due to lightening can be cured by surgical operations only. Temporary blindness can be treated by the following remedies :

GELSEMIUM : Blindness from excessive watering of eyes as by weeping.

LYCOPODIUM : Blindness at night.

PHYSOSTIGMA : Night blindness.

RANUNCULUS BULB. : Sudden blindness during day or at night in the pregnant woman.

BLISTERS

Blister is a fluid filled, thin walled structure on the skin.

ALLIUM CEPA : Blisters on feet or heels due to excessive walking or from pinching of shoes.

APIS MEL. : Blisters due to insect bites.

BAPTISIA TINC. : Blisters in typhoid fever.

CANTHARIS : Blisters due to excessive walking or burns.

GRAPHITES : Burning blisters.

HYPERICUM PERF. : Blisters from scalding with hot water, etc.

IGNATIA AMARA : Blisters in intermittent fevers when Nat-m. fails.

KALIUM MUR. 200 : White blisters in the mouth.

MAGNESIUM MUR. : Blisters on lips.

MEDORRHINUM 1M : Blisters on the inner surface of the lips and cheeks.

NATRIUM MUR. : Blisters on tongue. Blisters in the mouth or at the corner of the mouth. Specially during fever and menses.

NATRIUM PHOS. : Blisters on the tip of the tongue.

NITRICUM ACIDUM : Blisters and ulcers in the mouth, tongue and genitals which bleed easily.

RANUNCULUS BULB.	: Blisters formed on the skin by a slight pressure.
RHUS TOX.	: Blisters in fevers with much itching around.
THUJA OCC.	: Painful white blister in the mouth and on tip of the tongue.

BLOOD

Blood forms 7 to 8% of the body weight. Thus, an adult weighing 70 kg. has a blood volume of about 5 litres. Blood is composed of a fluid (plasma) in which floats red and white corpuscles, fats,various chemical substances,etc. Solids constitute about 22% and the rest 78% or so is water. It provides nutrition and respiration to the body tissues and transports wastes of the tissues to the excretory organs. It maintains body temperature. Various hematological disorders are discussed under separate heads like anemia, bleeding, blood clots, blood pressure, hemorrhage, hemophilia, leukemia, menses, thalassemia, etc. in this book.

BLOOD CLOTS
(THROMBOSIS)

AMMONIUM CAUST. Q	: It is a powerful cardiac stimulant. It should be given by inhalation in cases of fainting in heart diseases or in cases of hemorrhage or blood clots. Internally, 3rd potency.

ASPIDOSPERMA Q : Blood clots in pulmonary artery of the lungs are removed by the use of this remedy. 10 drops, 4 times a day.

CEANOTHUS A. Q : Materially reduces the clotting of blood.

CRATAEGUS OXY. : It has solvent power upon crustaneous and calcareous deposits in the arteries.

KALIUM MUR. 12X : It is stated to absorb the blood clots.

LILIUM TIG. : Frequent palpitation with a feeling, as if the heart is squeezed.

LYCOPODIUM : Great palpitation all the times even when asleep. Cramps in the chest.

MERCURIUS SOL. : Dying feeling due to weakness of the heart. Pain and palpitation in the cardiac region.

PITUITRINUM : Checks hemorrhages and aids absorption of blood clots.

SECALE COR. : It is indicated when there is numbness and coldness in extremities and in hypertension.

BLOOD PRESSURE

Thousands of persons die each year from the effects of hypertension. High blood pressure does not cause a feeling of uneasiness, dizziness or nervousness. As a result people with high blood pressure live for several years without knowing it and it silently leads to heart attack, stroke or kidney failure and even death. In blood pressure cases, diet plays an important part. In high blood pressure, the patient should avoid use of salt, alcohol, spices and fried foods. Non-vegetarian food is not useful. Raw green vegetables or boiled vegetables are a good diet both in high blood pressure cases and low blood pressure cases. Patient should avoid argument and anger. He should be advised to take a lot of rest and milk containing not more than 2% fats. Using less salt and eating more fruits and vegetables prevent development of high blood pressure. Magnesium suppliments have a small but significant effect on lowering the blood pressure. Blood pressure is measured and recorded in two numbers, as 128/82. The top reading is called 'systolic' and the bottom reading is called the 'diastolic' pressure. One's blood pressure is unique to oneself only. Systolic is the pressure against the walls of the blood vessels when the heart pumps. Diastolic is the pressure against the walls of the blood vessels between the heart beats. Systolic is related to strokes, but heart disease is related both to systolic and diastolic.

There is no best blood pressure but the chart below shows ranges accepted by the medical experts:

	Normal	Border line	High
Systolic pressure over	139 or less	140 -159	160 or more
Diastolic pressure	89 or less	90 - 104	105 or more

HIGH BLOOD PRESSURE (HYPERTENSION)

Measuring Blood Pressure

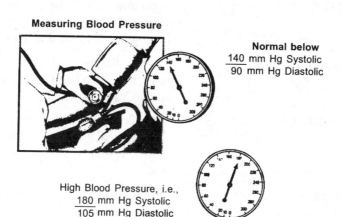

Normal below
<u>140</u> mm Hg Systolic
90 mm Hg Diastolic

High Blood Pressure, i.e.,
<u>180</u> mm Hg Systolic
105 mm Hg Diastolic

ADRENALINUM 2X : It causes a very prompt fall in blood pressure and is used as a palliative. It should be used carefully and the blood pressure should be measured before its administration so that the blood pressure does not fall, all of a sudden.

AURUM MET. : High blood pressure with low pressure of the pulse. The patient is disgusted with life but is afraid of death.

AURUM IOD. : High blood pressure of persons suffering from progressive paralysis with mental deterioration.

BARYTA MUR. 3X : It is a good remedy for high blood pressure of the aged. There is increased tension of the pulse. Systolic is high in comparison with diastolic pressure which is low.

CACTUS : Hypertension with heart trouble, with a feeling of constriction in the region of heart and pain.

CALCAREA CARB. : For fat, flabby and chilly patients. Sweat on head, palms and soles. Craves eggs.

CEANOTHUS A. Q : High blood pressure due to diseases and enlargement of spleen, for which it is an excellent remedy.

CONIUM MAC. 200 : Hypertension of bachelors and maids in old age.

CRATAEGUS OXY. Q, PASSIFLORA Q, RAUWOLFIA Q : During the intervening period when Lachesis is administered, take five drops each of these three medicines in a little water thrice daily and on the next day take the following (described below) treatment. These two treatments are to be taken on alternate days.

FERRUM PHOS. 6X, CALCAREA PHOS. 6X, KALIUM MUR. 6X : Two grains of each (total 6 grains) must be taken thrice daily for a day and on the next day, the mixture described above should be taken. And it should be repeated as stated above. This treatment will control and cure most of the recent cases. Even chronic cases are much benefited. It takes 15 days to 3 months for results. Blood pressure should be measured every week and it should not be allowed to fall much below the normal.

GLONOINUM : Throbbing of the heart. Each beat is heard in the ears. High blood pressure during menopause or due to suppression of menses. Headache is always present.

IGNATIA AMARA : Development of temporary hypertension following emotional shock.

LACHESIS 1M : Start the treatment with this medicine and repeat it after a month if the case is not cleared. No other medicine should be taken on this day. In most of the cases, this medicine cures the case.

LYCOPUS : Lowers blood pressure of patients having heart diseases.

NATRIUM MUR. 200 : Due to shock or grief. Thyroid malfunction, diabetes, etc. Craves salt.

PHYSOSTIGMA : Feeling as if a 'cap is gripping the head' has led to a marked relief in several cases of hypertension.

PITUITRINUM : Relieves the headache of patients suffering from high blood pressure; checks brain hemorrhage and dissolves blood clot.

PLUMBUM MET. : Hypertension may be due to gout or kidney troubles or from thickening of the arteries. Great paleness of the skin and red blood corpuscles are decreased.

VERATRUM VIR.	: Oppression, sighing, rapid respiration and gasping for breath are the guiding symptoms, for the use of this remedy. It induces fall of both systolic and diastolic blood pressure.
VISCUM ALB.	: Systolic blood pressure is high and diastolic low.
URANIUM NIT. 3X	: High blood pressure during dropsy. Great emaciation is evident.

NOTE: Raw onions and garlic in diet help to keep the blood pressure down.

LOW BLOOD PRESSURE (HYPOTENSION)

Low blood pressure can occur in shock and collapse, in hemorrhages, infections, fevers, cancer, anemia, neurasthenia, defective functioning of any organ, other wasting diseases and approaching death. So treatment should be according to the symptoms only. One should not be misled by the name low blood pressure. The following remedies will prove useful.

CACTUS 200	: Low blood pressure due to heart diseases. Characteristic constriction as if an iron band around the heart is the guiding symptom for the use of this remedy. Temperature is usually sub-normal.
CAFFEINUM 3X	: It is used when there is a general muscular weakness.
CALCAREA PHOS. 200	: In persons growing too fast.

CAMPHORA 1X	: Low blood pressure with subnormal temperature. 3 doses at an interval of 15 minutes. It should be given either in pills or on a lump of sugar, but not in water.
CARBO VEG.	: Low blood pressure due to low vitality.
CHINA OFF.	: Hypotension due to loss of vital fluids like blood or semen and due to dehydration on account of vomiting and diarrhea.
CRATAEGUS OXY. Q	: It is a great heart tonic and arrests further fall of blood pressure.
GELSEMIUM	: With irregular heart beats and palpitation. Feels as if heart would stop beating if does not move about.
KALIUM PHOS. 200	: Low blood pressure due to nervousness.
LYCOPODIUM 200	: It is indicated in irritable persons with urinary or digestive or wind troubles.
NATRIUM MUR. 200	: When this remedy is indicated, there will be a craving for salt. For such patients the heat of sun is not bearable.
RADIUM BROM.	: Low blood pressure due to severe pains in different parts of the body, on skin affections and particularly when there is a conspicuous increase in white blood cells.

SPARTIUM SCOPARIUM 1X : Produces comfort in cases of hypotension and increases the strength of the heart.

VISCUM ALB. 200   : Low blood pressure due to neuralgia's and rheumatism. Weight and oppression of the heart, as if being squeezed.

BLOOD PURIFIER

ECHINACEA Q   : Septic conditions call for the use of this remedy. It purifies the blood and stimulates the immune system.

GUNPOWDER 3X   : It is a great blood purifier in septic and skin troubles. Clears skin diseases which are obstinate to be cured.

BLOOD SPITTING
(SEE HAEMOPTYSIS)

BLOOD TRANSFUSIONS

In a large number of major surgical cases like hip replacement, hysterectomy (removal of uterus), prostrate, orthopedic, etc., blood transfusion is required to make good the loss of blood. Usually matching blood of other healthy persons is used for this purpose. This procedure is risky because the blood donor may have some serious diseases which may have escaped notice at the time of taking the blood. Homoeopathy has a solution to avoid the risks. Patients awaiting elective surgeries having no defect in blood ,can give their own blood which can be stored to be used later during the operation. This can be done 6-8 weeks before the day of operation. After giving blood, the patient should take a dose of NATRIUM CACODYL. 1X in the morning and a dose of LECITHINUM 1X in the evening daily. This will elevate his red corpuscles count and the amount of hemoglobin. A week before the operation more blood can be taken and stored, if needed. After the operation, FERRUM PHOS. 3X, should be taken four times a day in three grain doses. It will further make up for iron and hemoglobin loss, if any and will avoid the risk of fever also.

Blood taken from the umbilical cord of new born babies (cord blood) can be used in the bone marrow transplants even if it is not a perfect match. This blood is found in the umbilical cord and placenta after child birth. It is rich in stem cells which have the ability to become any kind of blood cell and can be used to replenish a damaged immune system. It is best for family members and possibly even for donation say doctor researchers.

BLOODY URINE
(SEE HAEMATURA)

BLOTCHES
(SEE ACNE)

BLUSHING

AMYLEMUM NIT.

: Blushing or flushing of blood to the face on least excitement either mental or physical. It cures permanently, cases of habitual blushing.

FERRUM MET.

: Face flushes from least pain, emotion, exertion and excitement.

BODY ODOR

CALCAREA CARB. 200

: Bad smell from the body due to fetid sweat, specially on the forehead.

GUAIACUM OFF.

: Bad odor from the body as if never changed. This odor can be felt even after a bath and change of clothes.

HEPAR SULPHURIS

: Body smells like old-rotten cheese.

MERCURIUS SOL.

: Breath, excretions and body smell is foul. Skin always moist. The odor from the mouth is very foul and can be felt all over the room.

PSORINUM 200

: Fetid body smell on account of fetid sweat. The skin is oily. Body has a filthy smell even after a bath.

SILICEA

: Bad smell from perspiration on

feet, hands and armpits. The patient is chilly.

SULPHUR 200 : Bad smell from the body with no perspiration, but dry skin. All discharges and exhalations are of an offensive character.

BOILS

ARNICA MONT. : Tendency to small boils which are painful. One boil is cured, when the other comes out. The boils come out in crops. Similarly, boils come in crops in Gunpowder also.

BELLADONNA : Throbbing, painful boils with redness. It should be used in the beginning.

BELLIS P. : Boils all over. They are sore and painful with swelling.

GUNPOWDER 3X, ECHINACEA Q : Either of these remedies may be given when boils resists other treatment. Both the remedies are antiseptic and blood purifier respectively. Gunpowder works better when there are crops of boils.

HEPAR SULPHURIS : Suppurative boils.

SEPIA : Boils in children.

THUJA OCC. 200 : Crops of boils on face, neck and nose. Give one dose a week.

TUBERCULINUM 1M : Crops of small boils, very pain-

ful, successively appear on the
nose. The pus is green and foul
smelling.

BONES

ACIDUM FLUOR., SILICEA : Give alternately to cure necrosis
of the bones of jaws.

ACIDUM SALICYLIC. : Caries of bones due to the
suppression of foot sweat.

ARISTOLOCHIA CLEM. : Pain in the bones of the ball and
socket joints.

ASAFOETIDA 3X : Unbearable pain and caries in
the bones. Pain in bones in syphilitic patients.

AURUM MET. : Pain in the bones worse at night.
It is a great solvent of enlarged
bones.

CALCAREA CARB. : Caries of the spinal cord. Rheumatism on account of defective
bony growths.

CALCAREA FLUOR. : Necrosis of the bone of upper
right jaw.

CALCAREA PHOS. : It is a remedy for weak bones
which are easily breakable. They
do not serve the purpose of
supporting parts, they are
supposed to do. It creates new
bone marrow.

CAUSTICUM : Deformation of the bones about
the joints. Tearing pains in the
bones and joints, worse at night

causing restlessness. Better by warmth. Sinking of strength and faint like feeling.

DROSERA : Tuberculosis of bone.

EUPATORIUM PERF. : Pain in the bones in fevers, etc. or without a visible cause. Pain in the wrists and spine. Bone pains of all descriptions with restlessness.

EUPHORBIUM OFF. : Burning pain in the bones and necrosis of the bones.

GRAPHITES · : Pain in the bones of the feet and ankles with great restlessness.

GUNPOWDER : Inflammation of bones, during menopause.

HECLA LAVA 3X : It has a marked action on many affections of the bones like swelling (ostitis), abnormal growth of the bones (exostosis), difficult teething,caries of bones, tumor of bones (osteosarcoma), inflammation of spine (rachitis), death of the bones (necrosis), jaw bones, neck bones, etc. Has to be used for a long time.

HYPERICUM PERF. : Severe nerve pains in the hip joints.

MERCURIUS SOL. : Pain in the bones of limbs worse at night. Patient is very sensitive to cold.

MEZEREUM : Bone pains accompany chilliness and the patient is very sensitive to cold air. Pain shoots upwards.

PHOSPHORUS	: Periosteum painful and swollen, ulcers affecting bones. Cures necrosis and caries of lower jaw, vertebra and tibia.
PHYTOLACCA DEC.	: Pain in the bones of patients suffering from syphilis.
RUTA G. Q	: Pain in bones due to an injury specially pain in the long bones.
SYMPHYTUM OFF. Q	: Inflammation and pains due to a fracture of the bone. It acts as a glue for bones in fractures.
TAMUS Q	: A paint on the hip or knuckle bones or any other part where there is a great pain, takes away the pain speedly. Use it orally also.
THERIDION	: Rachitis, necrosis and caries of teeth.
THIOSINAMINUM	: Wasting of spinal marrow.
VANADIUM	: It helps fixation of calcium in the bones.

NOTE: Regular moderate exercise builds bones and helps prevent fractures and osteoporosis.

Osteoporosis occurs when bones lose calcium faster than is replaced. The bone breakdown happens faster than bone formation, making the bone vary fragile.

Vertebrae
(spinal bone)

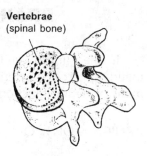

Five simple to help reduce risk of osteoporosis:

1. Know your risk factors.
2. Talk to your doctor about your risk factors and preventative steps you can take.
3. Ensure that your diet is rich in calcium and vitamin D.
4. Incorporate physical activity, including weigh-bearing exercise, into your lifestyle (30 minutes three times a week, or break into shorter segments to fit your schedule).
5. Limit caffeine and alcohol intake and quit smoking.

Cross-section of healthy bone

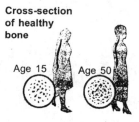

Age 15   Age 50

BORING OF NOSE

ARUM TRIPH.

: Inclination to scratch by boring fingers in the nose due to itching and tingling in the mucous membranes of the nostrils is cured by this remedy.

CINA

: Itching of the nose all the time. Wants to rub it and pick at it. Bores it till it bleeds.

BRAIN CONCUSSION

It is a clinical syndrome due to mechanical, usually traumatic, forces; characterised by immediate and transient impairment of neural function.

ARNICA MONT. Q   : A person falls unconcious as a result of a heavy and hard blow on the brain. Give 5 drops every 15 to 20 minutes and consciousness will return gradually. The patient may vomit.

KALIUM PHOS. 6X   : After the use of Arnica Q, use this remedy, giving a dose each hour. This will restore the person to normal health.

BRAIN FAG
(MENTAL FATIGUE)

AESCULUS HIP. 3X : Loss of memory. Sadness. Confused and bewildered.

AMBRA GRISEA   : Nervous and mental weakness due to shock of loss in business, death of a loved one, failures, etc. Dwells upon disagreeable happenings unnecessarily.

ANACARDIUM ORI. : Brain fag with marked loss of memory or due to over-study.

ARGENTUM NIT.   : Brain fag and general debility. Impulses to jump out of windows. Trembling. Vertigo. Fear of death. Headache with coldness. Feeling of strangulation in throat.

BELLADONNA : Brain fag after delirium.

CALCAREA CARB. : Brain fag on account of fear of failure, tension, depression or wounded pride.

IGNATIA AMARA : Changeable mood. Silent brooding. Mental and physical depression. Sad and tearful. Sighing and sobbing.

KALIUM PHOS. : One of the best remedies for prostration of brain, mental and physical depression. For sleeplessness use 200X, otherwise 6X potency.

LACHESIS : Brain fag in diphtheria.

NATRIUM MUR. 200 : Sleeplessness due to dwelling over unpleasant events of the past and thus tires his brain.

NUX VOM. : Fatigue caused by mental work or by worries.

PICRICUM ACIDUM : Mental fatigue due to headache. Mental fatigue in teachers who have to teach lengthy hours against their will. Mental fatigue of literary persons and writers who work for long hours.

SULPHUR : Brain appears tired on waking up in the morning.

ZINCUM PHOS. : Brain fag due to business worries. Weak memory. Attacks of vertigo which is better on rest and lying down.

BRAIN HEMORRHAGE (APOPLEXY)

ACONITUM NAP. Q : When brain hemorrhage is sudden, due to any cause, give 4-5 drops in water every 15 minutes. It is the first remedy to be employed in sudden and violent attacks.

ARNICA MONT. : Due to a fall or blow on the head, there is brain hemorrhage or apoplexy. The face becomes red and puffed up. This remedy gives relief. Bar-c. is also helpful in cerebral hemorrhage.

ASTERIAS RUB. : Threatened brain hemorrhage when blood seems to be rushing to the head.

BARYTA CARB. 3X : Use it for cerebral hemorrhage resulting in one sided paralysis.

CUPRUM MET. : Cannot speak properly and stammers before brain hemorrhage occurs.

FORMICA RUFA : It should be given when the case has been cured. It prevents recurrence.

GLONOINUM 3X : Threatened apoplexy due to sun stroke.

HYOSCYAMUS NIG. : Falls down suddenly with a scream and red face. Involuntarily urination and stool, due to brain hemorrhage.

KALIUM BROM. : Sudden rupture of blood vessels in brain with paralysis and coma.

KALIUM PHOS. 6X	: Brain fag due to excessive mental work.
LAUROCERASUS	: Sudden cough, suffocation, loss of speech and palpitation due to threatened brain hemorrhage or due to actual brain hemorrhage.
NATRIUM SULPH. 200, 1M	: Threatened brain hemorrhage due to falls and injuries to the head.
NUX MOSCH.	: Affections of the brain occurring in infants during attack of cholera.
NUX VOM.	: Threatened brain hemorrhage with giddiness, headache and fullness of the head and in alcoholics after heavy drinking.
OPIUM	: Coma and oppressed respiration. Lies down unconscious with eyes half open after brain hemorrhage.
PITUITRINUM 3X	: Cerebral hemorrhage will be checked by the use of this remedy. It also helps absorption of blood clots. Apoplexy due to hypertension. Give in 10 drop doses.
STRONTIUM	: Threatened cerebral hemorrhage from shock after surgical operations and high blood pressure or from sequel of chronic hemorrhage.
TABACUM 200	: Anemia of the brain.
ZINCUM MET	: Brain fag. Paralysis of the brain.

BRAIN INFLAMMATION
(ENCEPHALITIS)

ACONITUM NAP. : If the inflammation of the brain is accompanied by fever, restlessness, anxiety and thirst, use this remedy.

APIS MEL. : Oedema of the face. Patient cries in sleep or during unconsciousness.

BAPTISIA TINC. : Brain inflammation causes delirium of a low type and the patient is sleepy.

BELLADONNA : When the eyes and face are red. High fever with delirium. Congestion of the brain.

BRYONIA ALBA : Little delirium but much pain. The patient looks stupid. Nausea may be present and patient lies quietly, does not want to be disturbed.

BUFO RANA : Numbness of the brain, is cured by this remedy.

GELSEMIUM : Brain inflammation is indicated by headache, vertigo and pain in the neck and shoulders. Brain congestion may be with or without fever.

RUTA G. : Inflammation of the brain due to injuries.

STAPHYSAGRIA : Brain appears as if squeezed.

BRAIN TUMOR

General symptoms of a brain tumor are headache and vomiting without nausea. Vision is also affected. Any swelling on the head may be watched carefully.

CALCAREA FLUOR. 200	: A very useful remedy when the tumor is hard and stony. Creaking noise in head. Great depression. Sparks before eyes. Brain fag and vomiting.
PLUMBUM MET.	: Epileptic form of convulsions, giddiness and in some cases, coma. Pain as if a ball rose from the throat to the brain. Voices in the ears. This is a leading remedy.
SCIRRHINUM 1000	: A dose may be given at the start of the treatment. No medicine should be given for the next 48 hours.
SULPHUR 200	: It should be used as an intercurrent remedy once a month and no medicine should be given for the next 24 hours.

NOTE: Despite all the advances in cancer research, brain tumors remain one of the most elusive and challenging cancers to treat. This is the second most common form of childhood cancer and represents the second fastest growing cause of cancer deaths among those over 65.

BRAIN UNDEVELOPED

BARYTA CARB.

: Children born with an undeveloped brain, grow physically but not mentally. They behave like children even at puberty and beyond.

They are not able to look after themselves. Such persons are incapable of marriage and should not marry. This medicine may help development of the brain in some cases only.

BREAST (MAMMAE)

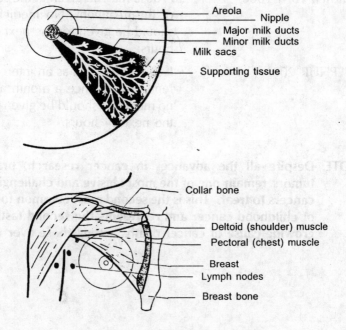

ARSENICUM ALB.	:	Hard tumor of the breast.
ARSENICUM IOD 3X	:	Cancer of the breasts after ulceration has started.
ASAFOETIDA 3X	:	Breasts swollen with appearance of milk in unmarried girls who were never impregnated.
ASTERIAS RUB.	:	Cancer of the breasts in ulcerative stage. Breasts are hard and painful. The patient has a red face. It acts on both the breasts but better on the left. It is a good remedy for cancer.
BELLADONNA 200	:	Tumors of the breasts. Breasts feel heavy and hard and become hot and red. Useful when the disease has not prolonged long.
BELLIS P.	:	Any trouble of the breasts after sustaining a bruise on it.
BROMIUM	:	Tumor or cancer of the breast.
BRYONIA ALBA	:	Breasts hard and inflamed.
BUFO RANA	:	A palliative medicine in cancer of breasts.
CARBO ANIMALIS	:	Tumor on the nipples.
CHIMAPHILA Q	:	Painful tumor of the breasts. Breasts very large.
CONIUM MAC. 1000	:	Breasts enlarge in boys at the time of puberty. Breasts look like that of a woman. Give a dose every fortnight till cured. Tumor of the left breast or hardness of the right breast.
CONIUM MAC. 1M, PHYTOLACCA DEC. 200	:	Use either of the remedy with due regard to the other symptoms for lumps of breast whether during nursing or otherwise.

HEPAR SULPHURIS 200, PSORINUM 200, CONIUM MAC. 30, SABAL SER. Q	: Two doses daily of the either remedy will develop the breasts which are developing slowly at the age of puberty. Sabal is valuable for undeveloped mammary glands.
CYCLAMEN	: Swelling of breasts after menses. There may be a milky secretion from the nipples.
GRAPHITES 200	: Scars left by abscesses on the breasts, soften up and go away by the use of this remedy. Lumps in breasts of suspicious appearance also go away under the action of this remedy.
HYDRASTIS CAN.	: Cancer of the breasts, before start of ulceration. Tumor of the breasts. Nipples retracted and drawn back.
IODIUM	: Dwindling mammary glands while other glands grow normally.
KREOSOTUM	: Dwindling mammae with small hard painful lumps.
LAC CAN., CALCAREA CARB.	: Breasts become tender and painful before menses.
LAC CAN. 200	: Breasts swollen, painful before and better on appearance of menses.
LACTICUM ACIDUM	: General trouble of the breasts like pain, enlargement, etc.
LYCOPODIUM 1M	: Breasts do not develop in young girls when they suffer from amenorrhea. This remedy cures

amenorrhea and causes the
breasts to develop.

NUX MOSCH.   : Breasts once rounded and beautiful become flat and out of shape.
Breast too small. Mammae develop too slowly. All this is cured
by the use of this remedy.

ONOSMODIUM 10M, CM : Breasts undeveloped with infantile uterus and ovaries. Aching of
breasts and itching of nipples.
Use one dose every 15 days to
restore the normal size or for
appearance of the breasts.

PHYTOLACCA DEC.   : Swollen breasts neither heal nor
suppurate, hard and very sensi-
tive. Tumor or cancer of breasts.
Breasts become irritable before
and during menses.

PITUITARINUM 3X   : Defective development of breasts
at puberty.

PLUMBUM IOD.   : Induration of the mammary
glands, specially when the ten-
dency to become inflamed appears and the breasts become
sore and painful.

RANUNCULUS BULB.   : Pain like pleurodynia in the chest.

RAPHANUS   : Pain between the breasts and
below the breasts.

SABAL SER.   : Undeveloped breasts or shrunken
breasts due to the diseases of the
uterus. Breasts undeveloped and
shriveled with infantile uterus
and ovaries. Debility both physical and sexual.

SABINA	: One breast smaller than the other.
SARSAPARILLA Q	: Nipples are short and flat and instead of projection, depression exists. 2 drops in water twice daily.
SCIRRHINUM 1000	: This cancer nosode may be used once only at the commencement of the treatment for cancer.
SCROPHULARIA NODOSA Q	: A powerful medicine for tumors and nodosities in the breasts. Can also be applied locally.
SILICEA	: Hardness of the left breasts. Sinuses of the breasts. Patient is always chilly.
TARENTULA CUB.	: Cancer of the breasts specially in the old age.
THYROIDINUM 2X	: Fibroid tumors of the breasts.
TUBERCULINUM 1000	: Benign tumor of the breasts. Menses are too early and too profuse.

NOTE: Breast tumors are some what linked to ovarian problems in many cases. Therefore treatment of the ovary and menses leads to the cure of breast cancer.

BREATH

ARNICA MONT.	: Fetid breath as of rotten eggs. Bitter taste. Mouth is dry and thirsty.

AURUM MET.	: Bad smell from the mouth of girls at puberty. Taste bitter and gums ulcerated.
BORAX	: The breath smells moldy. Mouth and tongue ulcerated. Mouth feels hot and tender.
CARBOLICUM ACIDUM	: Fetid breath and putrid discharge.
CROCUS SAT.	: The breath has an offensive, sickly smell.
ELAPS COR.	: Thick, offensive, dry, green yellow crusts form on the back of the mouth, producing very foul breath.
HELLEBORUS NIG.	: Horrible smell from mouth.
MERCURIUS SOL. 200	: Bad smell from mouth during fever or when suffering from pyorrhea. Gums swollen. Saliva increased and is fetid. Bad odour from the mouth fills the whole room in which he is sitting.
NITRICUM ACIDUM	: Putrid breath, great salivation.
NUX VOM.	: Bad odour from the mouth after dinner. Breath smells sour.
PETROLEUM	: Odour of onions from the mouth after eating raw onions or otherwise also.
PYROGENIUM	: Horrible breath like rotten dead fish. Taste terribly fetid.
QUERCUS 3X	: Smell of faeces or flatus, discharged from the bowels, in the breath.
SINAPSIS NIG.	: The breath is offensive and smells like onions.

NOTE: There are thousands of living organisms in the mouth and some of them produce fetid smell. A common bad breath producer is anerobic bacteria which lives in the tiny crevices of the tongue.

Experts have estimated that 1000-10000 live on the surface of a tooth in a clean mouth. People who do not clean their mouth, tongue and teeth properly have more of such bacteria. Saliva checks the growth of bacteria but during sleep,saliva production almost ceases and bacteria go on multiplying. Thus, many people complain that they have a bad breath in the morning on rising. Many mouth washs are available in the market. All of them contain alcohol. They help for an hour or two and their excessive use produces more bad smell than it was before their use. The best way to stop bad odour from the mouth is the immaculate oral hygiene by brushing the teeth properly twice daily along with cleaning of the tongue by a tongue cleaner. Homoeopathic remedies can do the rest of tne work to stop bad breath.

BREATHLESSNESS
(DYSPNEA)

ACTAEA SPIC. : Dyspnea from exposure to cold air.

AMBRA GRISEA : Dyspnea due to nervousness.

ANTIMONIUM ARS. : Dyspnea on account of destruction of air passages of the lungs and the inflammation of, lungs.

ARSENICUM ALB., CALCAREA CARB., CHININUM ARS., NATRIUM MUR., SEPIA : Use either of these remedies, taking into consideration the other symptoms if the dyspnea is aggravated from ascending stairs.

ASPIDOSPERMA Q	: Cardiac dyspnea.
BORAX 3X	: Out of breath when going upstairs. Arrest of breath when lying, is obliged to jump and catch breath which causes pain on the right side.
BROMIUM	: Inspiration very difficult. Cannot inspire deep enough.
CALCAREA CARB.	: Feels suffocated due to dyspnea in a closed room, wants windows and doors open particularly at night.
CHINA OFF.	: Dyspnea during pregnancy specially due to flatulence.
CHLORALOSUM	: Can inhale air without any difficulty but cannot exhale. Feeling of a plug in the larynx.
COCA 3X	: Dyspnea of aged, alcoholics and atheletes.
COCCULUS IND.	: Dyspnea due to constriction of trachea.
CRATAEGUS OXY. Q	: Extreme dyspnea due to heart troubles and least exertion.
IODIUM	: Weakness and loss of breath on going upstairs.
LACHESIS	: Dyspnea from least thing coming near the mouth or nose.
LYCOPODIUM	: Great dyspnea due to a neglected pneumonia with rattling of mucus in the chest and flapping of the wings of the nostrils at each breath.

MEDORRHINUM 200	: Breathing very oppressed. Dyspnea on a little exertion. Cannot exhale from the lungs.
NAPHTHALINUM 3X	: Dyspnea and sighing respiration due to any cause.
NATRIUM SULPH.	: Dyspnea aggravated during damp and cloudy weather.
STAPHYSAGRIA	: Dyspnea in males, after coition.
STROPHANTHUS HISP. Q	: Dyspnea in anemic persons with congestion of lungs and palpitations.

BRIGHT'S DISEASE
(SEE NEPHRITIS)

BRONCHITIS

AMMONIUM CARB.	: Chronic bronchitis of the old and weak patients. Weakness is so much, that he cannot raise the mucus.
ANTIMONIUM IOD.	: Frequent fits of cough. Yellow, thick mucus.
ANTIMONIUM TART.	: Wheezing and rattling of mucus but little is expectorated after a great effort.
BRYONIA ALBA	: Tickling cough, worse at night. Free expectoration in the morning and worse in a warm room.
CARBO VEG.	: Bronchitis of old people.

FERRUM PHOS. 6X	: Bronchitis of young children who are pale and weak.
IPECACUANHA	: Bronchitis of infants. Wheezy breathing with feeling of suffocation. Nausea.
KALIUM BICH.	: Acute or chronic bronchitis. Mucus is tenacious, tough and stringy and is difficult to raise.
KALIUM HYPOPHOS.	: Chronic bronchitis.
MULLEIN Q	: Removes bronchial irritation.
NATRIUM ARS.	: Bronchitis of children after 7 years of age and before puberty.
PHOSPHORUS	: Cough on speaking and laughing, which is worse at night. Cough when comes is strong and it hurts the body. The patient tries to suppress it as long as possible to avoid the hurting.
PULSATILLA NIG.	: Cough worse lying down, which compels the patient to sit up.
RHUS TOX.	: Bronchial cough of old people followed by eructations of gas. Expectoration of small plugs of mucus.
TEREBINTHINIAE 1X	: Chronic bronchitis.
VERATRUM ALB.	: Chronic bronchitis in the aged. Loud, barking, stomach cough followed by eructation of gas. It is worse in the warm room or on entering a warm room from cold air.

BRUISES

ARNICA MONT.
: Bruises on any part of the body or the whole body. Skin is black and blue.

BELLIS P.
: An excellent remedy for bruises, sprains and injuries to nerves and deep tissues. There is much muscular soreness.

CONIUM MAC.
: Ill effects of bruises and shocks.

HYPERICUM PERF. 3X
: Bruises of fingers, toes and spine.

LEDUM PAL.
: Black and blue bruises from blows. Black eye from a blow of a fist.

RUTA G. Q
: Bruises of bones, tendons and cartilages.

SULPHURICUM ACIDUM
: When bruising persists for an unduly long time or skin becomes livid on account of the mechanical injuries, use of this remedy. It is more beneficial then Arnica.

BUBO

Inflammatory swelling of one or more lymph glands especially in the groins is known as bubo.

BADIAGA
: Glands in the arm pit, neck, groins and breasts swollen, enlarged and inflamed. Bubo is syphilitic.

MERCURIUS COR.	: In acute cases of soft bubo.
MERCURIUS IOD.	: Syphilitic bubos.
MERCURIUS SOL.	: In chronic cases when the bubo has become hard.

BUNIONS

This condition is ten times more common in women than men. It is a painful enlargement at the junction of the big toe and the small toes. It is probably caused by wearing badly fitting shoes.

BENZOICUM ACIDUM	: Bunion of the great toe with tearing pain. This remedy may be of use, if urine has the bitter smell of bitter almonds. This smell can be felt in the whole room.
HYPERICUM PERF. 3X	: Bunion with tingling and burning pains. This remedy helps to reduce the pain of bunions.
RHODODENDRON CH.	: Gouty swelling of the great toe specially the right one. The pain is worst before thunderstorm and in damp weather.

BURNINGS

| ALOE SOC. | : Great burning with itching of the anus, compelling the patient to bore a finger in the anus. |

ARSENICUM ALB. : Burning sensation in fever, better from heat and warm drinks. Burning of soles better by applying cold water.

BELLADONNA : Burning in upper parts of the body during fevers but extremities are cold.

CAUSTICUM : Burning warts and wounds. Burning scars left after healing of wounds,etc. It is a remedy for burning, rawness and soreness anywhere in the body.

FLUORICUM ACIDUM 200 : Feeling of emission of burning vapours from pores of the body. Burning of the whole body without temperature. The patient is better by washing with cold water or in cold weather. He is able to withstand any amount of cold.

LYCOPODIUM : Burning between shoulders.

OPIUM : The patient finds his bed too hot to sleep upon.

PHOSPHORUS : Burning of hands. Cannot cover them. Burning between shoulders.

RADIUM BROM. : Intense burning of the skin as if on fire, relieved by a hot water bath and in open air.

SANGUINARIA CAN. : Burning of cheeks, palms, soles and other parts.

SECALE COR. : Burning sensation on the skin throughout the body. Wants parts uncovered though they are cold to touch. Feels better in cold. Aversion to heat.

| SULPHUR | : A remedy of first choice for sensation of burning anywhere in the body- eyes, nose, discharge, anus, soles, etc. and burning increases by washing. The patient cannot cover his feet. |

BURNS (SCALDS)

ACIDUM PICRIC. Q	: This dilution applied on lint is the best application for burns until granulation begins to form.
ARSENICUM ALB.	: If ulcers proceed towards gangrene.
CANTHARIS Q	: For burning pains of burns. It is a remedy for all stages of burns and scalds.
CAUSTICUM 6	: The patient is never well since burnt. Pain and shocks are removed by the use of this remedy. The burns are deep and the skin has been destroyed. Old burns which do not get well and for ill effects of burns.
HEPAR SULPHURIS	: If ulcers develop on the burnt parts, use this remedy internally.
URTICA URENS Q	: 5 drops in water given every half an hour relieves burning and pain.

NOTE: Immediately after a burn, when the skin is intact, bathe the burnt parts in icy cold water in which a few drops of Cantharis Q have been added. Keep the parts dipped in icy cold water till the burning disappears. No blisters will be formed and there will be no ill effects.

CANCER

Body cells have the property to die and regrow. When the cells lose their property of dying and continue to grow, they grow out of control and spread. That is a cancer. This is a result of a defective gene. It is not yet known as to why cancer cells evade destruction. Research is required as to how to trigger the immune system to kill tumors.

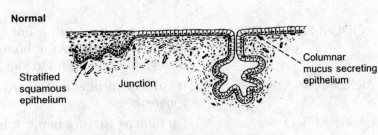

Normal

Stratified squamous epithelium

Junction

Columnar mucus secreting epithelium

Carcinoma in situ

No clear stratification; cells undifferentiated; mitoses

Altered cells filling crypts

ACETICUM ACIDUM	:	Epithelial cancer and cancer of layers lining the cavities of the alimentary canal.
ACIDUM PHOS 1X	:	It is useful in relieving pain of cancer and mental and physical debility.
ARSENICUM IOD. 3X, ASTERIAS RUB.	:	Cancer of breasts when ulceration has started.
ARSENICUM ALB. 1M	:	Cancer of the testicles. Give two doses a day, when no other

general symptom of the remedy
is present.

ASTERIAS RUB. 1X : It acts on cancer of both breasts
but better on left breast. Breasts
are hard and painful. Patient is
fleshy with a red face. It has a
great influence in cancer diseases.

BELLIS P. : Cancer of the stomach with
burning pain in the oesophagus.

CADMIUM PHOS. : Cancer of testicles.

CADMIUM SULPH. : Cancer of stomach with persistent vomiting of a black fluid and
constant bleeding. Also for
cancer of prostrate gland.

CISTUS CAN., : For cancer of prostrate gland.
CROTALUS H.

CALCAREA SULPH. : Fibroma of uterus with very offensive, yellowish bleeding and
cystic tumors.

CALENDULA OFF. Q : Has a remarkable power to produce local bleeding of a cancer
and helps to make acrid discharge healthy and free. Use it
as an inter-current remedy whenever healing is required after
exudation.

CARCINOSINUM 200, 1000 : It should be given in all the cases
of cancer in the beginning of the
treatment.

CARDUUS M. Q : Cancer of the liver. It reduces
pain of cancer and also reduces
the inflammation of the liver.
Diarrhea due to cancer,
especially that of the rectum.

CHININUM SULPH.	: Cancerous ulcers due to suppression of malaria.
CHOLESTERINUM 3X	: For cancer of the liver.
CHOLINUM Q	: It gives encouraging results in the treatment of bladder cancer.
CINNAMOMUM Q	: Used as an antiseptic agent for washing of cancer parts when the skin is intact. Use 3 to 4 drops in about 2 litres of water, orally 5 drops, few times daily. It is specially useful when an offensive odour is present. It also reduces pain of cancer. May be used for hemorrhage after delivery.
CISTUS CAN.	: Cancer of glands of the neck with sensation of coldness in various parts.
COBALTUM MET.	: Cancer of the lungs.
CONIUM MAC. 1M	: Cancer of breasts and testicles.
CONDURANGO Q	: Cancer of oesophagus and stomach. Relieves pain of cancer. Even touch of a finger on the affected site gives pain.
CROTALUS H.	: Cancer of stomach with vomiting of bloody, slimy mucus.
ECHINACEA Q	: 10-15 drops in a little warm water reduces the pain of cancer in the last stages. Bleeding is foul smelling.
EUPHORBIUM	: It acts as a palliative for reducing the burning pain of cancer. It also removes the bad odour coming out of the cancer. Ulcerating carcinoma and epithelium

of the skin with biting, burning pains in bones due to cancer.

FICUS REL. Q : Intractable bleeding from fibroids. A very positive remedy.

GALIUM APARINE : For cancerous ulcers and nodulated tumors of the tongue.

GRAPHITES : Cancer of pylorus and duodenum.

HECLA LAVA 3X : Cancer of the bones.

HEPAR SULPHURIS : When the patient becomes weak due to copious dischargeS from the opening of a cancer, this remedy in higher potencies dries the discharges and helps to remove the weakness.

HOANG NAN Q : It is useful in cancer of any gland whether bleeding or not. Start with 5 drops thrice daily and gradually increase the dose to 25 drops. It removes foul smell and revives the healing process.

HYDRASTIS CAN. : Cancer of breasts before start of ulceration. Cancer of the uterus. It can be used for douching; 10 drops in a tumbler of luke warm water.

HYDROCOTYLE A. Q : Palliative in pains of cervical cancer.

KALIUM ARS. : Skin cancer without any visible symptoms. Many small nodules under the skin.

KALIUM CYAN. : Cancer of the tongue.

KALIUM PHOS. : When cancer has been removed surgically and the healing process has started but the skin is drawn tight over the wound causing inconvenience, use of this remedy eases the patient.

KREOSOTUM : Cancer of the vagina and prostrate. Dribbling of urine. Cannot control the urge to urinate.

LEMON JUICE : Palliative in pains of cancer of the tongue. Use 5ml in 8 ounces of water.

MALANDRINUM 1M : It is efficacious in clearing the remains of cancerous deposits. Only 1 dose is given at the end of the treatment when cancer has been cured.

MORPHINUM : Pain of cancer is relieved when the patient is very sensitive and restless, jerks the limbs. Convulsions are threatened.

ORNITHOGALUM : Cancer of intestinal tract especially of stomach in its lower part and at the start of the intestines. Depression of spirits, complete prostration. Painful contraction and duodenal distention. Pains increase when food passes through the pyloric outlet. Cancer of abdomen. Give a single dose of 10-15 drops and repeat only after seeing results.

OVA TOSTA 3X : Relieves pain of cancer anywhere when backache is present.

PHOSPHORUS : Excessively bleeding fibroids and cancer specially in the stomach. Cancer of pancreas or of bones specially lower jaw and tibia.

RADIUM BROM. : Cancer of skin with itching, great burning and restlessness, better by hot bath and moving about.

SCIRRHINUM 1M	: To be given once only as an intercurrent remedy.
STRYCHNOS Q	: Removes offensive odour and hemorrhage of cancer.
SYMPHYTUM OFF.	: Cancer of bones, periosteum specially of joints.
TARAXACUM Q	: Cancer of the bladder.
TARENTULA CUB.	: It reduces pain of cancer.
TARENTULA CUB., SCIRRHINUM, LACHESIS	: Use any of these remedies for cancer of breasts, taking into consideration other symptoms of the remedy concerned.
THUJA OCC. 200	: Ill effects of vaccination resulting in cancer of face with rapid emaciation
USTILAGO MAY. Q	: Cancer of cervix with a sensation as if boiling water is flowing along the back. Bleeds easily.
VIBURNUM PRUN. Q	: For cancer of tongue.

NOTE 1: When the selected remedies do not produce relief, anti-miasmic remedies like Thuja, Medorrhinum, Syphilinum, etc. should be employed to induce the system to respond to the proper remedy. Besides the above, cancer nosodes like Carcinocinum and Scirrhinum have particular importance in vacating cancer miasm which therefore, need to be kept in mind during the treatment.

NOTE 2: Red hot peppers are loaded with antioxidants, bioflavonoids, plenolic acid and plant sterals that all help to protect against cancer. Research has shown that hot peppers can lower cholesterol and have anti blood clotting abilities,making them a smart choice for heart

health too. Red hot peppers contain 14 times more
vitamin A than that found in a fresh, green hot pepper.
Both are excellent sources of vitamin C.

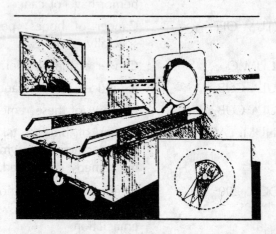

In a CAT Scan, a computer directs X-ray beams from a rotating disc at regular
intervals. The beams travel through the portion of the body being studied onto a
device that registers the beam's findings. The results are analyzed by a computer,
and the data appear as a three-dimensional image on a TV screen.

CARBUNCLES

Carbuncle is a deep seated pyogenic infection of the skin and
subcutaneous tissues, usually arising in several continuous hair
hats follicles, often preceeded or accompanied by fever, malaise
and prostration.

ACIDUM CARB. 200 : Carbuncles accompanied with
diabetes, which do not heal nor-
mally. The discharge is very offensive.

ANTHRACINUM 1000 : Carbuncles with burning and
high fever.

APIS MEL. : Carbuncles with burning and stinging pains,extremely sensitive to touch.

ARSENICUM ALB. : Intense burning and swelling. Pain is greater after midnight.

BELLADONNA : Intense pain and redness at the site of carbuncles. Swelling. Throbbing. This remedy may be used in the beginning.

CALENDULA OFF. Q, ECHINACEA Q : When the carbuncle has opened, a piece of lint soaked with either of the remedies should be applied to the ulcer. These have great antiseptic and healing powers.

EUCALYPTUS 1X : Urethral carbuncles which burn and cause tenesmus in the urethra.

HEPAR SULPHURIS 200 : There is 'throbbing pain and burning. The carbuncle is sore to touch. The carbuncle has burst and there is a thick discharge of pus. The patient is weak and speaks in a very low tone.

LACHESIS : Carbuncles with dark blue color, accompanied with fever.

MYRISTICA SEB. : It acts as a knife and breaks open the carbuncles. In healing its powers are greater than Silicea and Hep.

SILICEA 200 : Carbuncles on the back between the shoulders and under the nape of the neck. More indicated when suppuration has set in and the pus is thin. Fistulous openings

are usually present. Repeat
weekly. There is not much pain.

CARIES (NECROSIS)

ACIDUM FLUOR.	: Caries of long bones and their surrounding tissues and skull.
ASAFOETIDA 3X	: Ulceration and caries of the bones of the nose, specially in the syphilitic patients.
AURUM MUR.	: Caries of the bones of the nose, skull, palate and cervical bones specially in syphilitics.
BARYTA CARB.	: Caries of the long bones. Tearing, tension and boring in the bones.
CALCAREA CARB.	: Caries of vertebrae with curvature of spine.
CALCAREA CARB., SILICEA	: Caries of vertebrae.
CALCAREA FLUOR.	: A general remedy for caries of bones when there are no special indication for the use of other remedies.
CALCAREA PHOS.	: Caries of the soft bone.
COCA 3X, THERIDION	: Caries of teeth.
CONIUM MAC.	: Caries of bones of sternum.
HECLA LAVA 3X	: A general but a useful remedy for caries of any bone and its surrounding tissues.
HEPAR SULPHURIS, SILICEA:	Caries of the facial bones.
KREOSOTUM	: Caries of teeth. Very rapid decay

of teeth with spongy, bleeding gums. Teeth dark and crumbly.

PHOSPHORUS : Caries of lower jaw bones, bones of vertebra and tibia.

SILICEA : Caries of the bones of upper right jaw.

STAPHYSAGRIA : Syphilitic caries with painful ulcers.

STRONTIUM NIT. : Caries of femur bone.

CATARACT

Loss of transparency of the lens of the eye, or of its capsule is known as cataract.

CALCAREA FLUOR. 200 : One dose may be given weekly on days when Causticum is not administered.

CAUSTICUM 1000 : Use in the beginning of the disease and give one dose a month.

CINERARIA MAR. 3X : It is widely used as eye drops in cataract and corneal opacities and is reputed for its curative effect. 2 to 3 drops in each eye thrice daily. It should be continued with the above treatment. Has to be used for 3 to 6 months.

COLCHICUM AUTUM. : Soft cataract. Pupils unequal. Pupil of the left eye contracted. Dim vision after reading.

PHOSPHORUS : If the above two remedies fail to cure within three months and when there are black spots before the eyes, use this remedy. Great burning of the eyes.

SILICEA : Cataract in office workers. After effects of injuries and ulcers of the cornea.

SULPHUR : This should be used as an intercurrent remedy occasionally, in between the periods of treatment.

ZINCUM SULPH. 1000 : Not repeated frequently will clear up the opacities of the cornea.

NOTE :About half of these aged 65 to 74 and 70% of those 75 or older have cataracts. Such patients have a cloudy or fuzzy vision, fading in appearance of colors, problems with glare from lamps,sun or car headlights. Double vision. At the first instance a change in glasses,stronger bifocals or use of magnifying lenses may be sufficient along with the medication. If it does not help even after a lapse of sufficient period of treatment, surgery may be suggested.

Surgery : Surgery of cataract can be done at any stage of the disease. It is generally successful at the hands of a competent and reputed eye surgeon.

CATARRH

Catarrh is an inflammation of a mucous membrane with increased flow of mucus or exudate.

AGARICUS MUS. : Catarrh of the chest. It is accompanied by sneezing and cough.

CORALLIUM RUB.	: Post nasal catarrh. Profuse secretion of mucus dropping through the posterior nares.
ELAPS COR. 6	: Most effective remedy for chronic nasal and pharyngeal catarrh with greenish discharge.
HYDRASTIS CAN.	: Constant dropping of yellow mucus from the posterior nares. Catarrh of nose. Periostitis of the nasal bones.
KALIUM BICH.	: Discharge of stringy, tough and green mucus due to catarrh of nose.
KALIUM MUR. 6X	: It is a valuable remedy for deafness following catarrh and discharges from the ear.
LYCOPODIUM	: Catarrh of throat, creating difficulties in swallowing which is generally painful. Catarrh of chest in infants with rattling of mucus.
LYCOPODIUM, AMMONIUM CARB., HEPAR SULPHURIS	: Nose completely stopped up due to catarrh of nasal membranes. Has to breathe through the mouth.
MEDORRHINUM 1M	: Chronic nasal catarrh of children. Nose is always dirty with thick yellow mucus. Tonsils are enlarged and the child can breath through mouth only.
MENTHOLUM	: It has proved to be curative in acute nasal catarrh and in acute eustachian tube catarrh.
PHOSPHORUS	: Blowing of nose is accompanied with drops of blood. Handkerchief is always bloody.

PULSATILLA NIG.	: Discharge of yellow mucus. Crusts and pain at the root of the nose.
SPIGELIA	: Chronic catarrh of the nose with post nasal dropping of bland mucus.
SULPHUR	: Chronic catarrhs with a red nose.
TEUCRIUM MAR.	: It is the best remedy for nasal catarrh and atrophy. Offensive crusts and clinkers. Ozena. Loss of sense of smell.

CATHETER
(COMPLICATIONS OF USE)

ACONITUM NAP.	: A dose is given before passing a catheter into the urethra to remove the obstruction for passing urine, it will prevent pain and complications.
STAPHYSAGRIA	: When the urethra is stretched by passing a catheter, this remedy will remove subsequent complications. It will remove the pain or any ulcers caused in the process.

CHANGE OF LIFE
(SEE MENOPAUSE)

CHAPS
(CRACKS)

ACIDUM NITRIC.	: Chilblains in toes.
CISTUS CAN.	: Deep cracks and fissures on hands. Skin on hands dry. It suits persons who have to work hard with hands.
GRAPHITES	: Cracks and fissures at the ends of fingers.
NATRIUM MUR.	: Dryness of the finger tips. Has to moisten them often by putting them in the mouth. Cracks about finger nails.
PETROLEUM	: Cracks at the ends of the fingers and on the back of the hands. Skin is rough and bleeds sometimes. The disease is worse in winter.
SARSAPARILLA Q	: Chaps and cracks on the skin of hands and feet.
TAMUS	: Chapped hands.

CHEATING

COCA	: Inclined to cheating and lying as his sense of right or wrong is abolished. He can do any thing wrong without thinking that it is bad.
PULSATILLA NIG. 1000	: The patient is apt to make false representations. This medicine will rectify this habit.

CHEST

ACALYPHA IND.

: Constant and severe pain in the chest.

ACONITUM NAP.

: Constant pressure on the left side of chest. Oppressed breath on least motion.

ARNICA MONT.

: Pleurisy resulting from injury inflicted by a broken rib, yeilds to its use. Bryonia and Kali-c. work as supplements, if needed for removal of pain.

BRYONIA ALBA

: Stitches in the chest in the region of the heart.

CIMICIFUGA

: Pain on the right side of the chest.

COCCULUS IND.

: Cramps in the chest.

CONIUM MAC. 1000

: Gynecomastia. Abnormally large mammary glands in males making the breasts look like that of a women and sometimes may secrete milk. Give a dose every 15 days till cured.

GAULTHERIA Q

: Pleurodynia and severe pain in the epigastrium are cured by the use of this remedy.

ILLICIUM

: It has a special indication in every disease i. e. there is pain in the region of the third rib, about an inch or two from the sternum, generally on the right side and occasionally on the left side.

KALIUM CARB.

: Pain in the lower right chest through to back. Very characteristic stitching pains.

MERCURIUS SOL.

: Pain in the right side of the chest. Sweating without relief and peculiar mercurial tongue (with imprint of teeth) and mouth.

NAJA TRI.

: Oppression of the chest causing suffocation and choking. Inability to lie on the left side of chest. Stitches in the chest, in the region of the heart.

PHOSPHORUS

: The chest is shaped like that of a pigeon (pigeon chest). This remedy in 30/c potency, given three times a day for a period of three months, makes the chest appear normal.

RANUNCULUS BULB.

: Rheumatic pains in the chest. Bruised pain in the ribs. Muscular pains in the chest as if bruised. Pleurodynia. Pains worse inspiration, moving and in the evening.

RHUS TOX.

: Oppression of the chest. Cannot breathe due to sticking pains.

RUMEX CRIS.

: Raw pain under the collar bones and sometimes behind the sternum.

SULPHUR

: Oppression as if of a weight on the chest. Burning. Difficult respiration. Wants windows open.

CHICKEN POX

ANTIMONIUM TART.   : After 24 hours of the use of Variolinum, if fever is left, give it every two hours till the fever lasts. It takes generally two days.

CALCAREA PHOS. 6X   : After the patient has been completely cured, weakness always remains. Give this remedy every two hours to remove weakness.

RHUS TOX.,   : After the use of Ant-t., use these BRYONIA ALBA   remedies in alteration every three hours for removal of the residual symptoms like fever, cough, etc.

VARIOLINUM 200   : Give one dose at the start of the treatment to cut short the disease and averting its further dangers. It should be given at the end of the treatment when the disease has been cured and the weakness has been removed. It will remove the ugly scars left. When chicken pox is prevalent in a locality, all children not affected by the disease, should be given one dose in the morning and one dose in the evening for two days as a preventive to the disease.

NOTE: Chicken pox occurs in children between ages 1 to 15. It is seldom a life threatening disease. It is caused by Varicella zoster virus which remains in the infected person's sensory nerve roots for life. Sometimes in adulthood, it is reactivated and results in shingles. It is a communicable disease.

CHILBLAINS
(FROSTBITE)

Chillblains: erythema, itching and burning especially of fingers, toes, heels, nose and ears caused by vascular constriction on exposure to extreme cold; lesions can be single or multiple, and can become blistered and ulcerated.

AGARICUS MUS.

: Chilblains have a sensation as if cold needles were pricking. Itching is present alongwith swelling. The affected skin is red and pricky.

FRAGARIA VESCA

: Chilblains worse in summer.

HEPAR SULPHURIS, SILICEA

: Chilblains with pus in the cracks of the skin.

NITRICUM ACIDUM

: Ulcerated chilblains in toes.

PETROLEUM 200

: Fingers and toes become deep red and bluish with swelling, burning and itching due to cold or by taking out the hands from gloves or feet from socks and immediately placing them in cold water or on cold floor when they are still hot. Chilblains every winter.

PSORINUM 200

: Rough and chapped skin worse in winter.

PULSATILLA NIG.

: Chilblains with swollen veins. Burning and throbbing pains cause crying. Bluish, inflamed swellings and desire for sympathy.

RHUS V. Q   : Applied locally gives immediate relief to itching and burning in chilblains.

TAMUS Q   : Chilblains with discoloration of the skin with chaps. Takes away pain of chilblains speedly when it is painted on the affected part.

TEREBINTHINIAE   : Chilblains where the skin is not cracked.

NOTE: In such cases, the patient should be kept in a cold place, but should not be exposed to a current of air. He should be washed with ice cold water in the parts affected. This process may last for hours. During the intervening period, any of the above remedies may be given according to symptoms.

CHILD - ABNORMAL
(ALSO SEE HYPERACTIVITY)

AETHUSA CYN.   : Children get up in sleep, appearing frightened and start crying without any apparent cause.

AGARICUS MUS.   : Children are late in learning to talk and walk due to some mental defect.

ANACARDIUM ORI.   : Laughs on serious matters and serious on unimportant matters.

ARGENTUM NIT.   : Child looks withered and dried and looks like an old person. Does not want to go to school.

BARYTA CARB.   : Children are backward mentally

and do not grow and develop, take cold early. Aversion to strangers.

CALCAREA CARB. : Children are late in learning to walk due to some defect in bones.

CAUSTICUM : Under developed child - late in learning to walk and talk.

CHAMOMILLA : Asks for things and refuses to accept them when offered. Impatient and restless child. Cannot tolerate little pain. Girls have very sensitive breasts and an inadvertent touch of the breast, though not developed, causes sensation or pain.

CYPRIPEDIUM PUB. : Child cries out at night, is wakeful and begins to laugh and play.

GRAPHITES : Children who are impudent, disrespectful, teasing and who laugh at reprimands.

HEPAR SULPHURIS : Beats other children, wicked, slightest cause irritates him.

IODIUM : His hunger is never satisfied. Though eats well but still loses flesh. Greedy and irritable. Restless, cannot rest still. Generally has thyroid trouble.

JALAPA : The child is good all day long but screams and is restless and troublesome at night.

NATRIUM MUR. : Children are late in learning to talk.

PHOSPHORUS : Child is unmanageable, wild

	tempered with lean and pale constitution. He picks up a quarrel with everybody without a reason.
PULSATILLA NIG.	: The girl has a "weather cock" like character - easily consoled and unstable. Absent minded and fears the opposite sex.
SEPIA	: Sad and weeping tendency. Averse to work and family. Indifferent to family members. Emotional.
SILICEA	: Child is obstinate and head strong. Does not listen to parents.
SULPHUR	: Child hates to be washed. Tries to sit down everywhere though needed to stand. Standing is the worst position for such children.
TUBERCULINUM	: Child is rude, wild tempered and becomes violent on trifles. Extremely obstinate.

NOTE: My experience has shown that abnormal activity in a patient results from stressful psychic events, and disputes in the family.

CHLOROSIS
(ANEMIA DUE TO IRON DEFICIENCY)
(SEE ANEMIA)

CHOKING

BARYTA CARB.   : Spasm of the oesophagus as soon
                            as food enters it,causing gagging
                            and choking.

CACTUS 3X   : Strenuous respiration and subse-
                            quent choking due to a heart
                            trouble.

LACHESIS   : Choking on account of a feeling
                            of a plug in the throat on swal-
                            lowing warm things.

MEPHITIS   : Choking from drinking and
                            eating as the drink or the food
                            goes a wrong way to the wind
                            pipe or choking from one's own
                            vomits.

SPIGELIA   : Choking from copious mucus
                            falling from the posterior nerves,
                            blocking the wind pipe or from
                            continuous cough and asthma.

NOTE: In all cases of choking, the patient should hold his neck
with hands to indicate choking and the person nearby
must give a few hard strokes on the back of the patient
to restore respiration. If a person remains choked for
a few minutes, he can die. Choking does great harm
to the brain where oxygen supply is obstructed. Memory
is weakened by choking.

CHOLECYSITIS
(SEE GALL BLADDER)

CHOLERA

AETHUSA CYN. : Useful in cholera of children and infants. Milk is vomited in curds after taking. The patient is restless, cries and has colic.

ARSENICUM ALB. : The patient does not yield to the above treatment and the respiration becomes slow, deep and grasping and the symptoms of death are appearing, use of this remedy may save a life.

CAMPHORA Q : When cholera is epidemic, 2 to 3 drops on a lump of sugar will protect those not affected by the disease. If diarrhea has started and the patient has nausea, give 5-6 drops every 15 minutes on sugar. It is considered specific for the disease.

COLCHICUM AUTUM. 3X : When the abdomen is bloated with wind, it will give relief from flatulency and other symptoms of cholera.

CUPRUM ACET. 3X : If some person in the family is already suffering from the disease, the rest of the members should take a dose of this medicine morning and evening for protection against the disease.

HYDROCYANICUM ACIDUM : Rice colored stools.

IPECACUANHA : Nausea, very easy copious vomiting and sudden profuse rice water like stools. Forced discharge of stool. Loud noise in the abdomen like gurgling of water. Coldness and cramps in the body. It is valuable remedy in cholera.

PODOPHYLLUM   : Stools are profuse, offensive and gushing.

SEPIA   : Diarrhea and vomiting becomes worse by drinking milk.

VERATRUM ALB.   : If the patient is not relieved by Camphora or rather has become worse by this, use Veratrum album. It is very useful when cold perspiration is present on the forehead and the patient has cramps and rice water stools.

CHOLESTEROL

Cholesterol is usually measured in millimoles (mmol) in a litre (mmol/L). Reading is taken from the blood which is taken from finger tips. A serum cholesterol of 6. 21 mmol/L (240 mg) or above is considered risky and reading over 8. 58 mmol/L (300 mg) is dangerous. A reading of 5. 17 mmol/L (200mg) to 6. 21 mmol/L (240 mg/DL) is considered as a border line level. A serum cholesterol under 5. 17 mmol/L (200 mg/DL) is considered healthy. The lower is better.

Heart muscles are nourished by oxygen carried through thin vessels called the coronary arteries. If this circulation is severely reduced or blocked, the muscles quickly become starved of oxygen and cannot function normally - this is heart attack. Cholesterol forms thin layers inside the coronary arteries gradually reducing the inner space, consequently reducing the blood flow. When the arteries become sufficiently narrow a blood clot is formed which obstructs the blood flow causing insufficiency of vital nutrients and oxygen carried by the blood. A heart attack, thus follows. To prevent the heart attack, the level of cholesterol must be lowered. To achieve this, diet restrictions are needed. Butter, butter oil, meats (except that of a fish), ice creams, cheese and cream, egg yolks, fried articles, etc. increase the level of cholesterol. Alternative diets are available and should be used.

The following homoeopathic medicines reduce the level of cholesterol and may be used according to the indications. Diet restrictions must be kept in view. Cholesterol in blood should never be more than 200 mg per 100 cc of blood.

ALLIUM SATIVUM Q   : Acts specially on fleshy subjects who eat a great deal more, specially meat than they drink. 5 drops a dose, three times a day reduces cholesterol in about a month. It has been proved that it reduces total serum cholesterol level.

CRATAEGUS OXY. Q   : It has a solvent power upon crustaceous and calcareous deposits in the arteries and thus reduces the thickening of the arteries.

EMBELICA OFF. Q   : It is an excellent remedy for this purpose. It can also be taken as a (East Indian Amla) vegetable or jam, which are prepared from the fruit itself.

GINSENG   : Reduces cholesterol level.

LYCOPODIUM   : It lowers the level of cholesterol in aorta and liver.

OENOTHERA BIENN. Q   : It lowers the level of cholesterol in aorta and liver.

TERMINALIA ARJUNA,   : It is also an excellent remedy for
BALERICA Q   reducing cholesterol.
(East Indian Bahera)

**NOTE: In december 1998 the American Journel of Nutrition
reported the results of latest study of 45 participants by
Gene Spiller of California, Jenkins of Toronto and a
researcher in Verona Italy. They said that nuts and
almonds are better for lowering the level of bad
cholesterol. Nuts contain a high proportion of mono-
unsaturated fats which lower the risk of cardio-vascular
diseases.**

CHOREA

Irregular, spasmodic, involuntary movements of the limbs or
facial muscles, often accompanied by hypotonis is known as
chorea.

AGARICUS MUS.   : Twitching, jerking and restlessness in children with bluish face
and fingers.

ASAFOETIDA   : Chorea on account of nervous
disorder. Involuntary action of
the muscles. Pain and numbness.

AVENA SATIVA Q   : Chorea due to nervous disorders. Strength of the hands is
diminished. Give 15 drops thrice
daily in warm water.

CUPRUM ACET.   : Give it in cases which resist
treatment.

IGNATIA AMARA   : Chorea of emotional origin or
when accompanied by emotional
symptoms.

MERCURIUS SOL.	: Tremors of hands. Excessive perspiration which does not relieve.
MYGALE	: Jerking of arms and legs.
STRAMONIUM 200, OPIUM 200	: Chorea due to fear and fright. Give one dose a week.
ZINCUM PHOS.	: In worn out and weak patients, worse by cold.

CIRRHOSIS
(SEE LIVER)

CLAIRVOYANCE

It is a perception of objective events (past, present or future) not ordinarily discernible by the senses; a type of extrasensory perception.

ACONITUM NAP.	: Predicts that his beloved, living miles away, is singing a certain song.
AGARICUS MUS.	: The patient is inclined to make prophecies. Behaves as if he knows everything and every happening in advance.
IODIUM	: The patient is on the verge of insanity. Destroys things without reason. Becomes violent at occassions.

CLAUSTROPHOBIA
(DREAD OF CLOSED PLACES)

It is a morbid fear of being in a confined place.

ARGENTUM NIT. : Cures a person who is afraid of being confined to a closed place.

SUCCINUM : Its use removes the fear for closed places and trains.

CLIMACTERIC
(SEE MENOPAUSE)

CLUMSINESS

APIS MEL. : Numbness in the hands and finger tips, so that the patient cannot hold things properly and drops them easily. He is generally clumsy.

BOVISTA : Great weakness in all the joints and clumsiness with the hands, so he drops things easily.

COCCYX
(LAST BONE IN THE SPINE)

ANTIMONIUM TART. : Sensation of weight and a feeling that the coccyx is hanging down.

BOVISTA	: Itching in the coccyx.
CARBO ANIMALIS	: Burning in the coccyx on touching it.
CAUSTICUM, ARNICA MONT., RUTA G.	: Bruised pain in the coccyx.
CICUTA VIR.	: Tearing and jerking pain in the coccyx. Back is bent backwards like an arch. Pain is worse during menses. Vertigo, gastralgia and muscular spasms may accompany the pain.
EUPHORBIUM OFF.	: Pain like electric shocks in the coccyx.
HYPERICUM PERF. 12X	: Pain on account of a fall or an injury to the coccyx.
KALIUM BICH.	: Pain in the coccyx when sitting.
LACHESIS	: Pain in the coccyx and sacrum. Worse rising from a sitting position.
PAEONIA OFF.	: Ulcer at the end of the coccyx.
PLATINUM MET.	: Numbness in the coccyx.
SILICEA	: Sensation of pressure on the coccyx.
XANTHINUM	: Patient cannot sit on a hard surface and keeps a cushion below while sitting. Pain in the coccyx all the time.

COITION - MALE

ACIDUM PHOS. Q	: Sudden relaxation of the penis during the act before ejaculation

and the desire arises for intercourse once again.

AGARICUS MUS.	: Weakness after coition. This remedy covers many complaints arising after coition.
AMBRA GRISEA	: Asthma on attempting coition.
ANACARDIUM ORI.	: Want of enjoyment during coition.
BARYTA CARB., LYCOPODIUM	: Falls asleep during the act of coition.
BUFO RANA	: Convulsion during coition.
CALADIUM SEG.	: Penis relaxes during coition, there is no emission or orgasm even after a long time of coupling.
CALCAREA CARB.	: Coition followed by weakness and irritability.
CANTHARIS	: Coition followed by pain in the urethra.
DAPHNE IND.	: Coition followed by toothache.
GRAPHITES	: Aversion to coition due to impotency. Patient is constipated and fat.
GRAPHITES, LYCOPODIUM	: Aversion to coition. Legs turn cold after coition.
KALIUM CARB., CANNABIS IND.	: Coition followed by backache and weak vision.
MILLEFOLIUM	: No ejaculation at all on coition even after a prolonged act and then the penis relaxes.
MOSCHUS	: Coition followed by nausea and vomiting.

NATRIUM CARB.	: Coition followed by profuse perspiration.
NATRIUM MUR. 200	: Emission even after coition and already ejaculation.
PHOSPHORUS	: Irresistible desire for coition. Desire again for sexual intercourse after coition. Constant wish for coition forces the patient to vices.
SELENIUM MET.	: Coition followed by irritability and prostration. Increases desire, decreases ability.
STAPHYSAGRIA	: Coition followed by urging to urinate and breathlessness.
SULPHUR	: Ejaculation on attempting coition and before penetration.
TITANIUM	: Too early ejaculation of semen in coitus.
SABAL SER.	: Urination difficult after coition.
KREOSOTUM	: Burning in penis on coition or in coming in contact with the secretion of vagina.

COITION - FEMALE

ACIDUM PHOS.	: Dull headache after coition.
AGARICUS MUS.	: Any complaint after coitus.
AMBRA GRISEA	: Asthma during coition and on attempting coition.
ARGENTUM NIT.	: Hemorrhage after coition. Coition is painful.

BERBERIS VULG.	: Desire diminished on account of cutting pain during coition. Sensation of pleasure comes very late or is absent.
BROMIUM	: Absence of thrill during coition.
CANNABIS IND.	: Backache after coition.
COBALTUM MET.	: Weakness in legs and backache after coition.
HYDRASTIS CAN.	: The patient hates coition and does not even want to talk about love making.
KREOSOTUM	: Discharge is bloody and burning after coition.
LYCOPODIUM	: Chronic dryness of the vaginal cavity. Great burning in the vagina during and after coition.
NATRIUM MUR.	: Aversion to coition in anemic women with dryness of the vagina.
PLATINUM MET.	: Fainting during coition.
PLUMBUM MET.	: Aversion to coition.
PULSATILLA NIG.	: The patient does not allow the man to touch the parts. Clitoris is very sensitive to touch.
SALIX ALBA	: Excessive desire for sexual intercourse.
SEPIA	: Coition is painful. There is vertigo after coition and aversion to coition. The vagina is dry or leucorrhea is present. Constipation may be there.
STAPHYSAGRIA	: Coition painful in younger life. Breathlessness after and during coition.

STRYCHNINUM   : Great desire for sexual intercourse and the desire inflames
on touch of any portion of the
male body.

COLDNESS

AGARICUS MUS.   : It has a peculiar symptom, as if
pierced by icy needles. Very
sensitive to cold.

AMBRA GRISEA   : Sensation of coldness in the
abdomen.

AMMONIUM MUR.   : Sensation of coldness in the back
and between the shoulders.

BARYTA CARB.   : Children takes cold easily and
have swollen tonsils.

BELLADONNA   : It is associated with a hot red
skin from head to nates but his
extremities are cold even in high
fever. Hot in head, cold in legs.

CALCAREA CARB.   : Cold and damp feet. Feeling as
if wearing cold and damp
clothings. Coldness of legs with
night sweats. Internal and external coldness of various parts of
the head as if a piece of ice were
lying against it. Aversion to open
air, cold air goes right through
her. Sensation of coldness in a
single part unmistakably points
to this remedy.

CAMPHORA   : Icy coldness of the whole body,
even the breath is cold. Icy cold
feet with pain. Better by warmth.

CARBO VEG.	: Icy coldness of hands and feet. The skin appears blue on account of poor blood flow. The patient is better by fanning and from cold.
CHINA OFF.	: The person is very sensitive to cold draught.
CHININUM ARS.	: Coldness of hands and feet, knees and limbs.
CISTUS CAN.	: Sensation of coldness in various parts.
CORALLIUM RUB.	: The patient feels too cold when uncovered and too hot when covered. Coldness is relieved by artificial heat.
CUPRUM ARS.	: Icy coldness of the whole body with cramps and obstinate hiccoughs. Frequent vomiting and cold sweats.
HELODERMA 200	: Great coldness. Cold waves from occiput to feet or from feet to occiput. Coldness of the whole body externally and internally. Sensation of coldness of the whole body and the internal parts like heart, lungs, kidneys, etc.
HEPAR SULPHURIS	: Extremely sensitive to cold air. Closes all the doors and windows and sits as near as possible to the heater.
LOBELIA PURP.	: The patient feels too cold without shivering.
MANCINELLA	: Icy coldness of hands and feet.
MENYANTHES TRI.	: Icy coldness of hands and feet.

NATRIUM CARB.	: Icy cold from knees down. The hollow of knee is painful on walking.
NUX VOM.	: Chilliness on being uncovered, yet he does not allow being covered . Avoids open air. Body hot but uncovering makes him feel chilly.
PSORINUM	: Feels cold in the head. Wants warm clothing even in summer. He will take a quilt even during very warm nights.
PULSATILLA NIG.	: Sersation of coldness between shoulders. Pains are accompanied with constant chilliness. More severe the pain, the harder the chill.
RHUS TOX.	: Catches cold and cough by getting wet or due to change of weather.
SECALE COR.	: Coldness in the fingers and toes with sensation of burning. Rest of the body is also cold but burning sensation is present all over. Fingers and toes blue. The patient is better by cold, uncovering and rubbing.
SEPIA	: Patient feels cold even in a warm room. Chills easily.
SILICEA	: Icy cold hands and feet with warmth of the rest of the body. Want of vital warmth even when exercising. Sensitive to cold when uncovering head or feet. Hugs fire.

COLIC

ALLIUM CEPA	: Colic of little babies with cutting and tearing pains. Child screams and cries.
ALOE SOC.	: Colic before and after stool. Pulsating pain around the navel. Pains around navel worse by eating or drinking. Diarrhea may or may not be present. Great accumulation of flatus and the abdomen feels full, heavy, hot and bloated.
ARSENICUM ALB.	: Colic on account of eating decayed food.
BELLADONNA 200	: Gall stone colic. It withstands repetition at short intervals. Pains are violent, they come and go repeatedly.
BERBERIS VULG. Q	: Renal colic specially when the left kidney is involved.
BRYONIA ALBA. 200 OR 30	: Food lies like stone in the stomach. Stools hard, constipated. Desire to lie quietly.
CALCAREA REN.	: Pains around the navel which are burning.
CHAMOMILLA	: Colic from a fit of anger or colic in children from wind and flatulence.
CHELIDONIUM 1000	: Gall stone colic, in which it gives immediate relief.
CHININUM ARS.	: Chronic colic, periodical at certain hours of the day.

CHOLESTERINUM 3X : If there is no relief or little relief after taking Chelidonium, one may, give this remedy for gall stone colic. It can be repeated every hour till the colic goes.

CIMICIFUGA : Pain in the hypogastrium.

COLOCYNTHIS : Pain around the navel which is better by pressure and warmth. Colic from a fit of anger is relieved by the use of this medicine. Pain in the abdomen causes the patient to bend double.

DIOSCOREA : Severe colic. Pains radiate from the abdomen to the back, chest, arms. Better by walking about. Flatulent colic.

GRAPHITES : Pain in the upper part of abdomen. The patient is constipated and the stools are hard.

IGNATIA AMARA : Hysterical colic.

IPECACUANHA : Colic with diarrhea and vomiting or nausea.

JALAPA : Colic in children with diarrhea and vomiting. The child cries constantly.

KALIUM BICH. : Pain spasmodic, soon after eating.

KALIUM CARB. : Stitching pain, worse with movements, specially before menses.

LYCOPODIUM 1000 : Renal colic when the right kidney is involved.

MAGNESIUM PHOS. 12X : Colic. Pains are throbbing and burning in character and are

	relieved by pressure and warmth. The patient passes wind constantly during the pain.
MERCURIUS SOL.	: Colic on account of dysentery.
NUX VOM.	: After over eating and due to sedentary habits.
POLYGONUM SAG. 12X	: Colic on account of the suppurative kidney. The pain travels along the spine.
PULSATILLA NIG.	: Pain after discharging flatus, excessively after taking rich fatty food.
SENNA 6	: Very useful in the colic of infants. Child seems to be full of gas and is generally constipated. Stools may be hard and dark or fluid-yellowish with colic before passing.
STANNUM MET.	: Cramp like colic around the navel with a feeling of emptiness in the abdomen. It is relieved by lying on the abdomen or by a hard pressure on the abdomen. The child stops crying when carried with his abdomen on the shoulder.
STAPHYSAGRIA	: Colic after abdominal operation. Chronic colic of children with much prostration and better by motion and straightening of the body.
VERATRUM VIR.	: Colic with soreness above the pelvis.
VIBURNUM OP.	: Pain in the lower abdomen usually connected with menstruation.

COLITIS
(INFLAMMATION OF THE LARGE INTESTINES-COLON)

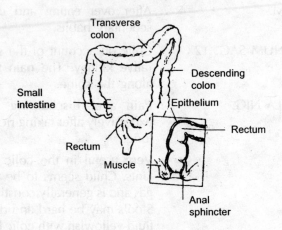

ALLIUM SATIVUM : Colitis with stools containing shreds of intestinal mucous membrane. Great hunger. Specially indicated in high fevers and fleshy persons.

ALOE SOC. : Constant bearing down in rectum. Bleeding. Rectum feels sore and hot, and is relieved by cold water. Lot of mucus and wind is expelled with stools and the pain remains in the rectum after passing stools. Gurgling in the abdomen.

ARGENTUM NIT. : Membranous stools. Flatus expelled with noise. Constipation. Pain in the region of spleen.

CADMIUM SULPH.	: Gelatinous stools. Cutting pains in the bowels and kidneys.
CANTHARIS	: Smell of food causes nausea and vomiting. Stools are membranous. Colic. Flatulence.
CHINA OFF.	: Yellowish watery stools. Absence of pain. Some flatus with stools.
COLCHICUM AUTUM.	: Distension of abdomen with wind. Pain in the region of liver. Stools contain white shreds.
COLOCYNTHIS	: Severe cutting pains in the abdomen forcing patient to bend double. Pains worse after anger. Bitter taste of the mouth.
FICUS IND. Q	: Hemorrhage before evacuation. Stools are bloody with pure red blood and colic.
KALIUM BICH.	: Chronic intestinal ulceration and perforation with cutting pain, soreness and burning.
LACHESIS	: Colitis with offensive diarrhea alternating with constipation. Abdomen very sensitive to pressure.
MAGNESIUM CARB.	: Abdomen distended. Diarrhea. Stools green, forced out.
MERCURIUS DULC.	: Stools are scanty and are mixed with blood, mucus and bile. Anus sore and burning.
SELENIUM MET.	: Colitis on account of tuberculosis of the peritoneum.
SEPIA	: Entero-colitis. The leading symptom for choice of this remedy is always worse after taking milk.

STAPHYSAGRIA 200 : Simple or ulcerative colitis after insults and injuries like after rape.

SULPHUR : Treatment should be started and ended with this remedy.

TEREBINTHINIAE : Entero-colitis with hemorrhage and ulceration of bowels.

THUJA OCC. 1M : Colitis on account of amoebic dysentery.

COLLAPSE

CAMPHORA Q : Coldness, external and internal. Symptoms after exposure to cold or cholera.

CARBO VEG. : A lowered vital power from loss of fluids, after drugging and diseases. In old people with venous congestion. State of collapse in cholera and typhoid. The patient appears lifeless with coldness of the body. Breath is also cold but the head is hot. Pulse is imperceptible and quickened respiration. Gasps for breath.

CUPRUM MET. : Collapse symptoms with cramps in epileptic fits.

GLONOINUM : Due to sun stroke.

HYDROCYANICUM ACIDUM : Blueness of the skin due to defective oxidation. Forceful, irresistible desire to sleep. Collapse symptoms in epileptic and hysterical convulsions.

STRONTIUM CARB.	: Collapse symptoms after surgery. Profuse perspiration is a strong indication for its use. The patient feels warm and comfortable after the use of this remedy.
VERATRUM ALB.	: Symptoms of collapse with cold perspiration on the forehead. It may be due to profuse drainage of discharges. It is a great heart tonic.

COLOR BLINDNESS

AGARICUS MUS.	: Reading difficulty. Deception of colors.
BELLADONNA	: Red objects appear yellow. Blinking of the eyes.
CARBONEUM SULPH.	: Black spots before eyes or sparkling before eyes. Jerking and twitching of the eyelids. Red and green look white.
CROCUS SAT., CALCAREA CARB.	: Blinking during and after reading.
DIGITALIS	: Yellow and blue look like white.
EUPHRASIA	: Constant blinking of the eyes due to any defect.
GRATIOLA OFF.	: Green objects appear white.
HYOSCYAMUS NIG.	: Objects look golden.
KALIUM BICH.	: Constant blinking in epileptic attacks.
PHOSPHORUS	: An excellent remedy. Usually cures color blindness.

STRAMONIUM : Red appears black and black as grey.

COMA

ALUMINIUM MET. 200 : Coma in diabetes because the amount of sugar in blood becomes negligible.

AMMONIUM CARB. : Fainting due to depression of spirits and with a weeping tendency.

AMYLENUM NIT. Q : Inhalation of this remedy during paroxysms of asthma, epileptic seizures, angina pectoris, migraine, etc. gives immediate relief.

ARNICA MONT. : Coma due to an accident, fall or injury.

ASAFOETIDA, SEPIA : Hysterical fainting.

BAPTISIA TINC. : Coma during typhoid fever.

BARYTA CARB. : Coma on account of brain hemorrhage.

CAMPHORA Q : In emergencies, it is a very good heart stimulant. It is also a satisfactory remedy for sub normal temperatures and low blood pressure. Three drop doses on a lump of sugar (never in water) repeated at 15 minute intervals produces the desired results. Smelling of this remedy is equally useful. Body is icy cold, but the patient does not desire to be covered.

DEXTROSE OR SUGAR	: Coma due to an over dose of insulin is cured by a few grams of sugar given dry on the tongue, to be sucked or it may be given dissolved in water. In such cases, urine is sugar free.
GELSEMIUM	: Coma in cerebro-spinal meningitis.
HELLEBORUS NIG	: Coma due to injuries or blows on the head.
HEPAR SULPHURIS	: Fainting due to pain.
HYDROCYANICUM ACIDUM	: Coma on account of brain congestion or after an epileptic fit.
LACHESIS	: Coma during labor.
MOSCHUS	: Fainting due to the slightest excitement.
NUX MOSCH.	: This remedy may be given to a person who faints easily and often due to a little exertion like standing or even evacuating.
OPIUM	: Coma on account of strenuous breathing,and due to shortage of oxygen. Involuntarily urination or when frightened.
RANUNCULUS BULB.	: Coma on account of too much use of alcohol.
VERATRUM ALB.	: Fainting due to least exertion with cold. Sweat on the forehead.

COMPLEXION

BERBERIS AQ. Q : Clears complexion and cures acne,blotches and pimples on the face. Use five drops in water thrice daily, orally. One gram mixed with one ounce of glycerine may also be rubbed gently on the face which has been previously washed with soap and water and dried.

IODIUM 1000 : One dose a fortnight makes the complexion fair. Give one dose fortnightly for six months.

SARSAPARILLA OFF. Q : Clears the complexion of the face. Skin which appears emaciated, shriveled, wrinkled and dry becomes fresh and clear. Use 5 drops in water, three times a day.

CONCENTRATION, LACK OF

ICHTHYOLUM : Forgetful, irritable and depressed. Cannot concentrate his thoughts.

IRIDIUM MET. : The patient cannot concentrate on his thoughts.

MEDORRHINUM : Loses the thread of conversation.

ONOSMODIUM : The patient feels that he lacks the power to concentrate. Coordination is poor.

OPIUM : Lack of self control and ability to concentration.

SKATOLUM : The patient finds it impossible to study and becomes depressed because of this. Desires to be with other people.

TEREBINTHINIAE : The patient feels very tired and is unable to think properly.

CONFIDENCE, LACK OF

ANACARDIUM ORI. : Aversion to work and an irresistible desire to swear and curse. The patient lacks confidence in himself and others.

AURUM MET. : Thinks that he cannot be cured. There is no medicine or treatment which can cure him.

BARYTA CARB. : Loss of self confidence.

CALCAREA SIL. : Absent minded, irritable and irresolute. Lacks self confidence.

LYCOPODIUM : Loss of self confidence. Afraid to be alone. Lack of confidence in physician and his treatment.

CONFUSION OF MIND

ANTIMONIUM TART. : Vertigo with dullness of the mind.

ANAGALLIS : Apathy and inability to concentrate. Depression.

BAPTISIA TINC. : Mental confusion. Falls asleep while being spoken to.

BRYONIA ALBA	: Vertigo and nausea. Faintness on rising.
CALCAREA ARS.	: Confusion and delusions.
GLONOINUM	: Confusion and dizziness.
SALICYLICUM ACIDUM	: Confusion in the head on rising suddenly.
STICTA PULM.	: Confusion of ideas. The patient needs to talk a lot.
TRIFOLIUM PRAT.	: Confusion and headache on waking.

CONJUNCTIVITIS
(INFLAMMATION OF THE EYES)

APIS MEL.	: Conjunctivitis with pain and burning. Eyelids are red and swollen. Washing the eyes with cold water relieves.
ARGENTUM NIT.	: Profuse purulent white discharge, and gluing of the lids which are swollen.
BELLADONNA	: In the beginning of the disease when eyes are red and eyelids are swollen,with watering of eyes.
EUPHRASIA 6	: Watering of the eyes. Sneezing. Margins of the lids are red and swollen. Discharge is thick and acrid. Use internally 6C and externally as eye drops, Euphrasia Q to 50 parts of rose water.
MERCURIUS COR.	: Acrid lachrymation. Severe burn-

ing and soreness of eyes. Eyelids
get glued together.

NATRIUM MUR.   : Burning in eyes. Lachrymation,
                                burning and acrid. Lids swollen.
                                Eyes appear wet with tears.

PULSATILLA NIG.   : Symptoms of Bell. but the dis-
                                charge is thick and yellow with
                                gluing of the lids.

RHUS TOX.   : For oedematous conjunctivitis
                                with acrid discharge. Worse
                                during rains and winter.

NOTE: **Symptoms of conjunctivitis are mostly covered by
Pulsatilla, Natrium muriaticum, Lycopodium and Lachesis
- grade wise importance. The remedies are particularly
useful in viral conjunctivitis. Pulsatilla cures about 80%·
of such cases.**

CONSOLATION

COFFEA CRUDA   : Mocks at consolation. Does not
                                want consolation.

IGNATIA AMARA   : Symptoms are aggravated by
                                consolation in hysterical patients.

LILIUM TIG.   : Consolation aggravates uterine
                                problems and insanity.

NATRIUM MUR.   : Patient is more irritated and dis-
                                turbed by consolation. Weeping
                                alternated with laughing.

PULSATILLA NIG.   : Nothing pleases a Pulsatilla
                                patient more than consolation.
                                She has a weeping tendency.

| SABAL SER. | : Consolation makes him angry. |
| SEPIA | : Does not want to be consoled. Consolation aggravates. |

CONSTIPATION

It is a condition in which bowel movements are infrequent or incomplete.

ALUMEN	: Constipation of the most aggravated kind. No desire for stools for days together. Violent ineffectual desire for stools. No ability to expel stools and if expelled, is like marbles.
ALUMINA	: No desire for stools. Great straining. Constipation in infants, old people and women with very sedentary habits. Rectum is inactive.
AMBRA GRISEA	: Chronic constipation in old people. Never get done feeling and unsatisfactory motions and frequent ineffectual desire to pass stool. Cannot pass stools when others are present.
ANTIMONIUM CRUD.	: Constipation and diarrhea alternating and in old people.
ASAFOETIDA 3X	: Chronic constipation. Eructations loud and difficult. Pressure of the wind is always upwards.
BRYONIA ALBA	: Dry and hard stools. There is no inclination to pass stools.

CASCARA SAG. Q	: 10-15 drops in water acts as a laxative in constipation and restores normal functions. It is an intestinal tonic and helps remove dyspepsia.
CHELIDONIUM	: Stools are hard and like round balls or like sheep dung. Hepatic and gall bladder disorders are usually present.
COLCHICUM AUTUM.	: Constipation with ineffectual desire for stools. Pressure does not relieve. Feels faeces in the rectum but cannot expel them.
COLLINSONIA CAN.	: Constipation during pregnancy or following labor.
FUCUS VES. Q	: Constipation in obese patients with thyroid disorders.
GRAPHITES	: Stools are knotty, large lumps and united by mucus threads.
HYDRASTIS CAN. Q	: Stools are felt in the small intestines but do not come down to the large intestines and anus. Enemas or glycerine plugs are useless and do not relieve. Constipation with a sinking feeling in the stomach and dull headache. 20 drops a dose, gives temporary relief.
LYCOPODIUM	: The patient is constipated since puberty or last confinement.
MAGNESIUM MUR.	: Constipation of infants during dentition. Passes only a small quantity of stool like sheep's dung.

MERCURIUS SOL.	:	Never get done feeling. Little stool passes on each occassion and the desire remains. There may be cutting colic before each stool which may be greenish, slimy and bloody.
NATRIUM SULPH.	:	On every attempt to pass a stool, only a little wind passes.
NATRIUM MUR.	:	Unsatisfactory motions. Stool is like sheep dung.
NUX MOSCH.	:	Stool is soft, yet he is unable to expel it even after long straining.
NUX VOM.	:	Constipation with an ineffectual desire for stools in persons of sedentary habits, accustomed to purgatives.
OPIUM	:	Constipation due to the inactivity of the intestines. Stools are dry, hard and ball like.
PHOSPHORUS	:	Constipation. Stool is long and dry like that of a dog.
PLATINUM MET.	:	Constipation of travellers who often change food, water and places.
PODOPHYLLUM	:	Constipation alternating with diarrhea in children and colic.
SENNA	:	Never get done feeling with abdomen full of wind and painful.
SEPIA 200	:	Constipation during pregnancy. Stools are hard and knotty.
SILICEA	:	Constipation before and during menses. Stool comes down with difficulty and when partially expelled recedes again.

SULPHUR 200	: Constipation on account of fear of passing the stool because stools are hard, knotty and difficult to expel, they cause pain in the anus while passing.
THUJA OCC.	: Chronic constipation. Stool like hard, black balls. Constipation with violent rectal pain, causing stools to recede.

CONSTITUTIONS

In homoeopathy, there are three types of constitutions:

1. Syphilitic   2. Sycotic   3. Psoric
1. Syphilitic constitution is found in patients having a syphilitic history in their family.
2. Sycotic constitution is found in patients who have a history of gonorrhea in their family.
3. Psoric - all other diseases of skin, fever, etc. are found in psoric patients.

The following are the remedies :

SYPHILITIC	: Mercurius, Iodium, Kaliums, Syphilinum, etc.
SYCOTIC	: Thuja occ., Nitricum acidum, Medorrhinum, etc.
PSORIC	: Sulphur, Psorinum, etc.

CONTRADICTION

AURUM MET.	: Ailments resulting from contradictions.
COFFEA CRUDA	: Headache from contradiction.
LYCOPODIUM	: Cannot bear contradiction.
MERCURIUS SOL.	: Cannot tolerate contradiction. Desire to kill those not agreeing with him.
SEPIA	: Irritable and easily offended on contradictions.
TARENTULA HIS.	: Anger from contradiction.

CONVALESCENCE

A period between the end of a disease and the patient's restoration to complete health is known as convalescence.

ACIDUM SULPH.	: Uncomfortable debilitating perspiration following slightest exertion or drinking hot water and after debilitating illnesses.
APOCYNUM CAN.	: For weakness after fevers like typhoid.
CURARE	: Weakness with shaky lower extremities during convalescence. The patient is surprised on his weakness.
LECITHINUM 1X - 3X	: After the cure of disease, some weakness remains during the period of convalescence due to

a decrease in red blood corpuscles. Three doses a day for a week removes such a condition. It has a favourable influence on the nutritive condition, blood, weakness and insomnia during convalescence.

PSORINUM : It is useful for weakness during convalescence.

SULPHUR : For immediate effects to finish the after effects of the cured illness.

TUBERCULINUM 200 : When convalescing from measles, suddenly loses flesh, gains high temperature, drenching sweat and prostration.

CONVULSIONS
(UNCONSCIOUSNESS WITH MUSCULAR TWITCHING)

Convulsions are violent spasms or a series of jerks in the face, trunk and extremities.

AETHUSA CYN. : Convulsions due to indigestion, colic and anguish. Milk is vomited in curds soon after drinking and the patient passes out during a convulsion.

AMYLENUM NIT. : Convulsions during normal delivery.

ARNICA MONT.,
HYPERICUM PERF. : Convulsion after giving birth to a child by a Cesarean section.

BELLADONNA	: Convulsions in children. Flushed face and throbbing temples. May be due to any cause.
CALCAREA PHOS.	: Convulsions due to rickets or during dentitions.
CHAMOMILLA	: Convulsions during teething in children. Stools are green and the child is fretful. Convulsions in children when mother becomes extremely angry while nursing the child. It is also useful for convulsions during dentition.
CICUTA VIR.	: After convulsions, the patient does not remember anything on regaining consciousness.
CINA	: Convulsions due to worms.
HELLEBORUS NIG.	: Convulsions due to suppression of measles or other skin diseases.
HYOSCYAMUS NIG., CICUTA VIR.	: Convulsions during labor.
NUX VOM.	: Convulsions from eating indigestible fruits.
OPIUM	: Convulsions of children, when mother is suddenly frightened during their nursing.
STRAMONIUM	: Convulsions due to dreadful dreams.
ZINCUM PHOS., AURUM MUR., CUPRUM MET.	: Use any of these remedies, according to the symptoms, for convulsions of epilepsy.

CORNS

ACIDUM PHOS.	: Very painful corns.
ANTIMONIUM CRUD.	: It is a general remedy for recent corns which are hard.
FERRUM PIC. 3, RADIUM BROM. 30	: These two remedies given alternately each week to cure corns.
GRAPHITES	: Corns with deep cracks.
HYDRASTIS CAN.	: Corns on toes which re-appear after cutting.
NITRICUM ACIDUM	: Inflammed and ulcerated corns.
RADIUM BROM.	: A dose of 30 potency a fortnight is effective in all kinds of corns.
SALICYLICUM ACIDUM Q	: A solution of salicylicum acid made with 1 part of the acid and five parts of water can be painted at bed time every third night. It often cures.
SELENIUM MET.	: Inflammed corns on the soles of feet.
SULPHUR	: Remedy for soft corns due to pressure of shoes.
VERATRUM VIR. Q	: Painted on inflammed corns gives rapid and perfect relief.

CORONARY THROMBOSIS

A clot of blood in the blood vessel or in the cavities of heart is very dangerous. In such cases, help of a surgeon is necessary. In the meantime, the following remedies may be used according to the indications as a "first aid".

ARNICA MONT. 200 : Bruised pains and tightness of the chest.

CACTUS Q : Constriction in the heart region as if squeezed with an iron band.

COLOCYNTHIS : When the disease is due to the effect of anger.

LACHESIS : There is threatened paralysis of the left arm and left leg accompanied by numbness. Patient cannot bear tight clothes on the neck and abdomen.

CORYZA (COMMON COLD)

ACONITUM NAP. : Give in the beginning, at the start of the cold when the weather is very hot or very cold and there is much sneezing. Give it for two days; three doses a day. If it fails then give Ferr-p. 6X.

ALLIUM CEPA : Allergic coryza from pollen. Much sneezing. Copious, watery and extremely acrid discharge. Coryza with cough and headache.

AMMONIUM CARB. : Discharge of sharp burning water. Stoppage of nose at night. Coryza of long standing.

ARGENTUM NIT. : Coryza with chilliness, lachrymation and headache. Ulcers on septum.

ARSENICUM ALB. : For a ripe cold. Thin, watery discharge which is hot and excoriating. Nose feels stopped up. Sneezing gives no relief. It is worse in the open air and better indoors.

ARUM TRIPH. : Acrid, excoriating discharge. Nostrils sore. Nose obstructed. Must breathe through the mouth. Irritation in the nostrils. Discharge may be bloody.

ARUNDO : A remedy for catarrhal states. Burning and itching of the nostrils. Coryza and sneezing due to pollen allergy.

BELLADONNA : Coryza, mucus mixed with blood. Tingling at the tip of the nose which is usually red and swollen. Cough may accompany, when it does, it is tickling, short and dry and worse at night. Continuous inclination to swallow mucus.

CALCAREA CARB. : The patient takes cold early especially at every change of weather. Nostrils are dry, sore and ulcerated. The nose is stopped up and the discharge is fetid and of yellow color.

CALCAREA SULPH. : Cold in the head with thick, yellowish, purulent secretion frequently tinged with blood. One sided discharge from nose.

DULCAMARA : Profuse coryza during rain or when the days are hot and nights are cold. Coryza in new born babies.

EUCALYPTUS : Thin, watery coryza with fetid discharge. Nose does not stop running. Water comes out even by bending the head forward and without any effort.

EUPHRASIA 6 : Cold fully established with watering of eyes. Thick discharge but non irritating.

FERRUM PHOS. 6X : During the second stage of coryza, when there is heaviness of the head also.

HEPAR SULPHURIS 1X : It will often start secretion and profuse discharge in stuffy colds. Two or three doses are generally sufficient for the purpose. Sneezes everytime he goes in the cold dry wind. Nostrils ulcerated.

IODIUM : Coryza when the discharge is of thick, yellowish color.

IPECACUANHA : Coryza with stoppage of nose and nausea.

KALIUM HYDRIOD. : A good remedy for thin, watery, profuse, acrid coryza.

LEMNA MINOR : Discharge, very abundant and foul smelling. Nose obstructed.

LYCOPODIUM : Fluent coryza. Ulcerated nostrils. Nose stopped up at night.

MENTHOLUM : It is curative of acute nasal catarrh with pain in the eye balls and frontal headache. Ears appear blocked up producing deafness with sore throat.

MERCURIUS SOL.	: Acrid discharge. Very thick greenish discharge, has to be blown out. Sneezing in sun. It is worse in damp weather. Nostrils become ulcerated.
PHOSPHORUS	: Periostitis of nasal bones. Chronic catarrh with small hemorrhages. Handkerchief is always bloody.
PHYTOLACCA DEC.	: Flow of mucus from one nostril and posterior nares.
PSORINUM 1M	: One dose often gives immunity from catching cold.
PULSATILLA NIG.	: Coryza with stoppage of right nostril.
QUILLAYA SAP.	: If given early in the beginning of coryza, it stops the further development of cold, sore throat, dryness of throat and cough with difficult expectoration.
RHUS TOX.	: Coryza from exposure to cold, wet winds and on getting wet while perspiring. Sneezings. Tip of the nose is red, sore, ulcerated and swollen.
SABADILLA	: Coryza with spasmodic sneezing, severe frontal pains, redness and watering of eyes, sore throat beginning left side and tough mucus. Symptoms better hot food and hot drinks; worse cold and cold drinks. No thirst.
SAMBUCUS NIG.	: Dry. Coryza of infants. Difficult breathing and noisy breathing startles the child. Snuffles of infants.

SAPONARIA OFF. 10M	: It breaks up the cold, coryza and sore throat. The patient behaves as if drunk.
SOLANUM NIG.	: Acute coryza, watery discharge from the right nostril, left stopped up, with a chilly sensation alternating with heat.
TRITICUM REP. 1X	: It is an excellent remedy for coryza when the patient blows his nose constantly even when the discharge does not come on each occassion.

COUGH

ACETICUM ACIDUM	: Cough of patients suffering from phthisis. Chronic cough, with purulent expectoration.
ACONITUM NAP., HEPAR SULPHURIS	: Violent, dry cough due to exposure to cold, dry wind.
AGARICUS MUS.	: Cough ending with a sneeze and worse after sleep. Mucus is expelled in little balls.
AMBRA GRISEA	: Eructations with violent convulsive cough. Asthmatic breathing with eructations of gas. Gets out of breath when coughing. Tickling in throat, larynx and trachea.
AMMONIUM CARB.	: Cough in old people with asthmatic breathing. Mostly at 3 A.M. and worse after sleep. It produces great weakness.

ANTIMONIUM TART. : Hoarseness. Great rattling of mucus but very little comes out. Dyspnea better by lying on the right side.

ARSENICUM ALB. : Cough worse after midnight and lying on the back. Burning in the chest. Wheezing respiration. Expectoration is scanty and frothy.

BADIAGA : Cough worse in the afternoon and better in a warm room. Wheezing. Thick, yellow mucus which flies out of the mouth and nostrils on coughing.

BELLADONNA : Paroxysmal dry cough in the evening and early night which turns the face red. Tickling in the throat. Dyspnea. Cough provoked by speaking and exertion. Pain in the hips on coughing. Expectoration may be bloody. Barking or whooping cough with pain in the stomach before attack.

BRYONIA ALBA : Dry cough worse on movement, with pain in the head and chest. Cough at night making the patient sit up to avoid suffocation. Cough with headache.

CALCAREA CARB. : Tickling in the throat, larynx and under the sternum brings on hacking cough, which is worse during and after eating.

CAPSICUM : Dry hacking cough expelling an offensive breath. Explosive cough with pain in bladder, ears, legs and in distant parts of the body with fetid expectoration and fetid breath. Cough causes tears in the eyes and pain in the legs and ears.

CARBO VEG. : Cough caused by itching in the larynx, hoarse spasmodic with smell of sulphur vapours in the throat. It is relieved by cold and cold drinks.

CAUSTICUM : Dry cough in the evening from tickling in the trachea and also induced by speaking. Involuntary urination on coughing and pain in the hips. Cough of old people. Cough with soreness of the larynx and chest. Mucus seems stuck in the throat and is hard to expel.

CHAMOMILLA 200, CYCLAMEN, NITRICUM ACIDUM : Dry cough during sleep. Rattling of mucus in the child's chest and suffocative tightness of the chest. Cough of children during sleep without disturbing the sleep.

CHELIDONIUM : Very quick and short respiration. Short exhausting cough. Sensation of dust in the throat, not relieved by coughing. Loose, rattling cough with difficult expectoration. Pain in the right side of chest and shoulders. Small lumps of mucus fly out from the mouth when coughing.

CINA : Dry, hollow, hoarse, cough in children with worms symptoms. Gurgling from throat to stomach after coughing.

COCCUS C. : Troublesome cough of drunkards. Accumulation of thick vis-
cid mucus, which is expectorated with great difficulty.
Whooping cough attacks end
with vomiting of this mucus.
Suffocative cough; worse first
waking, with tough, white mucus, which strangles.

COLCHICUM AUTUM. : Cough at night only with involuntary passing of urine.

CUPRUM MET. : Cough has a gurgling sound,
relieved by drinking cold water.
Suffocative attacks worse at
3 A.M.

CYCLAMEN : Cough at night while asleep without waking, especially in chil-
dren.

DROSERA : Cough is hoarse,barking and la-
ryngeal. Constriction of chest and
abdomen. Throughout the day
there is no cough at all but it
starts as soon as the head touches
the pillow at night. Whooping
cough. The paroxysms of cough
follow each other very rapidly.

DULCAMARA : Winter coughs. Must cough a
long time to expel phlegm.
Cough after physical exertion.

EUPATORIUM PERF. : Cough arising from irritation of
the liver. Cough at night loose
with hoarseness. Soreness of the
trachea and scraped feeling in
the bronchi. Cough with soreness of the chest, compelling the
patient to hold his chest with his
hands. Restlessness.

HEPAR SULPHURIS	: Choking cough. Dry, hoarse cough; worse dry, cold winds, and when any part of the body gets cold, uncovered or from eating anything cold.
IPECACUANHA	: Cough with nausea and mucus which is expelled after some efforts. Suffocative cough; child becomes stiff and blue in the face.
KALIUM BICH.	: It is of a great value in chronic catarrhal inflammations of the pharynx and cough. The expectoration is very stringy and it sticks to the pharynx and tongue. After coughing and raising the mucus, patient has a need to blow the nose and it gives a sense of relief. Cough is better from warmth and sometimes from lying down. Ant - t. follows well and completes the cure started by Kali-bi.
KALIUM CARB.	: Cough between 2 to 3 A.M. with stitches in the chest. Expectoration is scanty and tenacious, but increases in the morning and after eating.
LAUROCERASUS Q	: Spasmodic, tickling cough especially in the cardiac patients, is often magically influenced by this drug. Dose, 2 to 5 drops in water, thrice daily.
LYCOPODIUM	: Cough returning at the same hour every day. Expectoration may be bloody. Worse 4-8 P.M. Throbbing headache after every

paroxysm of cough. Expectoration gray, thick, purulent and salty.

MEPHITIS : Cough following influenza. Violent spasmodic cough, worse at night.

MERCURIUS SOL. : Burning in the throat on coughing. Cough with yellow mucopurulent expectoration.

MYRTUS COMM. : Obstinate cough, mostly dry with pain in the upper portion of the left chest to the left shoulder blade.

NATRIUM MUR. 200 : Cough with bursting pain in the head and stitches in the chest. Cough with flow of tears while coughing. Cough from tickling in the pit of stomach.

NITRICUM ACIDUM : Cough during day time only with taste of blood in the mouth. Dry, hacking cough, from tickling in the larynx.

NUX VOM. : Cough brings on bursting headache and bruised pain in the epigastric region.

OSMIUM : Very noisy, dry, hard cough shaking the whole body of the patient.

PHELLANDRIUM AQUA. : Cough with fetid expectoration, early in the morning.

PHOSPHORUS : Persistant cough from strong odours is cured by this remedy. Dry, hoarse and barking cough provoked by strong odours.

PHYTOLACCA DEC. : Dry hacking, tickling cough worse at night. Pain in the chest under the sternum on coughing. Cough from tickling in the throat; worse cold air, laughing and talking.

PSORINUM : Cough returns every winter.

PULSATILLA NIG. : Dry, hard cough with great weakness in the chest. Dry cough in the evening and at night; must sit up in bed to get relief. Loose cough in the morning, with copious mucus expectoration. Urine is emitted on coughing.

RHUS TOX. : Bronchial coughs of old people, worse on awakening and with expectoration of small plugs of mucus. Cough in fever and on getting wet when perspiring.

RUMEX CRIS. : Cough is caused by deep inspiration, accompanied with great fatigue. Stitches in the chest. Involuntary urination on coughing. Dry, teasing cough, preventing sleep. Touching the throat pit brings on cough.

SAMBUCUS NIG. : Suffocative cough, coming on about midnight, with crying and dyspnea. Child awakens suddenly, nearly suffocated, sits up, turns blue. Expectoration of small quantities of mucus, only during the day.

SENEGA : Cough with rattling, wheezing and difficult breathing. Great accumulation of mucus. Very useful for old people. Cough often ends in a sneeze. Bursting pain in the back on coughing.

SPONGIA

: Great dryness of the air passages. Cough dry and barking. Cough with a sound, as if a wood was being sawed. Cough starts after eating or drinking, especially warm drinks.

SQUILLA MAR.

: Cough with sneezing, watering of eyes and involuntary urination. Child rubs face with fist during cough. Stitches in the chest. Loose and rattling cough with much mucus. Sneezing with cough.

STICTA PULM.

: Cough after measles, worse towards evening and when tired.

STANNUM MET.

: Influenzal cough from noon to midnight with little expectoration. During the day, expectoration is copious, green and sweetish. Violent dry cough in the evening.

SULPHUR 200

: Cough with rattling of mucus in the chest, expectoration loose, worse after bathing and in the morning.

TUBERCULINUM

: Hard dry cough during sleep. Expectoration thick, profuse and easy. Suffocation even in plenty of fresh air. Longs for cold air. Rales all over the chest.

VERATRUM ALB.

: Cough followed by eructations of gas. Cough on entering a warm room from cold air.

VERBASCUM : Cough deep, hoarse, hollow which sounds like a trumpet.

CRAMPS

AGARICUS MUS.	: Cramps in soles of feet.
AMBRA GRISEA	: Cramps in hands and fingers specially when grasping anything. Cramps in legs.
AMMONIUM CARB.	: Cramps in calves and soles.
APOCYNUM CAN., CARBO VEG.	: Cramps in soles.
ARGENTUM MET.	: Cramps in hands and feet. Weakness in the right arm and tearing sensation in the wrist and finger tips.
ARNICA MONT.	: Cramps as a result of over exertion or from muscular fatigue. Limbs feel as if beaten. Cramps are better on starting to move and worse from prolonged movement, heat and light pressure.
BISMUTHUM 6	: Cramps in hands and feet.
CALCAREA CARB.	: Cramps of severe nature, specially in the calves,fingers and toes. Worse at night and on stretching.
CAMPHORA Q	: Cramps in the body with icy coldness of the limbs and body.
CARBOLICUM ACIDUM	: In the lower legs while walking.
CHOLAS TERRAPINA	: Simple cramps in muscles of the

calves and feet, with pain like rheumatism.

COCCULUS IND.	: Cramps in the chest.
CUPRUM ARS.	: Cramps in the calves of legs, worse after midnight. These are relieved by standing.
CUPRUM MET. 12	: Never fails in cramps of calves, feet or legs,soles,palms,fingers and toes.
CYCLAMEN	: Writer's cramps. Pain in the bones of the hands.
FERRUM MET. 6	: Cramps in calves, soles and legs.
GELSEMIUM	: Cramps in the muscles of fore-arm. Trembling and weakness in all the limbs. Specific for Writer's cramps.
MAGNESIUM PHOS. 6X,1M	: Writer's and Player's cramps in the wrists,hands and fingers due to excessive and long writing or use of fingers and hands. Numb-ness is usually present and there is relief by pressing the affected part, by warmth and massage.
NATRIUM PHOS.	: Cramps of feet,calves and hands on writing.
NUX VOM.	: The legs feel numb and almost paralysed. Cramps in calves and soles.
PETROLEUM	: Chronic or acute, persistant, violent and firm cramps, with cracking of joints.
PLUMBUM MET., LYCOPODIUM	: Cramps in calves and toes at night in bed.

PODOPHYLLUM	:	Cramps in the intestines.
RHUS TOX.	:	Cramps by swimming in cold water. Cramps in calf muscles and legs by stretching, specially at night. Cramps, worse rest and better by movement.
SCROPHULARIA NOD.	:	Cramps in palms or in any part of the body in the vicinity of an enlarged gland.
SECALE COR.	:	Violent cramps, better by cold and cold applications. Violent pain in finger tips. Icy coldness of extremities.
VERATRUM ALB.	:	One dose taken at bed time for 3 or 4 nights prevents cramps during night, specially in calves.
VIBURNUM OP.	:	Cramps in the abdomen and legs of pregnant women are controlled very quickly by this remedy. It is a general remedy for all cramps.

CRAVINGS

ALLIUM CEPA	:	Craving for raw onions.
ALUMINA	:	Cures craving for chalk, charcoal, uncooked rice, tea and coffee seeds.
ANTIMONIUM CRUD.	:	Cures craving for eating pickles and acidic things.
ARGENTUM NIT., THYROIDINUM	:	Craving for sugar and sweets.

CALCAREA CARB.	: Craving for eggs, lime, slate, pencils, chalk, clay, raw potatoes, sweets, ice cream and dirt.
CALCAREA PHOS.	: Cures craving for fried food, ham and smoked meats.
CAUSTICUM	: Young girls crave for marriage.
CICUTA VIR.	: Cures craving for eating charcoal and raw potatoes.
CALADIUM SEG.	: Modifies craving for tobacco.
CYCLAMEN	: Craving for eating fish.
GUAIACUM OFF.	: Craving for stretching limbs and body.
HEPAR SULPHURIS	: Cures craving for pickles and vinegar.
IODIUM	: Craving for meat.
KALIUM BICH.	: Longing for beer.
MAGNESIUM CARB.	: Craving for meat in children.
MANGANUM ACET.	: Desire to always lie down in bed.
MEDORRHINUM	: Craving for salt, sweets, fruits and ice.
MERCURIUS SOL.	: Craving to eat cow dung and mud.
NATRIUM SULPH.	: Craving for ice and icy cold water.
NITRICUM ACIDUM	: Cures longing for indigestible things like chalk, sand, etc.
NUX VOM. 10M	: A single dose usually takes away the craving for drugs.
PALLADIUM MET.	: Craving to be flattered. Flattery pleases the patient.

PHYTOLACCA DEC.	: Cures desire for biting teeth and gums.
RHUS TOX.	: Craving for milk.
SANGUINARIA CAN.	: Craving for toffees, gol gappas, ice creams, etc. but does not want bread.
SELENIUM MET.	: Mad craving for spiritous liquors.
SEPIA	: Desire in women for wine, vinegar and sweets.
SULPHUR, PHOSPHORUS PLUMBUM MET., ACIDUM SULPH.	: All these remedies are useful for removing craving for alcohol.
TARENTULA HIS.	: Cures cravings for eating sand and ashes, specially during pregnancy.
THLASPI BURSA	: Craving for buttermilk and for eating cheese.
VERATRUM ALB.	: Craving for eating his own stool, drinking his own urine.

CROUP
(ALSO SEE BREATHLESSNESS AND LARYNGITIS)

Any affection of the larynx in children, characterized by difficult and noisy respiration and a hoarse cough is known as croup.

ACONITUM NAP.	: This remedy should be given in the beginning when there is a dry, barking cough with restlessness and a desire for drinking cold water.

CHLORALOSUM	: The patient can inhale air easily but cannot exhale. Extreme breathlessness and constriction of the chest.
HEPAR SULPHURIS	: Croup during cold, dry winds. Dry, barking, choking cough and whistling respiration.
MOSCHUS Q	: Sudden constriction of larynx and trachea without cough, hoarseness or catarrh. Put a few drops on cotton and keep it near the nostrils of the patient to inhale. It gives relief and suffocation is avoided.
SANGUINARIA CAN.	: Cough with wheezing and whistling. Severe breathlessness and constriction of the chest.
SPONGIA	: Respiration is short and difficult with sensation as if the larynx is plugged. Cough with a sound as if wood is being cut with a saw.

NOTE : During the attack the patient should not be allowed to sleep to avoid choking and suffocation.

CURVATURE OF BONES

CALCAREA CARB., BARYTA CARB., ACIDUM PHOS.	: Curvature of bones of the spine.
KALIUM CARB.	: Curvature of bones of the hip joint.
SILICEA	: Curvature of bones. It covers inflammation, softening,

necrosis, fistula and abscess of the bones.

SULPHUR   : Curvature of the backbone and ribs.

THUJA OCC.   : Head sinks into knees while sitting on the floor or is bent backwards, cannot sit erect.

CYSTIC FIBROSIS

This disease is connected with glands specially those which secrete mucus, resulting in inefficiency of the pancreas, lungs, etc. Thick mucus produced in the body keeps the pancreas from providing digestive enzymes and the lungs from providing sufficient oxygen. The disease attacks youngsters and young adults. No reliable cure is available in any system of medicine. Homoeopathic remedies have proved useful as palliatives, guided by symptoms.

CYSTITIS
(INFLAMMATION OF THE URINARY BLADDER AND KIDNEYS)

ACONITUM NAP.   : In recent cases, accompanied with high fever and restlessness. Burning pain in the bladder and pain during urination.

APIS MEL.   : Frequent desire for urination or increase in the quantity of urine with burning. Urine contains blood. More indicated in women.

BERBERIS VULG. Q, CANTHARIS Q	: Great burning in the bladder and pain along the urethra. Worse before and after urination.
CANTHARIS	: Cystitis with a non-stop desire to urinate. Burning, cutting pains in the abdomen and aching in the small of back. Urine is voided in drops with burning and it may contain blood.
DULCAMARA	: Inflammation of the bladder. Urine is milky, thick with mucus and blood. It is specially useful for old persons.
EPIGEA REPENS	: Chronic cystitis with dysuria. Burning in the neck of bladder while urinating and tenesmus afterwards.
EQUISETUM	: Cystitis in old people with deep colored urine and pain while urinating.
NUX VOM.	: Despite a frequent need to urinate, a little urine can be voided and there is pain in doing so. Chill and irritability is generally present.
POPULUS T.	: Catarrh of bladder in old people, and cystitis after operations and pregnancy.
STAPHYSAGRIA	: Cystitis with a continuous burning sensation and a feeling that a drop of urine is constantly trickling through the urethra. The patient is restless and angry. Such a condition may result from sexual intercourse or catheterization.

TRITICUM REP. Q	: A good remedy for chronic cystitis. There is a constant desire to pass urine. Urination is painful and difficult.
TUBERCULINUM 1M	: In chronic cystitis, its use gives brilliant and permanent results.
XANTHIUM SPIN.	: Chronic cystitis in women.

CYSTS

AURUM IOD.	: Ovarian cysts.
BRYONIA ALBA, SULPHUR	: They absorb serous exudates.
CALADIUM SEG.	: Cysts on the eyelids.
CALCAREA FLUOR.	: Cysts on the eyelids.
CALCAREA SULPH.	: Cystic tumor after the pus has found its vent.
MERCURIUS SOL.	: Hard and large cysts on the tongue.
NITRICUM ACIDUM	: A cystic tumor in the region of ear lobe. Cysts on the eyelids, if above remedies fail.
OOPHORINUM 3X	: It is an important remedy for ovarian cysts.
SILICEA	: Vaginal cysts.
STAPHYSAGRIA	: Cysts on the eyelids, appearing after styes.
THUJA OCC.	: A cysts on the tip of the tongue. Small and soft.

DANDRUFF (SEBORRHEA)

ARMORACIA SAT. Q : Mixed with an equal quantity of mustard oil, cures dandruff when rubbed on the scalp.

ARSENICUM ALB. : Scalp is covered with white dry scales which itch intolerably, specially in weak persons.

CALCAREA CARB. : Dandruff. Roots of the hair painful on combing.

GRAPHITES : Dandruff due to skin troubles like eczema. Hair mattes together due to glutinous oozing of the scalp. Lots of itching.

KALIUM MUR. : Whitish and copious dandruff.

KALIUM SULPH. : Ringworm eczema of the scalp. Yellowish and copious dandruff. Itching worse by heat.

LYCOPODIUM : Dandruff with itching of scalp and headache, worse after hot water bath. Hair falls out in bunches on combing causing baldness in single spots.

MEDORRHINUM 200 : Dandruff, with dryness of hair and itching of scalp.

NATRIUM MUR. 200 : Dandruff worse margins of the scalp. Oily, greasy skin of the scalp. Dandruff causes hair to fall in bunches when combed or scratched.

PHOSPHORUS 200 : Dandruff resulting in falling of hair in bunches. Itching of scalp.

PSORINUM : Foul smelling dandruff.

SANICULA AQUA 200	: Scaly dandruff over hairy parts of the body like head, eyebrows, eye lashes, pubis, etc. Repeat weekly.
SEPIA	: Ring like eruptions on the scalp with dandruff.
SULPHUR 200	: Should be used at the beginning of the treatment and to end the treatment; also when other indicated remedies fail to act.
THUJA OCC.	: White dandruff, resulting in falling of hair and drying of scalp.

DEAFNESS

BARYTA CARB.	: If deafness is due to inflammation of the parotid gland and there is a crackling sound in the ears.
CALCAREA FLUOR.	: Hardness of hearing from calcareous deposits on the tympani.
CARBO VEG.	: Deafness as a result of measles.
CAUSTICUM	: Deafness is due to the paralysis of auditory nerve.
CHENOPODIUM AN.	: Deafness to the sound of voice only.
COCA	: Chronic deafness, with noises in the brain.
CONIUM MAC.	: Hearing is impaired due to wax in the ear. Useful for deafness in seniles.
CICUTA VIR. 200	: Deafness is due to diseases of the brain.

FERRUM PIC. 1X	: Chronic deafness and tinnitus due to gout. Ear is dry and the blood circulation to the ear is defective. Vascular deafness.
GRAPHITES	: Deafness in noisy places. Can hear better while riding a car or bus.
HEPAR SULPHURIS	: Deafness due to perforation of the ear drum or an abscess in the ear.
KALIUM MUR. 6X	: It is a general remedy for deafness, when the cause is not known.
LEDUM PAL.	: Deafness due to suppression of coryza or from otorrhea.
LOBELIA INF.	: Deafness due to suppression of a discharge or eczema of the ear.
MEDORRHINUM	: Total and chronic deafness. Burning and itching of the ears.
MEPHITIS	: Deafness from birth.
MERCURIUS SOL.	: Deafness as a result of tonsillitis. The patient feels that the eustachian tube is closed. It is also useful in deafness of advancing years.
MEZEREUM	: Deafness as a result of thickness of the membrane. It also cures deafness due to eczema of the ears.
NATRIUM SAL.	: Progressive deafness on account of loss of bone conduction.
PHOSPHORUS	: Deafness to the sound of human voice.
PILOCARPUS M., GRAPHITES	: Deafness better in noises and in running trains or flying aeroplanes, and if it is due to a defect in the internal cavity of the ears.

PULSATILLA NIG., IODIUM	:	Deafness due to obstructions in the eustachian tube and also after measles or scarlet fever.
SALICYLICUM ACIDUM 3X	:	Simple deafness with tinnitus and noises in the ears.
SULPHUR	:	Deafness as a result of small pox.
THIOSINAMINUM	:	Deafness due to thickness of the drum and fibrous changes in nerve.
VERBASCUM THAPS.	:	In deafness, if the patient complains that something is covering the ear drum. Use orally in 30 potency and instill 2-3 drops of its oil in the ears.

DEATH

ACONITUM NAP.	:	Predicts the day of death. Fears death and believes that he will die soon.
AGNUS CASTUS 6	:	Fear of death makes him sad. He apprehends fast approaching death. Lack of courage.
ANTIMONIUM TART.	:	Coma with a pale face and blue lips showing apparent death.
ARSENICUM ALB. 200,1M:		Removes restlessness. Calms and eases the last moments of life. A dose will ease the final departure.
AURUM MET.	:	The patient wants to commit suicide, but has a great fear of death.
CAMPHORA 1X	:	Apparent death when the cause is not known.

HELLEBORUS NIG.	: Predicts the day of death without any fear of it.
HYDRASTIS CAN.	: Sure of death and desires it.
PULSATILLA NIG.	: Rattling of the throat before death is eased by two doses. Also eases the final departure.
TARENTULA CUB. 200	: Soothes the last struggle and pain of death, eases the final departure.

DEBILITY

(SEE WEAKNESS)

DECEIVING

(SEE CHEATING)

DEHYDRATION

The process of dehydration occurs when the output of water exceeds the water intake. It may result from excessive vomiting, excessive urine, excessive perspiration or diarrhea. The clinical signs of dehydration are sticky mucous membranes, dry or sunken eyes and doughy skin. There are no sure indications to show the severity of dehydration. Whenever there are prolonged bouts of diarrhea, etc., treatment of the diseases may be given with the indicated remedies. In addition, the following rehydration salt formula may be given in as much quantity, as possible.

In many cases it will cure. The following remedies selected according to the indications will prove useful.

CHINA OFF., CHININUM ARS., PSORINUM, PHOSPHORICUM ACIDUM, PICRICUM ACIDUM, MAGNESIUM SULPH., SULPHUR AND NATRIUM MUR.

REHYDRATION SALT FORMULA

1. WATER   : 1 litre.
2. COMMON SALT   : 3. 5 grams.
3. POTASSIUM CHLORIDE: 1. 50 grams.
4. SODIUM CITRATE : 2. 09 grams.
5. GLUCOSE   : 20 grams.

Half a lemon of normal size can be substituted for potassium chloride and sodium citrate and sugar can be given instead of glucose.

DELIRIUM

Delirium is an altered state of consciousness, consisting of confusion, distractability, disorientation, disordered thinking and memory, defective perception, prominent hyperactivity and agitation.

ARNICA MONT.   : Delirium, with talk about death; raves at night, springs out of bed with great heat.

AGARICUS MUS.   : Makes prophecies during delirium. Although excited, he is sad. Talkative.

ARSENICUM ALB.   : Delirium due to fear and anxiety when left alone.

BAPTISIA TINC.	:	Delirium during diphtheria.
BELLADONNA	:	Violent delirium with blood shot eyes. Head is hot but extremities are cold. The patient tears clothes, strikes and bites.
BUFO RANA	:	Delirium during dysentery and diarrhea.
COCCULUS IND.	:	Delirium at the onset of menses.
CUPRUM MET.	:	Delirium in cholera and also due to suppression of menses.
HYOSCYAMUS NIG.	:	Delirium from accusations, insults or jealousy and suspicion. Sings obscene songs. A mild type of delirium with no violence.
LACHESIS	:	Muttering delirium during menopause and suppression of menses. Choking sensation in the throat.
OPIUM	:	Delirium due to fear of ghosts, devils and furious animals.
STRAMONIUM	:	Laughs incessantly without any cause. Sings and claps hands. Appears to be talking to invisible persons and souls.
VERATRUM VIR.	:	Delirium during child birth or septic fever.
ZINCUM MET.	:	Delirium during high temperature and unconsciousness. Jerking of limbs.

NOTE: When sleep puts an end to a delirium, it is a good sign.

DELIVERY

(SEE LABOR)

DENTITION

AETHUSA CYN.	:	Convulsions from teething. Child lies unconscious, dilated pupils, staring eyes, eye balls turned downwards, thumbs and fingers bent inwards, cold limbs and body convulsed.
ACONITUM NAP.	:	Fever with restlessness. Child cries due to pain.
ACTAEA RACE.	:	Sleeplessness during dentition.
BELLADONNA	:	Convulsions during the teething period, followed by sleep.
BORAX	:	Dentition with aphthae. Children startle at night on any sudden noise. Dread of downward motion.
CALCAREA PHOS.	:	In pale children, teeth appear late. During dentition flatulent diarrhea of greenish thin stools; child refuses to nurse or wants to be nursed all the time.
CHAMOMILLA, CALCAREA CARB.	:	Fever, restlessness, irritability, and diarrhea of sour, green and watery stools.
KREOSOTUM	:	Teeth often decay, after appearing. Very painful and difficult denti-

tion, worse during night, as a result the child gets little sleep and wants to be petted all the time. Constipation, stools very hard and dry, or diarrhea with dark brown, watery and very offensive stools.

MAGNESIUM CARB.   : Diarrhea, stools green and like chopped spinach.

MERCURIUS SOL.   : Great soreness of the gums.

PHYTOLACCA DEC.   : Child bites the teeth and gums together during dentition.

PODOPHYLLUM   : Child presses the gums together or tries to chew something hard. Diarrhea during dentition.

TEREBINTHINIAE   : During the period of dentition, urine is suppressed. Child screams and cannot sleep. Twitchings. Swelling of gums. Otitis.

DEPRESSION

AGNUS CASTUS   : Depression due to impotence.

ACONITUM NAP.   : Depression with anxiety.

AMBRA GRISEA   : Senile depression.

AMMONIUM CARB.   : Depression of spirits. Uneasy. Dyspnea due to weakness. Weeps, cries and has fainting fits.

ARSENICUM ALB.   : Sadness, restlessness, irritability, anxiety and fear. Thinks it is useless to take medicines for his depression. Depression on account of a hidden feeling of guilt.

AURUM MET. 200	:	Nervous breakdown. Thinks of committing suicide but fears death greatly. Disgusted of life and thoughts. Profound despondency. Peevish. Rapid and constant questioning without waiting for the answers. Oversensitive to noise.
CADMIUM SULPH. 200	:	Depression due to lack of confidence and grit.
CALADIUM SEG.	:	Depression due to impotence.
COCA	:	Depression due to over work and excesses.
COCCULUS IND.	:	The patient is sad, absorbed within himself. He broods, is moody, silent and sits in a corner, buried in thought.
CONIUM MAC.	:	Depression during menstruation, pregnancy and menopause. Excitement causes mental depression. Timid. Weak memory. Afraid of being alone.
GAULTHERIA Q	:	Depression causing pain in the stomach and vomiting.
GELSEMIUM	:	Depression from heat and due to impotence.
HELLEBORUS NIG.	:	Depression in women during puberty. When menses have not started or are suppressed. Sensation of depression. General muscular weakness. Sinking sensation, worse at 4-8 P.M. Mania of a melancholic type. Frequent sighing.
HYPERICUM PERF. 1X	:	Depression. Sadness and mood swings. Feeling of exhaustion.

Feeling that everything involves too much trouble. Does not want to get up in the morning. Feels as if an icy cold hand was touching his head. Feels as if lifted high in the air. Anxiety. Brain seems compressed and head feels longer.

IGNATIA AMARA : Depression due to grief and worry. Melancholic. Full of contradictions. Tearful. Blames herself for everything that goes wrong.

KALIUM BROM. : Depression after unsatisfying sexual intercourse. Fear of moral deficiency.

KALIUM PHOS. 200X : Mental and physical depression caused by excitement, overwork, worry and insomnia.

LYCOPODIUM : Depression of a student after failing in school examination.

MANCINELLA : Mental depression at puberty and at menopause.

MUREX PURP. : Great sadness. Very anxious and worried about the future and depressed.

NATRIUM MUR. : Depression due to hunger.

NATRIUM SULPH., THUJA OCC. : Depression due to the hidden feeling of guilt.

NUX VOM. : Depression after seminal emissions.

OCIMUM CAN. 3X : Stress and depression. Forgetful. Lack of concentration.

PHOSPHORUS : Great lowness of spirits. Easily offended. Fearful. Restlessness. Fear that he has an incurable heart disease.

PULSATILLA NIG.	:	Depression due to hormonal changes. There is an extreme tendency to cry and craving for sympathy, fresh air and cold drinks.
STAPHYSAGRIA 200	:	Depression on account of insults and anger. Depression without any cause or from sexual sins or of a forced sexual intercourse and rape.
TARENTULA HIS.	:	Prostration, restlessness and trembling.
TUBERCULINUM 1M	:	Irritable. Insomnia. Melancholia, worse in the morning after sleep. Uses foul language; curses and swears.

DIABETES INSIPIDUS (POLYURIA)
(PROFUSE URINE WITHOUT SUGAR)

ACETICUM ACIDUM	:	Polyuria with a lot of thirst and weakness.
ACIDUM PHOS. Q	:	The patient passes urine several times during night only. This cures diabetes of all kinds in early stages.
ALFALFA	:	Polyuria.
ARGENTUM NIT.	:	Frequent and profuse urination. May be passed unconsciously during the day and at night. Dribbling of urine. Urine may contain sugar or may not contain sugar. It is useful for polyuria in diabetes mellitus or diabetes insipidus.

MUREX PURP.   : Strong smelling urine passed sev-
                           eral times at night.

SQUILLA MAR.   : Urine is passed several times, day
                           and night. requent urging to
                           urinate. Involuntary spurting of
                           urine while coughing or sneezing.

DIABETES MELLITUS
(URINE CONTAINING SUGAR)

Diabetes is a disruption in metabolism, the way your body uses food. It is a disease in which the body does not produce or respond to insulin, a hormone that is essential for energy production and growth.

Normal metabolism:
Food passes through oesophagus to stomach and small intestine where digestion converts some of it into sugar (glucose), which enters the bloodstream, Sensing glucose increase, beta cells in pancreas secrete insulin, a hormone that enables glucose to enter body scells. Cells use glucose for energy or store as fat for later.

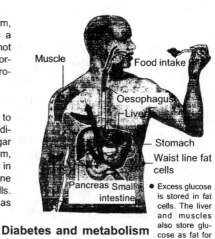

Diabetes and metabolism

Muscle

Food intake

Oesophagus

Liver

Stomach

Waist line fat cells

Pancreas Small intestine

● Excess glucose is stored in fat cells. The liver and muscles also store glucose as fat for later use.

Major forms of diabetes
● Type 1: One in about 20 people with diabetes is afflicted with this type. The pancreas produces no insulin or insufficient amounts and a person must receive insulin daily. This type usually strikes before the age of 30.

● Type 2: The most common form usually occurs after the age of 40 in overweight people. The insulin made by the pancreas is inadequate to prevent glucose from building up in the blood. Obesity increases resistance to insulin and is a major risk factor for developing Type 2 diabetes.

A) NON INSULIN DEPENDENT DIABETES

The onset in this type of diabetes is slow, and generally it is not accompanied by any symptom. It usually occurs over 40 years of age. Loss of weight and diet control often brings the blood sugar within normal range. With proper exercise, the indicated remedy will remove the discomfort.

B) INSULIN DEPENDENT DIABETES

It mostly occurs in children, young adults and is due to the lack of insulin or the patient's insulin does not work to convert sugar to glucose. Without insulin in adequate quantity and in proper form, glucose cannot enter the cells and remains in the blood. Eventually, it is spilled into urine which is passed frequently. To give proper treatment, urine and blood tests are necessary.

ACIDUM PHOS. 1X OR 2X : Diabetes in nervous patients. Soreness of the body due to grief, worry and anxiety. If given in the early stages of the disease, it cures.

ARSENICUM ALB. : Persistent unquenchable thirst. Sips water in small quantities and at short intervals. The mouth is generally dry. Itching of the body and pruritis. Here use Ars-br.

CANTHARIDINUM Q : Blood sugar increased, with high blood pressure. Give 10 drops in water, three times a day.

CEPHALANDRA Q : It works in both types of diabetes. Give 10 drops in water, thrice daily.

FENUGREEK Q : Mother tincture prepared from the yellow seeds and given 10-15 (east Indian methi) drops a dose thrice daily, controls diabetes and reduces sugar in blood and urine. Also controls simple polyuria.

GYMNEMA SYL. Q : 5-10 drops, four hourly. It is specially useful when the patient has an (Gur Mar)abolished taste of bitter things.

HELONIAS Q : It is useful for both mellitus and insipdus when there is excessive thirst, restlessness, melancholia and emaciation.

INSULINUM : It is a hormone, secreted by the pancreas, which is a ductless gland. It may be used in the beginning of the treatment, and thereafter, intercurrently. It helps in the production of an adequate quantity of insulin and in the proper form. Epileptic convulsions and mental derangements can be produced by injections of this hormone.

IRIS VERS. : Diabetes of patients suffering from disease of the pancreas, with burning in its region and vomiting. Acidity. Diarrhea or constipation.

LACTICUM ACIDUM : Persistent hunger and dry tongue. Copious urine, nausea, debility, great hunger and gastralgia.

MERCURIUS SOL. : Persistent, unquenchable thirst though there is much moisture (saliva) in the mouth.

PEPSINUM 1X - 3X : Diabetes due to diseases of the pancreas. Gout. Marasmus of children and emaciation.

PHASEOLUS L. : Diabetes with gout.

PHOSPHORUS : Diabetes in TB patients, or in patients suffering from rheumatism. The pancreas is diseased and does not function properly. Quantity of urine is increased and the patient desires cold water, on account of extreme dryness of the mouth. Useful in atrophy of the pancreas in diabetic patients.

RATANHIA PERU. : Diabetes but scanty urine.

SYZYGIUM JAMB. Q, URANIUM NIT. 3X : Both combined or given separately in alternation three hourly reduces sugar in blood and urine speedily. Usually the result is available in ten days. Uran-n. also controls high blood pressure.

TARENTULA HIS. : Rapid weight loss. Irritability with violent impulses. Copious urine.

THYROIDINUM : Diabetes mellitus when there is great weakness and a rapid change of symptoms.

URANIUM NIT. 3X : Diabetes due to a defective digestion. There is much thirst and an enormous appetite, yet the patient continues to emaciate.

NOTE 1: Normal blood sugar is 6-5% or 90 to120mg in 100ml of blood. 40% diabetics have hypertension.

NOTE 2: Conclusive diagnosis of diabetes can be found by testing of blood and urine in a clinical laboratory.

NOTE 3: Persons over 45 are at a risk of developing diabetes. With diabetes, the body cannot use or store properly the energy produced from the food eaten. It is because the pancreas either does not produce the required quantity of insulin or the insulin produced is not of a good qualitity. Failure to arrest the disease can result in damage of nerves and arteries, kidney failure and blindness. Risk factors include, being over weight, or inactive and having a family history of the disease. Early diagnosis, healthy eating, weight control and regular testing of blood and urine are essential.

DIABETES - ITS BAD EFFECTS

ABROMA AUG. Q	: Leucorrhea of diabetic ladies. Thick whitish discharge and dysmenorrhea.
ACIDUM PHOS. Q	: Reduced vision due to diabetes. Mental and physical debility. Impaired memory. Cannot collect his thoughts or find the right words to express himself.
ARGENTUM NIT.	: Useful in restoring power to the weakened ciliary muscles.
ARSENICUM ALB. 200	: Diabetic gangrene.
CEPHALANDRA Q-1, SYZYGIUM JAMB. Q	: For the cure of old ulcers in diabetic patients.
CARBOLICUM ACIDUM	: Carbuncle in diabetic patients.
COCA, MOSCHUS, CUPRUM MET. OR ACIDUM PHOS.	: Impotency due to diabetes.
CURARE	: Motor paralysis.
DOLICHOS	: Itching in diabetic patients without eruptions around the shoulders, knees and elbows. Worse at night.
GRAPHITES 200	: For various complications arising on account of diabetes.

HELONIAS	: Restlessness and thirst due to diabetes. It is also indicated in melancholia and emaciation.
HEPAR SULPHURIS	: Slightest injury suppurates. Stream of urine falls vertically and without force.
RANUNCULUS BULB.	: Diabetic coma. In such a case, give sugar in any liquid form immediately. When the patient regains consciousness, give the indicated remedy.
VANADIUM MET.	: It helps to stabilise blood sugar levels.
ZINCUM MET.	: Diabetes having an effect on the brain and spine resulting in convulsive twitching, troublesome uneasiness of the nerves and muscles of arms and legs with an irresistible desire to change their position. Involuntary urination when walking, coughing or sneezing. Involuntary motion of legs and feet, when asleep.

DIAPER RASH

BENZOICUM ACIDUM	: Diaper rash with urine smelling like ammonia.
MEDORRHINUM	: Diffuse redness all over the diaper area.
SULPHUR	: Diaper rash, worse after bathing, better in open air. It also cures rash caused by the use of certain drugs

such as bromide or iodine. It is also useful for red papular eruptions on the chin and anterior chest area of children seen during teething due to excess saliva pouring out of the mouth and coming in contact with the skin.

DIARRHEA

ACIDUM PHOS.	: Diarrhea of rachitic children. Stools are white, watery, involuntary and painless.
AETHUSA CYN.	: Diarrhea during dentition. Vomiting may be present.
ALOE SOC.	: Involuntary stools - may be solid and without the knowledge of the patient. Uncertain whether stool or gas will come. Stools lumpy and watery. Copious flatus. Patient is unable to control and has to run to the lavatory. Diarrhea from beer.
ARGENTUM NIT.	: Diarrhea caused by emaciation, sudden good or bad news, sorrow or anger. Watery and noisy. Diarrhea immediately after eating or drinking.
ARSENICUM ALB.	: Diarrhea with an unquenchable thirst.
BAPTISIA TINC.	: Stools are very offensive, thin, dark and bloody. Rumbling in the abdomen. Diarrhea during typhoid fever.

BOVISTA	: Diarrhea, before and after menses. Chronic diarrhea of old people. Worse at night and early morning.
CALCAREA PHOS.	: Diarrhea in children during dentition. Diarrhea from eating juicy fruits. Stools green, slimy, spluttering, fetid and contain undigested food articles.
CALCAREA PHOS., RHEUM, CHAMOMILLA	: Sour diarrhea during dentition.
CARBO VEG.	: Frequent, involuntary diarrhea of old people. Continuous oozing of moisture from the rectum.
CHAMOMILLA	: Diarrhea during the teething period, worse after anger. The child is cross and irritable.
CHAPARRO GRAPHITES, THUJA OCC.	: Use any of these remedies according to the other symptoms for chronic diarrhea.
CHININUM ARS.	: Diarrhea after taking fish and from eating eggs.
CHINA OFF., FERRUM MET., OLEANDER	: Diarrhea with undigested food in stools.
CHINA OFF.	: Painless diarrhea. Stools are frothy, pale and contain undigested food particles. Much flatulence. Worse after meals and in hot weather.
COLCHICUM AUTUM.	: Abdomen seems full of wind and water. Nausea. Vomits from the smell of food. Painful, transparent, scanty stools, which contain white shreddy particles.
COLOCYNTHIS	: Brown, watery stools after eating or drinking. Jelly like stools with musk like odour. Pain in the abdomen.

CROTON TIG.	: Gurgling in the intestines. Copious, watery stools are shot out forcibly. Constant urging to stool. Worse while drinking or eating.
DULCAMARA	: Green, watery, slimy, bloody with mucus. Worse in damp cold weather. Hill diarrhea.
FERRUM PHOS., KALIUM PHOS.	: Diarrhea during eating.
GRAPHITES	: Stools are brown, fluid and are mixed with undigested food particles. They have an intolerably fetid smell.
HYOSCYAMUS NIG.	: Painless, involuntary stool while urinating.
JATROPA, JALAPA	: Diarrhea with nausea and vomiting. Loud noise in abdomen like gurgling of water, or water coming out of a bung hole.
NATRIUM SULPH.	: Stools involuntary while passing wind. Great size of faecal mass. Early morning diarrhea.
NITRICUM ACIDUM	: Diarrhea after use of antibiotics. It is of a great value.
NUX VOM.	: Diarrhea due to over eating or dietic errors and indigestible foods. Pain in abdomen before stools. Stool contains undigested articles of food.
PHOSPHORUS	: Painless, copious, debilitating diarrhea. Very fetid stools and flatus. Discharge of blood from the rectum during stool. Green mucus or white, hard stools.

PODOPHYLLUM	: Diarrhea green, watery, fetid, profuse and gushing. Worse during teething and in the morning, while bathing or washing and in hot weather. Camp diarrhea. Diarrhea alternating with constipation. Prolapse of rectum before or with stools.
PULSATILLA NIG.200	: 2 or 3 normal stools a day. Diarrhea after measles. A remedy of great value in this condition. It cures diarrhea in opium eaters. Should be repeated after three hours, three doses a day. Stools contain undigested articles of food. Diarrhea due to food poisoning.
PYROGENIUM	: Diarrhea horribly offensive, brown black, painless and involuntary. Stools large or like black balls.
SEPIA	: Diarrhea after taking boiled milk.
SEPTICAEMINUM, PODOPHYLLUM	: Very useful in camp diarrhea.
SILICEA, NATRIUM CARB.	: Diarrhea on drinking milk.
SULPHUR	: Morning diarrhea. Patient rushes from the bed to the latrine. Painless diarrhea.
TANACETUM VULG.	: Diarrhea immediately after eating or drinking. In Arg-n., liquids go right through him and the case is worse after taking sweet dishes or sweet drinks.
TRIOSTEUM PERF., RHUS TOX., ARUM TRIPH., BAPTISIA TINC.	: Use any of these remedies according to symptoms, for diarrhea during typhoid.

TRIOSTEUM PERF. 6 : It is a very valuable remedy in diarrhea, attended with colicky pains and nausea.

VERATRUM ALB. : Diarrhea very painful, watery, copious and forcibly evacuated followed by great weakness.

ZINGIBER : Diarrhea after taking melons or polluted water.

DIET

Our life depends upon diet taken, knowing how much to eat and when to eat is what matters the most. It has been wisely said that eat to live and do not live to eat. It is rather difficult to lay down rules to suit all cases. Every individual case has its own requirements of food. The golden rule is that whatever is pleasing to your eyes to see, whatever is pleasing in taste to your tongue and whatever you feel pleased after eating, may be taken. So long digestion , body weight, strength and activities are normal, do not think about what to take and what not to take. Diet should be simple and better vegetarian rather than non-vegetarian. Milk and milk products not containing more than 2% fats is a must for every body. Infants under eight months should have nothing but their mother's milk. Failing this a wet nurse or a goats milk or cows milk diluted with 1/8 of water can be substituted. The milk should be boiled and brought to blood heat before serving. After this age, some good baby foods available in the market should be given. As the teeth develop, solid foods such as bread, butter and milk pudding may be given.

Some simple facts , which have emerged from worldwide surveys, are important. A consistent link between diet and health in old age has been found. A diet rich in fruits and fresh vegetables is associated with lowered incidence of such diseases as cancer, cataract and heart attacks. Not very long ago, vegetarians were considered second rate humans and inferior in health status to non-vegetarians. It is now recognised that vegetarians in general, live longer because they are less prone to high blood pressure, heart attacks and cancer. The main reason is that a vegetarian diet provides most of the antioxidants which offer protection against free radicals. Vitamins have their own role to play. A healthy balanced diet in correct proportion is necessary for a healthy life. However , some rules are necessary for not so healthy persons. Suggestions will be found in this book for such cases, where necessary.

DIPHTHERIA

Diphtheria is a specific infectious disease, marked by severe inflammation that can form a membranous coating, with formation of a thick fibrinous exudate on the mucous membrane of the pharynx, nose and sometimes the tracheobronchial tree.

APIS MEL. : There is edema of the throat with stinging pain and burning. Enlarged uvula. Scanty urine and puffiness about the eyes.

BAPTISIA TINC. : Delirium during diphtheria.

CALCAREA PHOS. 6X : Given thrice daily, removes the weakness remaining after the cure of diphtheria.

DIPHTHERINUM : Start the treatment with this remedy. Give it thrice, for only one day. It can be given in 200 potency, as a preventive of the disease.

GELSEMIUM : It is used when there is diphtheric paralysis of the pharynx.

KALIUM BICH.	: It is the best remedy for nasal diphtheria. Uvula is relaxed and there is a plug like sensation of plug in the throat.
KALIUM MUR. 6X	: Give it every hour, if diphtheria is accompanied with great prostration and there is characteristic glandular enlargement of the uvula and the entire soft palate. The improvement will be noticed next day.
KALIUM PERM.	: Gargling and rinsing the mouth with luke warm water, containing a few crystals of potassium permanganate, rapidly and surely removes the offensive odour of diphtheric breath.
LACHESIS 200	: The discharge from the nose is acrid. Membranes of the throat are dark red or bluish. Swallowing of saliva is painful.
MERCURIUS CYAN. 30X	: If given before exudation is deposited, it will prevent it to appear at all. Only 30X potency works. If the disease prolongs, the following treatment should be continued.
MERCURIUS IOD. 1X - 2X	: If there is a putrid sore throat and diphtheric patches are observed in the throat with pain on swallowing.
NAJA TRI.	: It is to be administered, when there is an impending paralysis of the heart. The patient is blue and awakened from sleep gasping. It is more indicated when the larynx is also affected.

PHYTOLACCA DEC. Q : Pain shoots from the throat to the ears. Dryness and sensation of a lump in the throat. Throat may be cleaned from time to time with Phyt. Q (5 drops in an ounce of water).

DIPLOPIA (DOUBLE VISION)

AGARICUS MUS. : Diplopia from overwork at the desk.

ARGENTUM NIT. : Sight fails for near objects, everything appears blurred or indistinct.

AURUM MET. : Diplopia or half-sightedness from overwork with the eyes or working in hot places; sensation in eyes as if they were being pushed out, with tension in them.

CAUSTICUM : Double vision when turning the eyes to the right.

GELSEMIUM : Double vision when turning the eyes to either side.

HYOSCYAMUS NIG. : Illusion of vision. An object appears double.

PHOSPHORUS : Paralysis of the eye muscles from excesses, accompanied by general loss of muscular tone.

SENEGA : Objects appear double when seen with both the eyes but appear normal when seen with one eye.

STRAMONIUM : Letters and objects appear double.

VERATRUM VIR. : Double vision. There is congestive headache.

DISLOCATIONS

ARNICA MONT. Q-1000 : Given immediately after fractures and dislocations, relieves nervousness and pain. Give a few doses in 1M potency every one hour internally and apply Q in cold water externally.

RHUS TOX. : If the pain remains give Rhus-t. 30 three times a day. The pain and swelling disappear in about 3 days.

DREAMS

ALOE SOC. : Dreams of passing stools.

APIS MEL. : Dreams of flying.

BELLADONNA : Dreams of fire.

CHELIDONIUM : Dreams of funerals.

KALIUM CARB. : Dreams of ghosts.

LAC CAN. 200 : Dreams of snakes and of urinating.

MERCURIUS SOL. : Dreams of animals.

NUX VOM. : Dreams of accidents. Sexual dreams causing emission of semen. Dreams from excessive mental exertion.

SILICEA : Dreams of thieves.

THUJA OCC. : Dreams of dead people and of falling from a height.

DROPSY

ACONITUM NAP.	: Simple dropsy with fever.
APIS MEL.	: Simple dropsy between the skin and flesh with fever. Unabsorbed effusions after inflammation of the serous cavities. Absence of thirst. Dropsy aggravated by heat.
APOCYNUM CAN. 3X	: A good and general remedy for dropsy between the skin and flesh. Dropsy with jaundice and other diseases of the liver. Abdomen distended. Digestion impaired. Dropsy aggravated by cold.
ARSENICUM ALB.	: Dropsy after scarlatina with albumin in urine and thirst. Disorders of the heart and lungs. Puffiness of the face and around the eye lids.
ARSENICUM IOD. 3X	: Dropsy due to heart diseases. Burning in gullet and stomach. Nausea, vomiting and diarrhea.
AURUM MET.	: Dropsy in syphilitic patients and syphilitic liver.
CALCAREA CARB.	: Dropsy aggravated by bathing.
CITRICUM ACIDUM, LEMON JUICE	: All forms of dropsy's are benefitted with a tablespoon full of lemon juice every 3-4 hours.
DIGITALIS	: Dropsy due to heart diseases. Nausea, vomiting and diarrhea. Urine scanty and contains albumin. Swelling of feet and genitals.
HELLEBORUS NIG.	: Cerebral dropsy with sensation of depression or as an after effect of head injury.

KALIUM CARB.	: Dropsy of throat and lungs.
MERCURIUS SOL.	: Dropsical swelling of feet and legs.
PHASEOLUS N.	: Dropsy due to kidney complications and heart diseases. It increases the quantity of urine thus reducing albumin and edema. It is a very good remedy in such circumstances.
SAMBUCUS CAN.	: It is a valuable remedy for dropsy in lower potencies. The chief indication is edema and dropsical swellings in legs, instep, feet, etc. Profuse sweat during the day only.
SQUILLA MAR.	: Acute dropsical swelling with suppression of urine.
TEREBINTHINIAE 1X	: Dropsy with hemorrhage from the kidneys, congestion and other infections of the kidneys.
URANIUM NIT. 3X	: High blood pressure during dropsy, specially of the abdomen.
VESICARIA COM.Q	: Edema due to complete failure of kidneys. Give 10-20 drops, 3 hourly.

DRUGS

Drug is a general term for any substance, stimulating or depressing, that can be habituating or addictive, especially a narcotic.

1. ALCOHOL
2. BARBITONES

3. CANNABIS SATIVA (MARIJUANA) HEMP	: Powder of leaves and flowers is used for smoking. Flowers of the female plant of Cannabis sativa (hemp) is usually used for smoking.
CANNABIS INDICA (HASHISH)	
4. COCAINE	: It is obtained from erythroxyln and is used for prolongation of the sexual act. According to the scientists at the University of Munich, cocaine can over stimulate the heart and may cause a heart attack.
5. HEROIN	: A narcotic derived from morphine or opium.
6. SLEEPING PILLS	
7. STRAMONIUM	: Its powdered seeds are used for smoking.
8. TESTOSTERONE (DOPE)	: It is a steroid derived from the male sex hormones. It is used by the athletes and sportsmen for increasing the stamina.

BAD EFFECTS OF DRUGS

ALCOHOL	: Its bad effects are removed by Sterculia Q and Ranunculus bulbosus Q (see Alcoholism).
BARBITONES	: Carbo vegetabilis removes its bad effects.
CANNABIS SATIVA, CANNIBIS INDICA	: Cannabis addiction may be treated and cured by Sulphur 200. A dose on alternate days in the morning, miraculously cures its bad effects

and addiction. For immediate effects, to remove intoxication, 5 ml of pure lemon juice mixed with 200 ml of water every 15 minutes. Studies prove that tetrahydrocannabinal or t. h. c. is the main active ingredient of marijauna and it is stored in the fats of the body, even if a person does not smoke himself but is only exposed to its smoke when the marijauna is being smoked by another person. Fat in the body is a natural storage area.

COCAINE : Conium maculatum 1M given infrequently removes its bad effects and bad habit.

HEROIN : Bad effects of its use are removed by the use of Avena sativa (common oats). Twenty drops in warm water should be given every half an hour till intoxication is removed. Black coffee also antidotes its intoxication. Berberis vulgaris is useful to counter its habit. Diarrhea of such addicts is cured by Pulsatilla and insomnia by Avena sativa Q - 20 drops a dose in hot water.

SLEEPING PILLS : Bad effects are removed by Coffea cruda 3X.

STRAMONIUM : Nux vomica 10M removes its bad effects and also the bad habit.

TESTOSTERONE : It is not habit forming and generally, no treatment is required. Zincum phosphoricum 3X antidotes it.

NOTE :

1.   A single dose of Nux vomica 10M removes the craving for drugs. It may be repeated on alternate days if required.

2.   Passiflora Q mixed with Avena sativa Q in equal parts and given in 20 drop doses, thrice daily, takes away the craving for heroin and cocaine.

3.   In all cases of drug addiction, give 40-50 drops of Passiflora Q at bed time. It will produce a healthy sleep without dreams and hallucinations.

DWARFISHNESS
(SEE ALSO BACKWARD CHILDREN)

Condition of being abnormally small may be hereditary which is mostly incurable. It may be due to a dysfunction of the pituitary, thryoid gland, etc. , when treatment of the affected gland may cure the disease. It can be due to the diseases of the skeleton mostly bones of the legs, where again a proper treatment can cure. If no such defect is located, the following treatment is suggested.

BARYTA CARB. 3X   : If the patient is plump (i. e. if he is moderately fat), give this remedy thrice daily for 30 days or repeat the treatment till the patient is cured.

BARYTA PHOS. 3X   : If the patient is thin and lean, use this remedy instead of Bar-c. 3X or repeat the treatment till the patient is cured.

COD LIVER OIL   : Nocturnal massage of this oil is also helpful in the treatment of dwarfish and emaciated babies.

MEDORRHINUM 1M : Children do not grow normally and remain dwarfish, under developed and under sized.

SYPHILINUM 1000 : After 24 hours of adminstration of Tuberculinum, give this remedy and again wait for 24 hours.

THYROIDINUM 3X : Arrested development of children - eats well yet looses flesh on account of thyroid trouble.

TUBERCULINUM 200 : Start the treatment with this remedy. No other remedy should be given for the next 24 hours.

DYSENTERY

A disease marked by frequent watery stools, with blood and mucus, and characterized by pain, tenesmus, fever and dehydration.

ALOE SOC. : Stools contain a lot of mucus or are jelly like. There is burning and pain in the rectum after stools. Burning, copious flatus. Insecurity of rectum. Patient is afraid of passing flatus as he is not sure whether the urge is for stool or flatus. Bleeding from the rectum.

ANTIMONIUM CRUD. : Stools composed entirely of mucus.

BAPTISIA TINC. : Dysentery of old people. Dysentery during typhoid fever.

CHAPARRO : It is an excellent remedy for chronic dysentery and diarrhea.

COLCHICUM AUTUM.	: Autumnal dysentery when days are hot and nights are cold.
MERCURIUS COR., MERCURIUS SOL	: Begin the treatment with Merc-c., if there is much blood or with Merc. if there is much mucus. Cutting pains are present and stools are scanty. Tenesmus, before and after stools. This generally cures the case.
NUX VOM.	: Stools contain much mucus. There are abdominal pains before stools and these are relieved after stools.
SEPTICAEMINUM	: It cures magically, the dysentery which is produced in camp life.
THUJA OCC. 200	: It is an excellent remedy for amoebic dysentery.
TROMBIDIUM	: Dysentery, worse by eating and drinking. Stools only after eating. Much pain, before and after stool. Burning in the anus.

DYSMENORRHEA
(PAINFUL MENSES OR DELAYED MENSES)

ABROMA RADIX 1X	: This remedy suits most of the cases of dysmenorrhea, unless symptoms definitely point out to another remedy. The use of this remedy proves very useful. 5 drops of it in a little warm water are given in a single dose on the first day of the flow and a similar dose is given every day during menses and after their

cessation for 7 days continuously, for cure. If it is not cured, repeat it 2 days before the starting of next period. It also brings about conception, in young sterile married ladies.

ALETRIS FAR. : Pains are like Chamomilla but the patient is constipated and weak.

CALCAREA CARB. 200 : Swelling and pain in breasts before the start of menses in fat ladies having thyroid and pituitary dysfunctions.

CALCAREA PHOS. 6X : Dysmenorrhea of young girls at puberty, during the first few monthly menses.

CAULOPHYLLUM : Severe labor like pains in the abdomen during periods.

CHAMOMILLA 200 : Labor like pain in the abdomen and hips. Menses are profuse. Diarrhea may accompany. Painful and delayed menses. Much irritability during periods.

COLOCYNTHIS : Menses start early and pain starts before the start of menses, compelling the patient to bend double because the pain is relieved by pressure. It is also benefited by applying hot water bottles on the abdomen.

CONIUM MAC. 200 : Swelling and pain in the breasts before start of menses. Scanty painful menses. It is specially useful in old maids and unmarried girls after puberty.

LAPIS ALBUS : Black clots on the first day of menses. Pains are very severe and the patient may become unconscious, because she cannot tolerate the pain. Pain subsides as the flow starts.

LOBELIA INF. : Vomiting before and after, start and cessation of menses. Pain in abdomen, ovaries and legs are so severe that the patient faints.

MAGNESIUM PHOS. 6X : It can be given in alternation with Abroma radix as it proves very useful. The pain is relieved by warmth and pressure like Colocynthis.

PULSATILLA NIG. 200 : Mild patients with weeping tendencies. Pain subsides on consolation or in open air.

SEPIA : Headache, accompanied with vomiting before start of menses which are profuse and early. Vomiting and acidity, after menses.

TUBERCULINUM 1M : Menses painful, too early, too profuse and last for a longer period. Pain increases as the flow starts and during menstruation.

VIBURNUM OP. 1X : It is a uterine tonic. The pain starts before the start of menses compelling the patient to bend double. Pain vanishes when the flow begins.

DYSPEPSIA
(INDIGESTION)

It is an impaired gastric function or "upset stomach" due to some disorder of the stomach; characterized by epigastric pain, sometimes burning, nausea and eructations.

ACIDUM PHOS.	: Food remains in the stomach for a long time after taking. Sour vomiting.
AETHUSA CYN.	: Milk is not digested and is vomited out in curds as soon as it is taken. Regurgitation of food about an hour after eating. Dyspeptics want to get relief by eating. They are always munching something which gives them temporary relief. A time comes when the stomach becomes over worked and refuses to perform its duty. Such a dyspepsia is relieved by occassional fasting and by taking Aeth. 3 times a day.
ALFALFA Q	: A few 10 drop doses, tones up the appetite and digestion.
AMMONIUM MUR.	: Pain in the stomach, immediately after eating. Regurgitation of food after eating. Nausea. Alternating diarrhea and constipation.
ANACARDIUM ORI.	: Dyspepsia of nervous people. Heartburn relieved by eating.
ANTIMONIUM CRUD.	: Tongue coated white, as if white washed. Belching with fluid coming in the mouth and tasting of ingesta.

BRYONIA ALBA : Feeling of a stone in the stomach. Sharp pains in the chest and back. Bilious vomiting. White tongue. Headache. Constipation.

CALCAREA CARB. : Heartburn, waterbrash. Abdomen distended and hard. White stools. Great hunger and white coated tongue.

CARBO VEG. : Acidity. Loose bowels. Flatulence and belching. Heartburn. Pain in the chest. Regurgitation of watery fluid from the stomach.

CARICA PAPAYA 1X : It furthers digestion, especially in those whose stomach can't tolerate meat and milk. Dose, one gram four times a day.

CHAMOMILLA : Bilious dyspepsia. Tongue yellow, taste bitter. Aversion to warm drinks.

COFFEE : A spoon or two of strong expresso coffee will often immediately relieve an acute indigestion from over eating and when the food taken remains in the stomach for a long time without digestion.

GRAPHITES 6 : Aversion to meat. Sweets nauseate. Hot drinks disagree. Nausea and vomiting after each meal. Morning sickness during menstruation. Burning in stomach causing hunger. Pain in the stomach temporarily relieved by eating and drinking hot milk.

IPECACUANHA : Gastric symptoms from and after indulgence in rich food as pastry,

	pork, sweets, ice-creams, etc. Constant nausea and vomiting.
IRIS VERS.	: Nausea and vomiting of watery and extremely sour fluid, especially early in the morning. Burning in the whole alimentary canal.
KALIUM BICH.	: Cutting pain in the stomach, soon after eating. Food lies in the stomach without being digested, giving a sensation of heaviness and load in the stomach.
KALIUM CARB.	: Dyspepsia of old people. Abdomen distended after eating a little. Heartburn.
LYCOPODIUM	: Great flatulence in the abdomen. Feels sleepy after dinner. Waterbrash. Tongue coated white.
MAGNESIUM PHOS.	: Sleeplessness on account of indigestion.
NATRIUM CARB.	: Old dyspeptics always belching. Very weak digestion. A slightest error of food causes indigestion.
NATRIUM MUR.	: Indigestion of smokers. Bitter taste. Blistered tongue, loss of taste. Heartburn with intense thirst. Constipation.
NUX VOM.	: Indigestion from indigestible food and alcohol. Cramping and spasmodic pain. Vomiting. Constipating. Flatulence in hysterical women especially during pregnancy.
PULSATILLA NIG.	: Indigestion from eating fried food and meats. Tongue moist and thickly coated white.

PLUMBUM MET.   : Lead dyspepsia is people suffering already with numbness of the extremities. Excessive colic, radiating to all parts of the body. Abdominal wall feels drawn by a string to the spine.

ROBINIA   : Indigestion due to acidity.

SANGUINARIA CAN.   : Tongue yellowish white. Foul eructations. Nausea not relieved by vomiting. Saliva increased. Bitter vomiting.

SEPIA   : Dyspepsia of tabacco eaters and smokers. Everything tastes salty.

VANADIUM MET. 6   : Indigestion after gastroenteric inflammation. Three doses a day for a few days, improves digestion quickly. It has the same effect in early TB.

DYSPHAGIA
(SWALLOWING DIFFICULT)

APIS MEL.   : Swallowing difficult and painful on account of edema of the mucous membrane of the throat which appears as if stung with a bee. There is an inability to even swallow a single drop of water.

ARGENTUM NIT.   : Difficulty in swallowing with a splinter like sensation in the throat.

BAPTISIA TINC.   : Can swallow liquids only, due to vomiting and spasm of oesophagus.

BELLADONNA	:	Swallowing difficult on account of bright red swelling in the throat with dryness and burning.
CAPSICUM	:	Swallowing difficult on account of burning with constriction of the throat.
CARBOLICUM ACIDUM	:	Almost impossible to swallow and regurgitation on swallowing liquids due to inflammation of fauces or diphtheria.
CAUSTICUM	:	Food enters the larynx instead of oesophagus due to a disease of the pharynx causing difficulty in swallowing.
CROTALUS H.	:	Cannot swallow any solid substance due to spasm and constriction of the oesophagus.
HEPAR SULPHURIS	:	Difficulty in swallowing with a sensation of a plug and a splinter in the throat.
HYOSCYAMUS NIG.	:	Cannot swallow liquids. Uvula is elongated and muscles of the throat and pharynx are stiff.
IGNATIA AMARA	:	Stitches in the throat between acts of swallowing. Swallowing difficult on account of inflamed, swollen and ulcerated tonsils.
LACHESIS	:	Swallowing of both liquids and solids difficult due to the dry, intensely swollen throat.
MANCINELLA	:	Dysphagia from constriction of the throat and oesophagus.
NATRIUM PHOS.	:	Dysphagia due to blisters on the tongue, soft palate, etc.

PLUMBUM MET. : Cannot swallow solids due to constriction in the oesophagus and due to pressure and tightness in the stomach. Constant vomiting.

NOTE: It is one of the imperatives in medicine that if a person in middle life complains of 'dysphagia', one must not rest until carcinoma of the oesophagus or other organic causes have been excluded.

EARACHE (OTALGIA)

ACONITUM NAP. : Earache due to extreme heat or extreme cold. Very useful in the early stages.

ACTAEA SPIC. : Throbbing pain in the ears, while sneezing or blowing the nose.

AETHUSA CYN. : Otalgia is relieved by boring a finger in the ear.

BELLADONNA : Sudden unbearable pain with redness of the external and middle ear.

CAPSICUM : Otalgia due to rupture of the eardrum. Pains, worse at night.

CHAMOMILLA : A great remedy for earache in children. Otalgia is intolerable.

GELSEMIUM : Otalgia during menopause.

HEPAR SULPHURIS : Otalgia due to an abscess in the ear. Patient does not allow anyone to touch the ear, as touch increases the pain. Otalgia due to exposure to cold dry winds.

LACHESIS 200 : It cures the tearing pain in the ear caused by the fungus in the ear, which is generally black or white.

MAGNESIUM PHOS. Q : Give 3 grains with warm water every half an hour when the pains are relieved by hot application and by placing a hand on the ear.

MERCURIUS SOL. : Otalgia, worse warmth of bed; at night, sticking pains.

PLANTAGO Q : It gives relief from the earache. Instill a few drops in the ear. May be mixed in equal quantity with Verbascum oil for instilling in the ear.

PULSATILLA NIG. : External ear swollen and red. Otalgia worse at night.

VERBASCUM THAPS. OIL 30 (MULLEIN OIL) : Earache with a sense of obstruction of the ear. Dry scales and itching in the middle ear. Use oil externally and 30 potency orally.

EARDROPS

OLEUM MULLEINI : A little cotton plug lightly drenched with it should be inserted into the ear holes. It will cure itching and dry scaly conditions. Also makes hearing somewhat better.

PLANTAGO Q : Otalgia. A few drops warmed to the body temperature should be instilled in the painful ear. It relieves the pain.

EAR FUNGUS

LACHESIS : Bluish black fungus on the ear drum.

SILICEA : Whitish fungoid growths on the ear drum.

EAR NOISES
(TINNITUS)

ALUMINA, NITRICUM ACIDUM : Cracking noises in the ears, while chewing.

ARNICA MONT. : All sorts of noises in the ears after an accident or a blow on the ears.

BARYTA MUR. : Whizzing and buzzing in the ears. Echoing of sounds and voices. Humming, as from telegraph wires. Cracking noises, while chewing.

BELLADONNA : Hearing, ones own voice in the ears.

CAUSTICUM : All sorts of noises like roaring, tickling, humming, etc. Noises during deafness. Own voice sounds in the ears.

GLONOINUM : Beats of the heart are heard in the ears.

KALIUM MUR. : Noises of moving trains and chirping of birds in the ears.

LEDUM PAL. : Noises like ringing of bells, roaring like strong winds and storms.

MANGANUM ACET.	: Whistling noises in the ears.
NATRIUM SAL.	: Ringing and other noises in the ears. It is a very good remedy, if there is a progressive deafness.
PETROLEUM	: Ringing and crackling noises.
PICRICUM ACIDUM	: Humming, as if from the telegraph lines.

NOTE: **Researches at Buffalo (USA) Medical Center have identified the source of tinnitus as originating in the auditory cortex in the brain. When the inner ear is damaged, by blows, loud noises, etc, the brain "rewines" itself to conpensate for the loss of function. This "rewining" generates electrical signals, that the brain interprets as noises.**

EAR WAX

CONIUM MAC.	: A little wax is necessary in the ear. It is very poisonous and instantly kills any insect straying into the ear. However, abnormal secretion of wax is cured by the use of this remedy. Wax should also be removed manually.
LACHESIS	: It removes the irritation caused by hard and dry ear wax. The wax can also be softened by instilling a few drops of mullein oil and then removed manually.
WIESBADEN	: Copious secretion of ear wax which is soft, slimy, thin almost fluent and pale brown. Much itching in ears after its flow is cured by the use of this remedy.

EARS

AMMONIUM MUR.	:	Burning in the ears in cold weather and in cold air.
AURUM MET., AGARICUS MUS.	:	Burning, redness and itching of the ears. Use either of the remedies.
BARYTA CARB.	:	Ear lobes inflames on wearing any earring except gold.
CAUSTICUM, SULPHUR	:	Use either remedy, when the external ears burn and are very red.
FORMICA RUFA	:	Checks further formation of polypi in the ear and has a deterrent influence on their formation.
GLONOINUM	:	Beats of the heart are heard in the ears.
MERCURIUS SOL.	:	Burning of the ear drum (tympanum). Boils in the external canal.
NATRIUM SAL..	:	Diseases of the inner ear like loss of conduction of voice by the occicles producing deafness, vertigo and all sorts of noises and gradual deafness.
SANGUINARIA CAN.	:	Burning redness of the ear and cheeks.
STANNUM MET.	:	Ulceration of ear lobes on wearing earrings.
STREPTOCOCCINUM 200	:	A dose cuts the ear infections. About 30% of ear infections are caused by strepto-pneumonia. It removes the septic conditions and has a rapid action to cure fever.

ECZEMA
(ALSO SEE RINGWORM)

ACIDUM SULPH. : Livid, red, itching blotches and eczema. Relieves itching. Eczema due to staphylococcal and streptococcal infection.

ALUMINA : Dry irritating eczema.

ANTIMONIUM CRUD. : Eczema of the face, genitals and anus. Severe continuous itching. Eczema with gastric troubles. Burning is worse at night.

ARSENICUM IOD. 3X : Eczema of the beard with oozing of a watery discharge. Itching, worse by washing. Dry scaly itching.

ARSENICUM ALB. : Eczema with burning and restlessness. Itching produces burning, worse cold and cold applications. Eczema between fingers and cracks on the tips of the fingers. Best normally for chronic eczema, if there is great burning and itching.

BACILLINUM 200 : Ringworm. Eczema of eyelids.

BORAX : Itching on the back of the finger joints and with loss of nails.

CHRYSAROBINUM 6 : Vesicular eruptions, associated with foul smelling discharges and crust formation. Violent itching of thighs, legs and ears. Dry, scaly eruptions, especially around eyes and ears. Locally and externally, 10 drops in vaseline should be applied gently and not rubbed. Eczema behind ears.

CICUTA VIR. 200	: Eczema of chin in males. Eczema of the scalp. Whole head is covered with eczema, like a cap.
CLEMATIS ERECTA	: Pustular eczema. Vesicles with watery secretions, followed by formation of scales and crusts. Inflammation increases with the increasing moon and decreases with the decreasing moon.
CROTON TIG.	: Eczema of the face, genitals and testes. It reveals itching of all eczema's permanently and rapidly.
GRAPHITES 200	: Eczema of palms, hands and around the anus. Weeping eczema. A sticky fluid comes out on scratching. Eczema of the eyelids, face, genitals and anus. Cracks in the skin. Moist, scabby eruptions on the scalp, face, bends of joints, between fingers and behind ears.
GUNPOWDER 3X	: Where other remedies are hard to decide, give it in chronic eczema, 3 doses a day till cured.
HEPAR SULPHURIS	: Moist eczema with itching in the folds of skin. After scratching, pimples form on the skin. Eczema is worse during cold dry winds and better in damp, rainy weather and warmth. Eczema of genitals and scrotum.
HYDRASTIS CAN.	: Crusty, burning eczema on the neck.
HYPERICUM PERF.	: Eczema on hands and face with intense itching. Herpes zoster.

JUGLANS C.	: Pustular eczema on the lower extremities, sacrum and hands.
KALIUM BICH.	: Eczema of the scalp with thick, heavy crusts; which ooze a yellow, thick, gluey liquid.
KALIUM MUR.	: Moist eczema. It is especially useful in chronic and obstinate forms of eczema. Vesicles contain thick white matter. Eczema of the face and head of children.
LACHESIS 200	: It is of great value when the slightest touch, even of cloth, causes maddening irritation of eczema. If the affected skin has a bluish, purplish appeerence, this remedy is sure to help.
LEDUM PAL.	: Eczema of face and cheeks. Skin is red in color and is worse, scratching and at night. Putting feet in cold water gives relief.
LYCOPODIUM 200	: Eczema with violent itching and fissured eruptions. Skin becomes thick. Such patients usually have digestive and urinary troubles.
MERCURIUS SOL.	: Weeping eczema in the bends of knees and elbows. Vesicular and pustular eruptions. Itching, worse from the warmth of bed.
MEZEREUM	: Eczema on the hairy parts, with intolerable itching. Head covered with thick, leathery crusts with pus underneath. Hair becomes glued together. Bad smell from crusts and pus.

NATRIUM MUR.	: Crusty eczemaous eruptions on the margins of hair. Eczema behind the ears. Eczema of hair follicle. Eczema with thick scales, oozing pus.
OLEANDER	: Eczema of the scalp.
PETROLEUM	: Has yellowish green thick crusts on the face and neck. On scratching, a liquid comes out and it often bleeds. Eczema disappearing in summers and reappearing in winters. Eczema with fissures on hands and behind the ears. The discharge is thin and watery. It is specially suitable for eczema behind the ears.
PHOSPHORUS, SEPIA	: Eczema on lips. Apply Capsicum Q on the eczematous parts once a day. It cures.
PSORINUM	: Crusty, scaly, dry eczema of the scalp and face. Hair falls out. Terrible itching, worse from the warmth of bed. Oily skin. Eczema behind the ears and bends of joints.
RANUNCULUS BULB.	: Bluish eruptions and vesicles with burning and intense itching. Eczema on the palms.
RHUS TOX. 200	: Eczema blister like with a lot of itching. Restlessness. When blisters disappears, the skin becomes red. Offensive secretion. Burning. eczematous eruptions in winter and damp weather.
SELENIUM MET.	: Vesicular eruptions between fingers. Itching about finger joints

and between fingers. Itching of palms, ankles and folds of skin.

SEPIA : Eczema in circular spots at isolated places. Ringworm. Worse in bends of elbows and knees, and in spring weather.

SKOOKUM CHUCK 3X : An antipsoric remedy. Obstinate eczema of the dry skin.

STAPHYSAGRIA : Eczema of head, ears, face and body. Thick dry scales which itch violently. Scratching changes location of itching.

STREPTOCOCCINUM 1M : Repeated reappearance of eczema after cure. Scratching gives pleasure.

SULPHUR : Dry rough skin. Much itching. Eczema in the folds of skin. Eczema of the hairy parts. Pruritis, worse washing. Bad odour from the body. Eczema caused by the use of hair dyes.

THUJA OCC. : Simple, acute, general or local eczema in psychotic patients. Eczema, after suppression of gonorrhea or as an effect of vaccination. Eruptions only on the covered parts, which are very sensitive to touch.

TUBERCULINUM 1M : Chronic eczema of the whole body. Severe itching at night.

URTICA URENS 3X : Recent eczema on the back of hands. Burning of skin.

NOTE: The patient should be advised :-

1.   To reduce the number of baths. Excessive bathing and hot water actually removes moisture from the skin, making it dry.

2.   To avoid strong soaps, solvents or other products and while handling detergents, to wear rubber gloves.

ELECTRIC SHOCKS

ACIDUM FLUOR., CIMICI-: Pain like electric shocks.
FUGA, COLCHICUM
AUTUM.

AILANTHUS G.   : Sensation as if of an electric current is passing from the head to feet.

EUPHORBIUM   : Pain like electric shocks.

PHOSPHORUS 200   : Bad effects of electric shocks.

STRYCHNINUM   : Electric shocks are felt on touching any metallic thing like door handles and after walking on a synthetic carpet.

VERATRUM VIR.   : Sensation of violent electric like shocks in limbs.

ELEPHANTIASIS

CALOTROPIS Q   : Has been used with marked success in this disease by increasing the circulation of skin and producing perspiration.

ELAEIS Q	: The skin is thickened and hardened. Itching of the skin. Give 10 drops, thrice daily.
HYDROCOTYLE A.	: Dry eruptions on the skin. Great thickening of epidermoid layer and exfoliation of scales.
MYRISTICA SEB.	: The treatment may begin with this remedy, as it becomes of no avail in the later stages of the disease.

EMACIATION

Emaciation is becoming abnormally thin from extreme loss of flesh.

ABROTANUM	: General marasmus. Legs mostly affected , emaciation from below upwards. Appetite is good. Ill effects of suppressed diseases.
ALFALFA Q	: Acts as a fat producing agent. Corrects tissue waste.
AMBRA GRISEA	: Emaciation in mentally deficient children who are nervous and easily excited.
ANTIMONIUM CRUD., STAPHYSAGRIA, ARGENTUM MET.	: Emaciation of penis and testicles.
ARGENTUM NIT.	: Progressive emaciation. Craving for sweets. Flatus is expelled with a noise.
ARSENICUM ALB.	: Diarrhea, soon after drinking or eating. Burning in the stomach. Rapid emaciation due to fever.

AURUM MUR.	: Emaciation after syphilis.
BARYTA CARB. 200-1M	: Emaciation with glandular swelling and enlargement of the abdomen. Patient is shy.
CALCAREA CARB.	: Emaciation of skin with a large abdomen. Skin is folded. Bones do not grow rapidly and normally.
CALCAREA PHOS. 6X	: A good tonic during the disease. Skin is dry, wrinkled and withered. Can be given in alternation, with the indicated remedy. Childs face is wrinkled. Sweat on head and hands during sleep.
CAUSTICUM	: Emaciation due to long standing, worries or due to a disease.
CONIUM MAC., NUX MOSCH.	: Mammae develop too slowly at the age of puberty.
HYDRASTIS CAN.	: Emaciation after measles.
IODIUM 200, 1000	: Increases weight and flesh, while 2X and 3X reduces weight, flesh and obesity. Iodium in high potency is indicated when the patient only feels well by eating, but goes on emaciating. Glandular atrophy.
LYCOPODIUM	: Emaciation of the neck and face. Eats and drinks everything warm. Flatulence.
MAGNESIUM CARB.	: Emaciation with indigestion of milk. Craves meat.
NATRIUM MUR. 200	: Chilliness with an earthy complexion and constipation. Emaciation starts from neck or upper limbs and spread downwards.

ONOSMODIUM CM, CHIMAPHILA	:	Breasts absent or dwindled, due to atrophy.
PEPSINUM, NATRIUM PHOS.	:	Marasmus of children, who are fed on artificial food.
PHOSPHORUS	:	Emaciation after menstrual disorders.
PICRICUM ACIDUM	:	Emaciation though the appetite is good.
PLUMBUM MET.	:	Emaciation due to anemia. Wasting of muscles and paralysis.
SARSAPARILLA Q	:	Nipples depressed instead of projected. Neck emaciated. The skin of the neck is in folds. 2 drops in water, twice daily.
SILICEA	:	Emaciation due to defective assimilation. Patient is chilly.
SYPHILINUM	:	Extreme emaciation of the skin.
TUBERCULINUM 200	:	Rapid emaciation. Patient is always tired. Motion causes intense fatigue. Emaciation of the neck due to dehydration. Rapid emaciation in wasting diseases like TB, etc.
FERRUM PHOS. 6X, CALCAREA PHOS. 6X, NATRIUM MUR. 6X	:	Two tablets of each and all the three mixed-one dose should be given early in the morning along with another indicated remedy at an interval of three hours.

EMISSIONS
(SPERMATORRHEA)

ACIDUM PHOS. Q : Emissions at night and at stool. Sexual power deficient. Parts relax during an embrace. Inflammation of seminal vesicles. Semen ejaculated too soon in coitus. Sudden relaxation of penis preventing emissions.

ACIDUM PICRIC. : Erections very strong with great desire and emissions without relaxation of the penis.

AGNUS CASTUS : Seminal emissions without erections. Scanty emissions without ejaculation and on straining in persons who have been masturbating frequently. Suitable to old people who are physically impotent.

ANACARDIUM ORI. : Seminal emissions without dreams. Desire is increased and there is much itching of the penis. Prostratic fluid escapes during stool.

ARGENTUM MET. : Seminal emissions without any excitment, with polyuria.

CALADIUM SEG. : Emissions occur with or without dreams, in old age. No emissions and orgasm in coitus for a long time.

CALCAREA CARB. : Emissions with burning pain. Sweating and weakness after coitus. Emissions delayed. Pertains to both the sexes.

CARBO VEG.	: Emissions too soon and then head-ache.
CAUSTICUM	: Seminal emissions mixed with blood.
CONIUM MAC.	: Emissions on thinking of a sexual act or at the sight of an attractive women. Emissions due to suppression of sexual desire. Just an embrace is sufficient to discharge the semen.
DAMIANA Q	: Absence of sperms in semen and chronic prostratic discharge.
DIGITALIS	: Emissions with palpitations of the heart. Emissions without its feeling.
DIOSCOREA 12	: It is an excellent remedy for seminal emissions in weak persons. 2 or 3 emissions occur every night and on the following morning the patient feels very weak, particularly, about the knees.
ERYNGIUM AQUA. 2X	: Discharge of a prostratic fluid from the slightest cause. A remedy of first importance in spermatorrhea when it is without erections.
GELSEMIUM	: Nocturnal emissions even without dreams and slight or no excitement.
GRAPHITES	: Absence of emission during sexual intercourse for an abnormally long time, too early ejaculation otherwise.
KALIUM BROM.	: Emissions too frequent and without sexual intercourse. Depression after each emission.

LUPULINUM 1X	: Headache following a nights debauch and seminal emissions. It is a very good remedy for seminal emissions.
LYCOPODIUM	: Emissions in impotent people, too early if able to penetrate somehow.
LYSSINUM	: Emissions, too late or absent.
MEDORRHINUM 1M	: Emissions at night, followed by great weakness which may lead to impotence.
NATRIUM MUR. 200	: Emission even after ejacuation during coitus or retarded emissions which may not occur, at all.
NUPHAR LUT.	: Seminal emissions while passing a hard stool or on straining. Complete absence of sexual desire. Parts relaxed. Penis retracted. After spermatorrhea, pain in the penis and testicles.
NUX VOM.	: Frequent emissions. Bad effects of masturbation. Headache and impaired digestion.
ONOSMODIUM	: Deficient erections and speedy emissions.
SELENIUM MET.	: A very good remedy for seminal emissions. Emissions are too soon with long lasting thrill. Vertigo on rising in the morning. Dribbling of semen and prostratic fluid, during sleep.
SEPIA	: Emissions with insufficient erection in men and without any sexual excitement in women.

STANNUM MET.	:	Emissions with excessive prostration. Orgasm is easily produced, even by scratching the arm. In women, it transmits a sensation of great pleasure in the uterus leading to an orgasm.
STAPHYSAGRIA	:	Bad effects of masturbation. Great emaciation with blue rings around the eyes. The boy is shy and gloomy. It is very useful for removing weakness caused due to excessive spermatorrhea.
SULPHUR	:	Emission even before erection is complete.
TRIBULUS TER. Q	:	Debilitated states of sexual organs. Ready emissions and weak semen. Specific for early ejaculation. It corrects sperms and semen, and also ill effects of masturbation and spermatorrhea. Give 15 drops thrice daily.
THUJA OCC. Q	:	Nocturnal emissions are controlled by taking a dose consisting of 6 to 7 drops in water at bed time.
TITANIUM	:	Too early an ejaculation in coitus.

EMPHYSEMA

(DYSPNEA DUE TO DESTRUCTION OF AIR PASSAGES IN THE LUNGS)

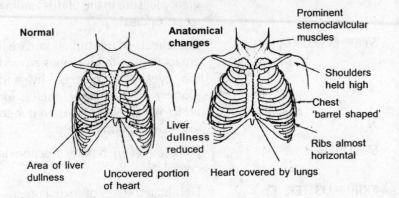

Normal

Anatomical changes

Prominent sternoclavicular muscles

Shoulders held high

Chest 'barrel shaped'

Liver dullness reduced

Ribs almost horizontal

Area of liver dullness

Uncovered portion of heart

Heart covered by lungs

Pulmonary pathology

At post mortem, the lungs are voluminous and pale. They contain little blood.

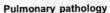

Bullae like bubbles may be formed at the periphery

Areas of lung between affected portions are often dark, congested and depressed

Edges of lungs are rounded

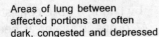

In this disease, lungs are enlarged. This comes gradually. It is believed that the disease is the late effect of chronic infection or the irritation of bronchial tubes. The patient may have been suffering from cold or cough for the past few years and begins to feel shortness of breath on exertion in the morning or evening or both. Sometimes, this symptom is confused with asthma or a heart disease. Weak and inflamed lungs interfere with passage of blood through the small blood vessels of the lungs. When the interference grows, the heart has to work harder to pump blood. The heart may also enlarge under the stress and may fail to work in the end. A high percentage of the people who suffer from this disease, are cigarette or drug smokers. Polluted air can also cause it. The following medicines, selected according to symptoms, afford relief to many and lengthen their life.

ANTIMONIUM ARS. : Head remedy. Excessive dyspnea and cough with much mucus secretion, worse on eating or lying down. Asthma like condition.

ANTIMONIUM TART. : Emphysema of the aged. Coughing and gasping, consequently. Great rattling of mucus in the lungs. Rapid, short, difficult breathing.

ASPIDOSPERMA Q : Tonic for the lungs. Removes temporary obstruction to the oxidation of blood by stimulating respiratory centres. Want of breath during exertion is a guiding symptom. Give 10 drop doses.

BRYONIA ALBA : Frequent desire to take a long breath; must expand lungs. Dry, barking cough worse at night. Quick; difficult respiration with pain in the chest.

CARBO VEG. : Emphysema due to ill or incomplete treatment of pneumonia and chronic hoarseness.

CHININUM ARS. : Asthma like attacks which occur periodically. Great prostration.

COCA : Emphysema. Want of breath or shortness of breath. Especially useful for aged sports men and alcoholics. Hoarseness or loss of voice and dyspnea. Give 5-6 drop doses every two hours, in severe cases of emphysema.

CURARE 6 : Threatened ossation of respiration on falling asleep. Short breath. Short, dry cough. Very distressing dyspnea.

NAPHTHALINUM : Dyspnea and sighing respiration. Emphysema of the aged with asthma. Long and continued paroxysms of coughing. Unable to breathe. Tenacious expectoration.

SENEGA : Chronic emphysema in old asthmatics with congestive attacks of oppression and weight on chest.

STRYCHNINUM : Respiration increased. Excessive dyspnea. Sharp, contractive pains in the muscles of chest. Persistent cough.

ENCEPHALTIS
(SEE BRAIN INFLAMMATION)

ENDOCARDITIS
(INFLAMMATION OF THE LINING MEMBRANE OF THE HEART)

ACONITUM NAP. : Palpitations with anxiety. Tingling in the fingers. Pain in the chest and left shoulder.

ARSENICUM ALB. : Dyspnea. Palpitation. Blueness of the skin and restlessness.

DIGITALIS : The least movement causes violent palpitation and sensation as if the heart would cease beating.

Very weak and slow pulse.

NAJA TRI.   : Feeling of weight on the heart.
                           Pain in the chest extends to the
                           neck, left shoulder and left arm.
                           Pulse irregular. Extremities cold.

TERMINALIA ARJUNA   : When no definite symptoms of the
                           heart can be determined and there
                           is palpitation and pain, give 5-10
                           drops every hour in acute cases
                           and after 3-4 hours in chronic
                           cases.

ENDOMETRIOSIS (METRITIS)
(INFLAMMATION OF THE UTERUS)

Endometriosis is a chronic disease that can occur in any women of child bearing age. In some cases it causes severe pelvic pain, especially during menstruation, but in other cases there are no symptoms at all. The tissue lining the uterus is called endometrium and inflammation of the endometrium is called endometriosis or metritis. When a woman becomes pregnant or enters menopause, she may experience an improvement in her endometriosis. However, at the end of the pregnancy, the symptoms may return. Sometimes endometrial tissue may come outside the uterus through the fallopian tubes and may cause symptoms of endometriosis. The best way to confirm the diagnosis is by laparoscopy. In this method a thin tube is inserted in the abdomen to see the pelvic cavity. This will reveal the exact location of the disease. Thus it becomes easier for a homoeopath to administer the oral homoeopathic medicines for treatment of the patients to avoid surgery.

APIS MEL.   : Metritis with stinging and burning
                           pains; worse heat, touch and pres-
                           sure.

| ARSENICUM ALB. | : | Sticking pains in the pelvis extending down the thighs, worse in wet weather, after midnight, from cold and cold drinks, and right side. Better from heat and warm drinks. |

BRYONIA ALBA   : Intermenstrual pain with great abdominal and pelvic soreness worse with warmth and motion, better lying on the painful side, pressure, rest and cold things.

CIMICIFUGA   : Pain in the ovarian region shooting upwards and towards the frontal surface of thighs. Pain across the pelvis from hip to hip and immediately before menses. Worse, morning and cold. Better, warmth and eating. An important symptom is that more the menstrual flow, more is the suffering.

GELSEMIUM   : Labor like pains, extending to the hips and back. Worse, during damp weather and bad news. Better, bending forward and by profuse urination.

HYDROCOTYLE A. 3X   : It is indicated, when the cervix or the neck of the bladder is involved. There is dull pain in the ovarian region and redness of the cervix. Heat is felt in the vagina. Granular ulceration of the uterus is generally present. In such circumstances, this remedy is of great use.

SEPIA   : It is indicated when the vagina is involved and there are bearing down pains. Sticking and violent pains from the vagina to the uterus and are worse bathing, dampness and left side; better by pressure and warmth.

TILIA EUROPA   : Metritis after child birth . Intense sore feeling about the uterus and bearing down sensation. Profuse hot perspiration which does not give relief.

ENURESIS

(BED WETTING)

ACIDUM BENZ.   : Strong smelling urine of low specific gravity. Bed wetting several times during sleep. Urine smelling of ammonia, like horse's urine.

ALOE SOC.   : Enuresis in old people due to an enlarged prostrate gland.

BELLADONNA   : Restless sleep in nervous, excitable children who wet the bed. Involuntary passing of urine in sleep at during night.

CALCAREA CARB.   : Another good remedy for enuresis in children who arc plump, eat dirt and other indigestible things.

CAUSTICUM   : Involuntary spurting of urine on sneezing and coughing. Involuntary urination in children and aged at night during the first sleep.

CINA   : Enuresis due to the presence of worms in children. The child scratches the tip of his nose often.

EQUISETUM	:	Principal action on the bladder. A remedy for enuresis. Painful urination. Constant nocturnal bed wetting. The urine looks cloudy. Enuresis with dreams and nightmares.
KALIUM MUR. 6X, MAGNESIUM PHOS. 6X	:	3 grains of each mixed together can be prescribed in routine, when a definite indication of the other remedies cannot be found.
KALIUM PHOS. 6X	:	Enuresis with dark yellow urine. Incontinence of urine with an inability to retain urine.
KREOSOTUM	:	Enuresis in the first part of night with dreams as if urinating in the urinals. Otherwise also, must hurry when the desire comes or the urine escapes. It is specially useful in heavy sleepers who wet the bed in the first sleep.
LAC CAN. 200	:	Nocturnal enuresis. The patient dreams as if passing urine in the regular urinal. Wakes up after this.
LYCOPODIUM	:	Polyuria at night. Flatulence. Involuntary urination during sleep.
MEDORRHINUM 200	:	Nocturnal enuresis. A general remedy.
PLANTAGO 200	:	Nocturnal enuresis. Profuse flow of urine.
PSORINUM 200	:	Bed wetting of psoric patients. Wets the bed especially during full moon. Use it when the well selected remedies fail to act.
PULSATILLA NIG.	:	In girls, who wet the bed during the day as well as at night. Poor

		sleepers and in patients who eat too much. Increased desire.
SECALE COR.	:	Enuresis in old people due to enlarged prostrate glands.
SENEGA	:	Involuntary passing of urine in sleep during day.
SEPIA 200	:	Enuresis in sickly girls during the first sleep. A very effective remedy. Urine is very offensive.
SULPHUR	:	Enuresis, especially in untidy children. Must hurry to urinate, when there is a sudden call.
VERBASCUM THAPS. Q	:	Nocturnal enuresis of long standing, resisting treatment. Five drop doses, night and morning.

EPILEPSY
(ACUTE)

ABSINTHIUM	:	Petit mal.
ARGENTUM NIT.	:	Epilepsy in people suffering from indigestion. Loud belching during the attack or before it. If given half an hour before the attack, in such conditions, it prevents the attack. The patient is withered and dried in constitution.
BELLADONNA 1X	:	Recent epilepsy of young persons. Spasms followed by nausea and vomiting. Skin hot. Face flushed.
CICUTA VIR.	:	Violent convulsions. Fearful distortion of the eyes. Fingers

clenched. Bending of the head, neck and spine backwards. Moaning and howling.

IGNATIA AMARA : From emotional disturbances. Effects of grief and worry.

KALIUM BROM. : Attack at new moon. Prostration with congestion in the head. Anemia, gastric disturbances and problems of liver and digestion.

KALIUM CYAN. : Convulsions are violent. Face turns blue. Breathlessness before and during the attack.

OENANTHE CROC. 3X : Violent convulsions. Body becomes stiff. Foam in the mouth. Attack is worse during menstruation and pregnancy. Convulsive facial twitching.

OPIUM : Fits come at night in constipated persons. Much drowsiness, before and after the attack. May be due to fright.

STRAMONIUM : Recent epilepsy caused in stammering people on account of fright. Raises head frequently from the pillow.

EPILEPSY
(CHRONIC)

AGARICUS MUS. 1000 : Fits after every seven days. Before an attack, patient is talkative and yawns.

AMYLENUM NIT. Q	: It temporarily relieves epileptic convulsions. A few drops on cotton kept near the nostrils of the patient to inhale, will give immediate relief.
ARTEMISIA VULG.	: Epilepsy of childhood in girls at puberty. Petit mal without an aura. Attack is after fright, emissions and masturbation. Several fits come together.
BUFO RANA	: It is of use in feeble minded children or prematurely seniles. Seizures occur at night during sleep, more or less connected with the sexual sphere. It is of use in many cases of epilepsy.
CALCAREA CARB.	: Persons of scrofulous type. Children grow fat with large bellies and a pale face.
CIMICIFUGA	: Aura of a wavy type is felt in the brain before an attack. Opening and shutting sensation in the brain.
CUPRUM MET. 3X	: Aura begins in the knees, ascends to the hypogastrium, followed by unconsciousness, foaming at the mouth and falling. Constant protrusion and retraction of the tongue like a snake.
HYDROCYANICUM ACIDUM 200	: It is considered as a specific remedy for the cure of epilepsy.
HYOSCYAMUS NIG.	: Fits followed by nausea and vomiting.
INDIGO TINC.	: It is a useful remedy when the aura begins from a painful spot between the shoulders with flashes of heat from the abdomen to head.

MILLEFOLIUM : Epilepsy from suppressed menses.

PASSIFLORA Q, : 5 drops of Oenanthe Q or 100
OENANTHE CROC. Q   drops of Passiflora Q in half a cup
of cold water, given at bed time
usually prevents the nocturnal
attacks of epilepsy.

PLUMBUM MET. : Epilepsy in patients with unhealthy
skin, obstinate constipation and
mental depression.

PSORINUM 200 : It is used as an intercurrent remedy, when other symptoms of this
medicine are present.

SILICEA 200 : Fits during sleep. Nervous irritability. Ill effects of vaccination. Feel-
ing of coldness before an attack.
Children with a large head and
large abdomen.

SOLANUM NIG. : Convulsions of epilepsy of idio-
pathic type where the disease has
begun beyond the age of childhood. Hysterical epilepsy. Use 20-
40 drops of Q as a dose.

SULPHUR 200 : It should be used as an intercurrent
remedy.

TARENTULA HIS. : Hysterical epilepsy with intense
sexual excitement.

ZINCUM PHOS. : Removes the mental weakness in
epileptics.

DIET : **Epileptics should take more fats
like butter, etc. and less proteins.**

**NOTE 1: According to the recent estimates by the World Health
Organization, about 40 million people worldwide are
suffering from epilepsy.**

NOTE 2: Famous people who had epilepsy include, Charles Dickens, Beethoven, Vicent Van Gogh, Julius Caesar and Alexander, the Great.

NOTE 3:Researchers at the Institute of Neurology in London (England) say that the fertility rate in women suffering from epilepsy is lower than other women.

EPISTAXIS
(BLEEDING FROM THE NOSE)

AMBRA GRISEA	: Bleeding mostly in the morning and there are crusts of dry blood in the nostrils.
AMBROSIA Q	: 10 drops of this in water during and after the attack of epistaxis stops bleeding and generally stops its recurrence.
AMMONIUM CARB.	: Bleeding from the nose when washing face and hands. Dark blood which does not coagulate easily.
ARUM TRIPH.	: Epistaxis with constant picking of the nose.
BRYONIA ALBA	: Frequent bleeding from the nose when menses should appear.
CARBO VEG.	: Daily attacks of epistaxis. Patient becomes pale after bleeding.
ERIGERON Q	: Cures epistaxis when there is congestion in the head and the face is red.
FERRUM PHOS. 1X	: Epistaxis when no cause is known. As a general remedy for recurrent bleeding.

FERRUM PIC.	: It is almost specific for epistaxis.
FICUS REL. Q	: A few drops of it in water taken every 20 minutes stops bleeding.
IPECACUANHA	: Blood is bright red and nausea is usually present.
MILLEFOLIUM Q	: Its action is the same as of Trillium pendulum.
PHOSPHORUS	: Epistaxis when blowing the nose. Quantity of blood is very small and in drops. Handkerchief is always stained with blood.
SILICEA	: Nose bleeds when removing hard and dry crusts from the nostrils. Nasal bones are sensitive.
STRONTIUM CARB.	: Epistaxis with bloody crusts in the nose.
TRILLIUM PEND. Q	: A very good remedy for the disease. May be used internally and externally. A cotton plug drenched in it should be inserted into the nostrils and it will stop bleeding in seconds. Blood is bright red.
VIPERA	: Chronic epistaxis, even life long is cured by the use of this remedy. It is considered as specific for epistaxis.

ERECTIONS

ACIDUM PHOS. Q	: Erections painful after coition. Erection while standing.

AGNUS CASTUS	: Erections wanting.
AMMONIUM CARB.	: Erections in the morning.
ARGENTUM NIT.	: Erections fail on attempting coition.
BARYTA CARB.	: Great desire. During erections, shivering. Erections may be wanting.
FLUORICUM ACIDUM	: Strong erections during sleep.
LECITHINUM 3X	: Weak erection is usually on account of less supply of blood to the penis. Use of four doses of this medicine for 8 weeks raises the level of blood generally, and increases its supply to the penis on sexual stimulation.' It strenghtens the erection and man power.
LYCOPODIUM 200, GRAPHITES 200	: Erections incomplete during coition.
PHOSPHORUS	: Violent erections day and night. Erections incomplete during coition. Desire strong.
PULSATILLA NIG.	: Frequent erections with dribbling of prostratic juice.
RHUS TOX.	: Erections with urging to urinate.
SEPIA	: Erection remains after orgasm.
THUJA OCC.	: Erections without any desire for sex.

NOTE 1: See chapter Impotency.

NOTE 2 : A study has shown that 2 men in 5 have problems getting on an erection at age of 40. Nearly 7 in 10 do at the age of 70. It was estimated in early 1998 that the number of men coping with impotency is 140 million world-wise. Use of homoeopathic remedies give excel-

lent results in such cases. While taking cases of erectile dysfunction, the homoeopathic physician should know that the dysfunction can be on account of physical and psychological difficulties. Physical difficulties include aging, diabetes, high cholesterol and prostrate surgery. Such cases are incurable.

Psychological factors can be depression, anger, male dominance and use of drugs including tobacco. Such cases repond to the homoeopathic treatment. Not being able to have sexual intercourse is a great concern for some men as it is believed that unsatisfying sexual act is detrimental to sexual intimacy. In old age and in impotent persons, the flow of blood to the penis decreases causing feeble or no erection at all. Most men experience the problem at some stage of their lives and erection also decreases with advancement of age. Some patients use a vacum device for a successful sexual intercourse. It involves placing a hollow tube over the penis and inducing the erection with a vacuum pump. The erection is maintained by placing a band at the base of the penis. Such devices are available at some surgical stores.

NOTE 3 :Latest surgical methods have made erectile dysfunction of the penis reversible. A tiny suppository silicon bar is inserted into the penile shaft. It provides a permanent erection. When needed the bar is bent into an upright position and is lowered when done or when not required. It is important that this is done by a person who specializes in the art.

NOTE 4 : Five percent of erectile dysfunction cases are caused by irregular levels of sex hormones. Medication can solve the problem.

ERUCTATION (BELCHING)

Eructation is voiding of gas or of a small quantity of acid fluid from the stomach through the mouth.

ABIES NIG.

: Eructations with sensation of a painful lump in the epigastrium. Belching and pain in the stomach after eating.

AGARICUS MUS.

: Empty eructations, tasting of apples.

AETHUSA CYN.

: Regurgitation of food after about an hour of eating. Vomiting relieves the distress.

ANTIMONIUM CRUD.

: Belching with taste of ingesta. The tongue is coated white. Indigestion and constant belching.

ARGENTUM NIT.

: Belching is explosive in flatulent states. Person presents dried up looks and constitution.

ASAFOETIDA 3X

: Great difficulty in bringing up the wind. Hysterical eructations which are loud enough. The pressure of wind is always upwards.

CALCAREA CARB.

: Loud belching with heartburn. Frequent sour eructations.

CARBO VEG.

: Distention of abdomen with eructations tasting of food taken. Heartburn may or may not be present. Sensation of heaviness and fullness in the stomach. Rancid, sour or putrid eructations, after eating or drinking with temporary relief.

CARBOLICUM ACIDUM	:	Constant belching with nausea and vomiting, dark olive green. Belching with a bad taste and breath.
CHAMOMILLA Q	:	A few drops of it in warm water, taken during the attack gives immediate relief after 2 or 3 doses.
CYCLAMEN	:	Hiccough like eructations, worse after taking fatty food. Taste salty.
FERRUM MET.	:	Eructations after taking food. Belching gives a sense of relief.
LAUROCERASUS	:	Eructations tasting of bitter almonds.
LYCOPODIUM	:	Eructations rise upto the pharynx, where they burn for hours.
NATRIUM CARB.	:	Old dyspeptics always belching.
NATRIUM PHOS.	:	Sour eructations and taste.
NUX MOSCH.	:	Belching in nervous patients. Abdomen is bloated. Hiccough. Stomach is bloated.
OSMIUM	:	Eructations of the taste of raddish, taken a while ago. Smell is foul.
PHOSPHORUS	:	Belching large quantities of wind after eating.
PSORINUM	:	Eructations tasting of eggs although eggs were not eaten.
PULSATILLA NIG.	:	Nausea, with a bitter taste.
ROBINIA	:	Intensely acrid eructations.
SULPHUR	:	Eructations with particles of food coming into the mouth. Taste is very sour. Great acidity. Drinks much and eats little. Putrid eructations. Empty belching, worse after taking milk.

THUJA OCC.   : Rancid belching after taking fatty food.

ERYSIPELAS

(HOT, RED, EDEMATOUS, BRAWNY AND SHARPLY DEFINED ERUPTIONS)

AMMONIUM CARB.   : Erysipelas of seniles.

APIS MEL.   : Erysipelas of the new born near the navel and due to an injury.

ARSENICUM ALB.   : Erysipelas accompanied with low fever.

CALENDULA OFF.   : Erysipelas due to an injury.

CHINA OFF.   : This generally aborts the diseases if given at the onset. Curative in simple and recent cases.

CROTALUS H.   : Erysipelas which threatens to become gangrenous.

GRAPHITES 6   : It is a preventive for recurring erysipelas, discharging a glutinous fluid which is thin and sticky. The erysipelas threaten to suppurate.

HEPAR SULPHURIS   : Useful when suppuration occurs.

RHUS TOX.   : The skin at the point of erysipelas and around is very red. The patient is restless and thirsty. Fever may accompany the swelling and itching. Erysipelas commencing from the left side and spreading towards the right side.

SILICEA   : Chronic erysipelas which refuse to heal.

ESCAPE

BELLADONNA   : The patient desires to escape from a host of fearful hallucinations. He hides here and there without any success.

MERCURIUS SOL.   : The patient wants to escape from the world being weary of life, but he cannot do it on account of lack of will power.

OPIUM   : The patient wants to run away from all offers and wants. He wants to escape from the world but without any thinking of death.

VERATRUM ALB.   : In stages of insanity, the patient wants to escape his sufferings and wanders away from his home aimlessly.

EXCITEMENT OF SEXUAL DESIRE

MUREX PURP.   : Least contact of the parts of a woman will excite her sexual desire violently, after a dose of this medicine.

PHOSPHORUS   : It excites the sexual desire both in male and female. They want to have sex immidiately.

YOHIMBINUM Q   : It stimulates the sexual desire in a natural way and is a sex tonic.

EXERTION (STAMINA)

STERCULIA A. Q : It gives power to endure prolonged physical exertion without taking food and without feeling fatigued. 10 to 100 drop doses, 3 times a day. This is a better remedy than 'dope' or 'testosterone' used by the athletes and sportsmen for increasing their stamina.

EXPOSURE

ACONITUM NAP. : This remedy cures effects of sudden exposure to cold. It should be given at once, as soon as the exposure occurs.

BELLADONNA : The neck becomes rigid and stiff on account of exposure to a draught of wind. It may be used after Acon.

BELLIS P. : Affections due to cold winds. Exposure due to cold drinks when the body is heated.

BRYONIA ALBA : If Bell. does not suffice to remove the pains, etc. of the neck, this remedy will cure the case.

CAUSTICUM 10M : Facial paralysis from exposure to cold winds.

DULCAMARA : Stiffness and lameness across the neck and shoulders after getting cold and wet.

HEPAR SULPHURIS : For ill effects of exposure to dry cold winds, like cough, loss of voice, backache, etc.

RHUS TOX.   : For ill effects of exposure to humid
                          and damp winds.

EXPULSION OF FOREIGN BODIES

ACONITUM NAP.   : It expels foreign bodies like sand
                          and dust from the eyes.

SILICEA   : It promotes expulsion of foreign
                          bodies from the tissues of the body.
                          A fish bone embedded in the throat,
                          a needle or a coin swallowed
                          inadvertently is expelled by the
                          use of this remedy. It expels thorns
                          from the skin.

EYES

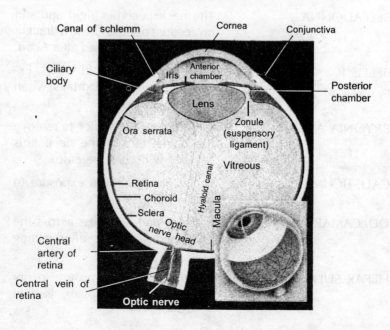

ACIDUM PHOS. Q	:	Blue rings around the eyes.
ACONITUM NAP.	:	Removes foreign bodies like sand and dust, from the eyes.
AGNUS CASTUS	:	Intense itching in the eyes. Pupils dilated. Photophobia.
ARGENTUM NIT.	:	Aching, tired feelings in the eyes. Better closing or pressure on them. Useful in restoring power of the weakened ciliary muscles.
ARSENICUM ALB.	:	Swelling around eyes. Burning. Corneal ulceration. Photophobia.
BADIAGA	:	Blueness under the eyes.
BERBERIS VULG.	:	Face pale, eyes sunken and blue rings around the eyes.
BISMUTHUM	:	Blue rings around the eyes with yellow appearance of the face.
CALADIUM SEG.	:	Cysts of the eyes.
CHINA OFF.	:	Dark rings around the eyes. Blueness of the margins of the lids. Eyes sunken. Face pale due to loss of vital fluids.
CINA	:	Blue rings around the eyes, specially with worm symptoms.
CROCUS SAT.	:	Vision of electric sparks before the eyes.
DIGITALIS	:	Blueness of the eyelids and their margins.
DUBOISIA HOP.	:	Red spots before the eyes.
EUPHRASIA 6	:	Watering of eyes all the time. Burning and swelling of lids. Sticky mucus on cornea compelling him to wink often, to remove it.

GRAPHITES	: Ulcers with thin and sticky discharge from the eyes.
KALIUM CARB., STAPHYSAGRIA	: Bag like swellings on the eyelids.
MENTHOLUM, RHODODENDRON CH.	: Pain in the eyelids.
MERCURIUS SOL	: Ulcers with fetid discharge from the eyes.
MERCURIUS SULPH. RUB.	: Ciliary neuralgia. Pain around the eyes running towards the temples. Redness of the whole eye and eyelids.
NATRIUM MUR.	: Headache from eye strain due to hard studies.
ONOSMODIUM	: Pain in the eye balls between the orbit and the ball, extending to the left temple.
PHOSPHORUS	: Dark circles around eyes due to nervous tension.
PILOCARPUS M.	: Eye strain from any cause. Eyes get tired easily from the slightest use. Vertigo and nausea, after the use of eyes. Pain in the eyes. White spots before eyes.
PLATANUS OCCI. Q	: Tumor of the eyelids. Apply tincture. It cures both acute, chronic or neglected cases, even when there is destruction of tissue and deformity.
RHUS TOX.	: Intensive ulceration of the cornea due to old injuries to the eyes.
RUTA G. Q	: Eyes strain from studies.
SAPONARIA OFF.	: Pain in the eyes and eye brows, worse left side. Pains are violent, sticking and deep in the eye balls.

SAPONINUM : Hot stitches deep in the eyes and left temple. Photophobia.

SEPIA : Yellowness of the face and blue rings around the eyes.

SILICEA, HEPAR SULPHURIS : Abscess and perforating ulcers of the cornea after an injury. Sharp pain in the eyes, worse when closed or touched.

SPIGELIA : Sparkling before the eyes.

STAPHYSAGRIA : Itching of lid margins. Affections of inner angles. Incised or lacerated wounds of cornea.

STRAMONIUM : Sensation of dirt or dirty fluid in the eyes.

SULPHUR : Black spots before the eyes.

TILIA EUR. : Muscular weakness of eyes. Sensation of a veil or gauze before the eyes.

VIOLA ODORATA : Pain immediately above the eyebrow.

BLACK EYE

ARNICA MONT. Q : A blow on the eyes produces a black and blue skin around the eyes. If there is only discoloration of the skin and swelling but the skin is intact, apply a lotion of 10 drops of the Q to an ounce of cold water with cotton and continue repeating it, till the soreness ceases. It may be given orally also.

CINERARIA MAR. : A lotion of 5 drops of this remedy in an ounce of distilled water should be instilled into the eyes thrice daily, in case of traumatic injuries to the eyes.

HAMAMELIS Q : If the skin is broken, a lotion of it is prepared with 5 drops in an ounce of cold water and may be applied as above.

LEDUM PAL. 200 : In the above cases, removes chances of tetanus and helps removing the discoloration. Contused wounds to the eyes.

SYMPHYTUM OFF. 200 : For traumatic injuries to the eyes and eye balls, no remedy equals this remedy. It is to be used when there is great pain in the eyeball itself, from a blow.

LIDS

BORAX : Inward diversion (entropion) of the eyelashes and falling of eyelashes.

CLEMATIS ERECTA : Chronic redness and irritation of the margins of eyelids.

EUPHRASIA Q : In all the above cases, a lotion of 10 drops in an ounce of rose or distilled water instilled into the eyes is very useful. 2-3 drops in each eye 3 times a day.

GRAPHITES 6 : Inflammation and much redness of the lid margins, and dandruff on the eyelashes.

HEPAR SULPHURIS 6 : Irritation and formation of much matter.

KALIUM CARB. : Bag like oedematous swelling of the eyelids, specially the left. On account of this guiding symptom many affections are cured.

MERCURIUS SOL.　　　　: Sticking together of the eyelids in the morning.

THIOSINAMINUM Q　　　: Diversion of the eyelids. A good remedy for ectropion (outward rolling of the eyelid margin.)

LIDS PARALYSIS (PTOSIS)

GELSEMIUM 6　　　　　: Drooping of the upper eyelids due to paralysis. Eyelids are heavy and the patient can hardly open the eyes.

PETROLEUM　　　　　　: Loss of eye lashes.

BLINKING

CROCUS SAT.　　　　　: Blinking after eye strain and reading a lot.

EUPHRASIA　　　　　　: Constant blinking of the eyelids when the cause is not known.

LYCOPODIUM　　　　　: Blinking due to nervous debility.

SEVERE INFLAMMATION OF THE EYES (OPHTHALMIA)

ACONITUM NAP.　　　　: Redness of the eyes, sensation of sand in the eyes and irritation of eyes is cured by this remedy, if used within two days of the onset of the disease.

ARGENTUM NIT.　　　　: Pus like discharge from the eyes glues the lids together. Mucus is felt in the eyes needing frequent wiping, indicates this remedy.

BELLADONNA : When the eyes are very red and inflammed, the use of this remedy will be found fruitful, specially when the nose is running and watering of the eyes is also present.

EUPHRASIA 6 : If the flow from the nose and eyes is acrid with symptoms of Belladonna, use this remedy.

MERCURIUS COR. 6 : In acute or chronic inflammation of the eyes, the use of this remedy three times a day is very effective and beneficial.

EYE DROPS : A lotion of 10 drops of Euphrasia Q in an ounce of distilled water should be instilled in the eyes 3 or 4 times a day, 3-4 drops at a time.

TWITCHING OF EYES

MAGNESIUM PHOS. : Twitching around the eyes and cheeks specially on the right side. Such frequent spasms produce a hinderance on focusing the eyes on an object, producing blurred vision.

AGARICUS MUS. : Jerking, twitching, trembling and itching of the eyes. Reading becomes difficult. Twitching of lids and eye balls.

RAPHANUS : Twitching of eye lids continuously with edema of the lower eye lids.

MEZEREUM : Twitching of the eye lids with ciliary neuralgia specially after

	operation of the eyes. Right cheek may also be affected. Constant twitching.
GELSEMIUM	: Contraction and twitching of the muscles of eye lids.
ESERINUM 6X	: Twitching of the lids, either right or left.
BADIAGA	: Twitching of the upper left lid.
HYOSCYAMUS NIG.	: Twitching of the lids.
IGNATIA AMARA	: Twitching all over the body, with spasm of lids.

FACE

ACONITUM NAP.	: Face, red and hot. On rising after lying down, the face becomes deathly pale. Chewing motion of the lower jaw. Tingling in the cheeks and numbness.
AGARICUS MUS.	: The facial muscles feel stiff and twitch, with itching and burning. Face red.
AMYLENUM NIT.	: Face flushed.
ANTIMONIUM ARS.	: Face bloated.
ARSENICUM ALB.	: Face swollen, pale, yellow and sunken.
BELLADONNA	: Face red, bluish red, hot and swollen. Facial neuralgia with twitching of muscles and a flushed face.
BERBERIS VULG., BISMUTHUM, CINA	: Pale face, sunken eyes surrounded by blue rings.

CACTUS : Pain in the face.

CANTHARIS : Itching vesicles on the face, burning when touched.

CARBO VEG. : Cold sweat on the face. Face puffy, cyanotic. Mottled cheeks and red nose.

CAUSTICUM 10M : Paralysis of the right side of face.

CHAMOMILLA, ACONITUM NAP., IPECACUANHA : One cheek red, the other pale.

CHINA OFF. : Face is pale, sickly, white with a bluish appearance around the mouth and the eyes.

CINA : Intense circumscribed redness of the cheeks. Face otherwise pale and hot with blue rings around the eyes. Cold perspiration on the face.

COLCHICUM AUTUM. : Swelling and tingling in the face. Pain in the muscles of the face. Cheeks, red and hot.

FERRUM MUR. 6X : Circumscribed red spots on cheeks.

GRAPHITES : Face red with anemia.

HELLEBORUS NIG. : Chewing motion of the jaws. Horrible smell from the mouth.

LUPULUS H. : Scarlatina like eruptions on the face.

LYCOPODIUM : Yellowish brown spots on the face.

MANCINELLA : Blue circles around the eyes.

NATRIUM CARB. : Pale face and blue rings around the eyes. Yellow spots on the face.

NATRIUM MUR. : Face greasy and shiny. Earthy, unhealthy look on the face.

PETROLEUM	: Blotches and roughness of the facial skin in winters or during cold weather.
PHOSPHORUS	: Circumscribed redness on one or both cheeks.
PHOSPHORUS, VERATRUM VIR.	: Pale, sickly complexion. Blue rings under the eyes. Circumscribed redness on one or both cheeks.
PLUMBUM MET.	: Face yellow, like that of a corpse.
SANGUINARIA CAN.	: Circumscribed redness and burning of cheeks, pain extends in all directions from the upper jaw.
SEPIA	: Yellow face or yellow spots on the face. Yellow saddle across the nose.
SILICEA, CALCAREA FLUOR.	: Disfigurement due to acne scars or scars left by ulcers and boils.
SPIGELIA	: Neuralgia of the face. The eyes, cheeks, teeth and temples are hot. They are very sensitive to touch and seems icy cold to the patient. Symptoms improve in the evening.
SULPHUR	: Face very red.
VARIOLINUM 200	: For the removal of scars left by small pox and chicken pox.
VERATRUM VIR.	: Convulsive twitching of the facial muscles.
VIPERA	: Face excessively swollen.

FACIAL PARALYSIS

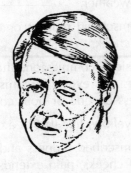

Note drooping and loss of facial expression on paralysed side. Facial muscles pull across the mid line — mouth is distorted.

CAUSTICUM 1M : Facial paralysis specially of the right side due to exposure to cold winds or from getting wet.

SENEGA 200 : Paralysis of the left side of face. Burning sensation on the face.

FAINTING

AGARICUS MUS. : Fainting after coition.

ALUMINA : Fainting from compelled standing.

AMMONIUM CARB. : Fainting from depression of spirits.

ARNICA MONT. 1M : Fainting on account of accidents, falls and blows. Sudden realization of financial loss.

ASAFOETIDA 3X : Fainting of hysterical women after emissions.

CAMPHORA : Tendency to unconsciousness. Feeling as if he would die. Fainting due to a shock.

CHAMOMILLA 200	: Fainting due to severe pain or after anger.
CHINA OFF.	: Fainting due to weakness, loss of blood and other vital fluids.
COCCULUS IND.	: Due to loss of sleep or riding in a carriage.
COFFEA CRUDA	: Due to excessive joy.
FERRUM PHOS. 6X, KALIUM PHOS. 6X	: 3 grains of each mixed together and administered with hot water, 3 times a day will remove tendency to fainting due to any cause.
GLONOINUM 3X	: Due to sun stroke.
IGNATIA AMARA	: Due to disturbed emotions and disappointments.
LACHESIS	: Due to jealousy, suppression of discharges and hot stuffy air.
MOSCHUS	: Fainting on a little excitement. Patient is inclined to hysterical attacks.
NUX MOSCH.	: Fainting from standing long. Fainting from the sight of blood. Fainting on passing a hard stool.
OPIUM	: Fainting due to fear and fright.
PHOSPHORUS	: Due to nervous excitement, fear and tension.
SEPIA	: Fainting in pregnancy due to weakness. Flashes of heat.
SPIGELIA	: Fainting due to heart problems.
VERATRUM ALB.	: Fainting on exertion with cold sweat on the forehead. Body cold and blue.

NOTE: Smelling of spirit ammonia, Camphora Q or Amylenum nitrosum relieves fainting. A little cotton drenched may be placed over the nose of the patient to inhale. It will cut short the fainting spell.

FALLOPIAN TUBES

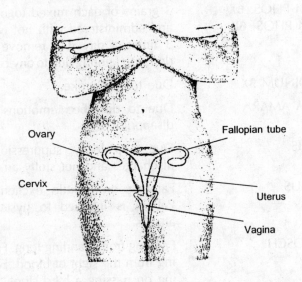

Ovary

Fallopian tube

Cervix

Uterus

Vagina

EUPIONUM 3	:	Removes blockage on both sides of the fallopian tubes.
LACHESIS	:	Removes blockage of the fallopian tubes, specially that of the right side. Burning in the ovary.
SELENIUM MET.	:	It is also useful in removing obstruction of the fallopian tubes.
TRITICUM REP.	:	Removes obstruction of the fallopian tubes in women.

FALLS

ARNICA MONT.	: The patient always sustains some bruises on the skin, on account of falls. This remedy will remove the soreness and discomfort.
HELLEBORUS NIG. 200	: If there are any bad effects from injuries to the head, this remedy will cure such after effects. It may be given in increasing potencies.
HYPERICUM PERF. 3X	: When the spine is shaken or bruised, this remedy should be given and repeated every two hours to prevent future complications.
MILLEFOLIUM 3X	: If there are any bad effects of a fall from a height, this remedy will remove those effects.
NATRIUM SULPH. 6X	: If there are any head symptoms and mental troubles from injuries to the head. It may be used in increasing potencies 6X to 1000.

FALSE LABOR PAINS

CAULOPHYLLUM	: False labor pains start about 10 days in advance of the date of actual labor. 2-4 doses will relieve such pains.
CIMICIFUGA	: False labor pains across the pelvis and from hip to hip.
PULSATILLA NIG. 200	: One dose, usually is sufficient to avoid false labor pains.

FATIGUE (TIREDNESS)
(SEE TIRED FEELING)

ANACARDIUM ORI.   : Mental fatigue from higher studies.
                             Fatigue of literary persons.

ARNICA MONT.   : Fatigue on account of over use of
                             muscles and brain. Mental and
                             physical fatigue. Limbs and body
                             ache as if beaten. It removes fa-
                             tigue of the brain and also of the
                             body.

ARSENICUM ALB.   : Fatigue after strenuous exercise,
                             stress or worry. Restlessness.

CALCAREA CARB.   : Physical and mental fatigue due to
                             overwork. There is a lot of anxiety
                             and inability to sleep with burning
                             headache.

CHINA OFF.   : Fatigue after travelling by air.

COCA   : Fatigue from journey and travel-
                             ling, especially during hot weather.

COFFEA CRUDA   : Fatigue due to hunger.

KALIUM PHOS.   : Tired feeling with trembling. There
                             is nervous exhaustion from over-
                             work or stress. Severe muscular
                             and mental fatigue, anxiety and
                             irritability . It is a remedy for
                             chronic fatigue syndrome.

MUREX PURP.   : This remedy is specially indicated
                             to nervous, lively and affectionate
                             women. The patient is greatly
                             fatigued, weak and run down.
                             Fatigue remains for several days,
                             the indicative and peculiar symp-

tom is that she feels more fatigued while sitting or at rest and feels alright on walking. Fatigue re-appears on sitting down.

NUX VOM. : Feeling of fatigue after sleeplessness or unrefreshing sleep. He is irritable and feels very chilly.

PICRICUM ACIDUM : Brain, spinal, nervous and general prostration with a feeling of tiredness all over the body and heaviness of the legs. The patient can hardly lift the legs. Slightest exertion of the brain causes headache.

RHUS TOX. : Fatigue from over straining, lifting and exercise.

SELENIUM MET. : Weakness of all parts of the body caused by hot weather. Debility causes a desire for sleep and strength rises as the sun sinks. Easy fatigue from any labour, mental exertion, night watching, etc.

SEPIA : Fatigue of weak women, is cured by this remedy. She feels fatigued even after a short walk or after any hard work such as 'laundry work' during pregnancy or lactation.

STERCULIA A. : This remedy gives power to sustain prolonged physical exertion without taking food and without the feeling of fatigue.

TUBERCULINIUM : Motion causes intense fatigue, aversion to work, wants a constant change.

NOTE : Feeling of fatigue is often the result of a lack of sleep, physical and psychological stress or exhaustion. Sexual fatigue is also caused by stress, anxiety and of course, aging. It causes an irritable and impatient nature. Rest, avoiding alcohol and caffeine, and physical exercise along with the medication brings back the good humour and feeling of well being.

FATNESS
(SEE OBESITY)

FEAR (PHOBIAS)

ACONITUM NAP.	: Fear of death and future. Fear of a crowd. Fear of crossing a street. Sweating, vexation and vomiting due to fear. Fear of an aeroplane, flying above over the head.
ANACARDIUM ORI.	: Fear of examination. Fear he is being pursued and persecuted.
ARGENTUM NIT.	: Apprehension, before an event. Fearful, nervous and melancholic. Lack of self confidence. Impulsive, wants to do things in a hurry. Great desire for sweet things. Diarrhea, from fear. Fear of crowds as in the temple, church or in a cinema. Gets nervous easily.
ARSENICUM ALB.	: Fear of death.
BELLADONNA	: Fear of dogs and animals. Fear of

fantastic illusions. Wants to escape.

BORAX

: Fear of downward motion. Fear of a thunder and sound of a firing gun, even far away.

CALCAREA CARB.

: Fear of night and solitude. Fear of remaining alone any time. Fears loss of reason and misfortune. Apprehensive. Forgetful.

CAUSTICUM

: Child is afraid of going to bed alone.

DROSERA

: Dislikes solitude. Always likes some one besides him, constantly. He wants company everywhere even when driving his car. Fear of being alone.

GELSEMIUM

: A sudden thunder of clouds or thunderstorm produces involuntary urination or diarrhea. In pregnant women, it produces symptoms of miscarriage. Emotional excitement leading to physical illness. Fear of examination and stage appearance.

HYOSCYAMUS NIG.

: Fear of being pursued. Fears that all the people around have turned against him. Fear on account of suspicion of others. Fear of being poisoned.

KALIUM CARB.

: Full of fears of imagination. Hates being left alone.

LYCOPODIUM

: It is a wonderful remedy for the anticipatory fear of examination, in students.

MANCINELLA

: Fear of becoming insane.

MEDORRHINUM 1M	:	Fears that she will go insane. Fear of dark and someone behind her. Fears that she cannot recover from her illness.
ONOSMODIUM	:	Fear of upward motion.
OPIUM	:	Fear causes diarrhea.
PHOSPHORUS	:	Fear when left alone. Fear of illness. Fears that something will go wrong. Fear of imaginary things. Fear of darkness. Very sensitive.
PULSATILLA NIG.	:	Fears being alone, darkness and ghosts, worse in the evening. Likes sympathy. Weeps easily. Timid and irresolute.
SEPIA	:	Dreads to be alone. Fear of evening and darkness.
SPIGELIA 200	:	Fear of knives, forks and all pointed things.
SUCCINUM, ARGENTUM NIT.	:	Fear of trains and closed rooms (claustrophobia).
VERATRUM ALB.	:	Passes urine, stool or wind on account of sudden fear of thunder of clouds or lightening.

FEET - BURNING

ARUNDO	:	Burning and swelling, mainly of soles.
CALCAREA SULPH.	:	Soles burn and itch.
CANTHARIS	:	Cold sweaty feet with burning soles.

HYPERICUM PERF.	:	Crawling in the hands and feet.
LYCOPODIUM	:	One foot, usually at night, feels hot while the other feels cold.
MEDORRHINUM	:	Feet are hot and tender. The soles feel sore, legs and feet become restless.
SULPHUR	:	Both the soles and hands burn specially during night.

FEET - COLD

ACONITUM NAP.	:	Numb, tingling, cold feet with hands hot.
BARYTA CARB	:	Cold, smelly feet, the toes and soles feel sore.
BELLADONNA	:	Cold legs and feet while the rest of the body is hot.
CALCAREA CARB.	:	Cold, damp feet with sour smelling sweat. Cramps in calves. Even the knees feel cold. Feels as if damp stockings were worn.
CAMPHORA	:	Icy cold feet, which feel sprained.
COLCHICUM AUTUM.	:	Swollen cold legs and feet.
DULCAMARA	:	Icy cold feet better warmth.
NATRIUM PHOS.	:	The feet are icy cold during the day but burn at night.
PICRICUM ACIDUM	:	Feet cold, cannot get warm.
SECALE COR.	:	Cold, dry hands and swollen feet with tingling in the toes and violent cramps, worse from warmth.

| SILICEA | : | Icy cold feet with offensive sweat. The foot feels sore from top to sole. |
| SQUILLA MAR. | : | Cold hands and cold, sore feet from standing too long. |

FEET – PAINS

ACIDUM TART.	:	Pain in the soles and heels.
EUPATORIUM PERF.	:	Swelling and pain in the left great toe.
HELONIAS	:	Feet go to sleep and feel numb when sitting.
LITHIUM CARB.	:	Pain in the soles of the feet and joints with a burning sensation. Pain in the hollow of the foot extending to the knee.
MEDORRHINUM 200	:	Soles tender and painful.
SQUILLA MAR.	:	Soreness of feet from long standing like that of sales girls, who have to stand at the sales, counter for long hours.

FEET — SWOLLEN

| APIS MEL. | : | Edematous swellings with stiffness and redness of feet. Dropsical effusions. |
| ARSENICUM ALB. | : | Swelling after injuries and overuse. |

BOVISTA	: Edematous swelling even after a sprain.
COLCHICUM AUTUM.	: Edamatous swelling and coldness.
DIGITALIS	: Swelling with numbness and coldness of the fingers.
MERCURIUS SOL.	: Dropsical swellings.
NATRIUM SULPH.	: Swelling with a burning sensation.

FEET - SWEATY

ARUNDO	: Copious and offensive foot sweat.
CALCAREA CARB.	: Sour foot sweat with burning of soles.
CARBO VEG.	: Sweaty. Feet with a tendency to cramps. The legs are cold from the knees downwards.
IODIUM	: Cold hands and feet with an acrid foot sweat.
LYCOPODIUM	: Profuse foot sweat with pain in the heels while walking and pain in the sole.
SILICEA	: Icy cold feet with an offensive sweat. The foot feels sore from the top through to the sole.

FEVERS

ACONITUM NAP.	: During the first stage of fever. Simple fever during very hot

weather or very cold weather. High temperature. Shinning, red, hot skin. Chilly, when uncovered or touched. Restlessness is always present.

ARSENICUM ALB. : High temperature, septic fevers, cold sweats and restlessness. Great thirst. Drinks often but little. Accumulation of dead skin scales on the lips, during fever. Fever worse during night. Malaria.

BAPTISIA TINC. : Debilitating fever. Soreness all over the body. Chill at about 11 A.M. Heat all over with occasional chills. Low type of fever. Fever while travelling in ships.

BELLADONNA : Fever without thirst. Feet icy cold, upper body steaming hot. Temperature high. Fever due to heat of the sun.

BRYONIA ALBA : Fever with full, hard, tense and quick pulse. Chill with external coldness, dry cough and stitches in the chest. Easy, profuse perspiration. Gastric symptoms may accompany.

FERRUM PHOS. 6X : In all early stages of fever. It stands between Acon. and Bell. Face flushed. Pulse soft. No restlessness.

GELSEMIUM : Much muscular soreness. Chilliness up and down the back. Wants to be held, because he shakes. Pulse low, full and soft. Heat and sweat stages debilitating. Great

	headache. Thirstless. Patient does not want to be disturbed.
NUX VOM.	: Fever with gastric symptoms. One important indication for the use of this remedy is that the patient feels chilly when uncovered and yet he does not allow to be covered.
PYROGENIUM 200	: Septic fevers. Coldness and chilliness during high temperature. Temperature rises rapidly. Great heat and sweating does not reduce the temperature. Wonderful fever remedy after child birth. Usually one or two doses cure.
RHUS TOX. 200	: Fever with weakness, restlessness and trembling. Diarrhea. Dry cough. Accumulation of dead skin scales on the lips. Fever with skin eruptions.
STAPHYLOCOCCINUM 200	: Fever on account of acne, abscesses, furuncles or where staphylococci is the chief bacterial factor. Septic fevers.
STREPTOCOCCINUM 200	: Reduces the temperature in all types of fevers. Rapid in action.

MALARIAL FEVER

CHINA OFF.	: Fever may return, every week. Chill generally in the afternoon, thirst before chill, drinks little but often. Easy perspiration. Symptoms, worse every alternate day.
CHININUM ARS.	: In prolonged malarial fevers with neuralgia. It cures such fevers.

CHININUM SULPH.   : Chill daily at 3 P.M. Painful swelling of various veins during chill. Shivering even in a warm room or with blanket on.

EUPATORIUM PERF.   : Heavily coated tongue. Bitter taste. Great pain in the bones. No thirst, during chill. Frontal headache. Violent shivering.

FERRUM ARS. 6   : In the later stages of malaria when the liver and spleen are enlarged.

MALARIA OFF. 200   : A dose given in the beginning when the fever is not high, either cures malaria or cuts short its course and avoids further complications.

NATRIUM MUR. 200   : Fever returns from 9-11 A. M. Continued chill and constipation. It should not be given during fever, else the fever will increase. Before fever when the temperature is not more that 98°F, a dose or two at an interval of an hour reduces the chances of fever, coming on.

TUBERCULINUM 200   : Post critical temperature of a remittent type. Repeat every two hours.

TYPHOID FEVER

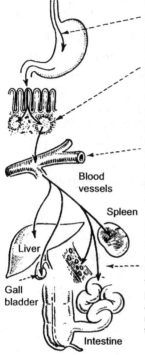

Ingestion of S. typhi (contaminated water or food).

Diagnostic test

Phase I
Invasion of intestinal lymphoid tissue and proliferation of bacteria. This phase lasts for 2 weeks and is virtually asymptomatic.

Positive blood and urine cultures obtained during febrile peroid.

Phase II
Invasion of blood stream causing bacteremia. General toxemia is caused with rise of temperature. Immunological reaction occurs leading to the next phase in 10 days' time.

Antibodies to S. typhi appear in blood.

Widal Test positive at end of this phase.

Phase III
Localisation of bacteria in intestinal lymphoid tissue, mesenteric nodes, **GALL BLADDER,** liver, spleen and sometimes the bones. Local necrosis, probably due to antigen-antibody hypersensitivity reactions, results in characteristic lesions.

Widal Test rising titre.

—— Culture of feces.

Blood vessels

Spleen

Liver

Gall bladder

Intestine

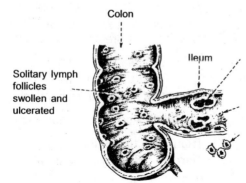

Colon

Ileum

Solitary lymph follicles swollen and ulcerated

Oval Peyer s patches become greatly swollen. Necrosis occurs with ulcer formation. The ulcers are brownish-black with undermined edges.

Solitary lymph follicles and mesenteric lymph nodes are also affected.

ABSINTHIUM : If there is sleeplessness, along with fever.

ACIDUM MUR.	: It is used in very grave conditions when there is bleeding from the rectum or the patient becomes unconscious.
ARSENICUM ALB.	: It does good in all sorts of fevers provided its symptoms of restlessness, unquenchable thirst, drinks often but little, sweat, etc. , are present. Appearance of dead scales of skin on the lips is also a good indication for its use. The patient feels chilly.
ARUM TRIPH.	: If there is delirium or diarrhea, or both.
BAPTISIA TINC., ECHINACEA Q	: Diarrhea or dysentery during typhoid fever. Stools very offensive with rumbling in the abdomen.
BRYONIA ALBA, BAPTISIA TINC.	: Given in alternation every two hours, often helps cure and does not allow complications to develop.
CUPRUM MET. 200	: When there is unconsciousness. One dose every 12 hours. Urine may be suppressed. Weakness. Restlessness.
GELSEMIUM	: To be used in the early stages, when there is a lot of headache.
PHOSPHORUS	: If complicated with pneumonia.
RHUS TOX.	: Triangular tip of the tongue and diarrhea. Restlessness is always present.

FIBROIDS (FIBROMA)
(SEE TUMORS)

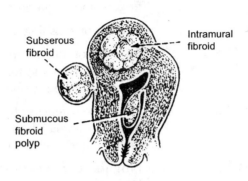

Subserous fibroid

Intramural fibroid

Submucous fibroid polyp

FINGERS

ACTAEA SPIC. 3X : Rheumatism of the finger joints. The joints swell after a little exertion.

AGARICUS MUS. : Fingers becomes weak, unable to hold things properly and the things fall unconsciously.

APIS MEL. : Numbness of the hands and tips of the fingers.

ARGENTUM MET. : Paralysis of fingers due to paralysis of the forearm.

BERBERIS VULG. : Neuralgia under finger nails with swelling of the finger joints.

BORAX 3X : Itching on the back of finger joints. Feeling of stinging in the fingers.

CAULOPHYLLUM 3X : Changing pain in fingers and toes. Stiffness of the joints and fingers. Cutting pains on closing the hands.

CINA	:	Boring of fingers in the nostrils.
ELAPS COR.	:	Skin peels off on the tips of fingers.
GRAPHITES	:	Cracks and fissures on the ends of fingers and between toes.
HYPERICUM PERF. 3X	:	Injuries or crushing of fingers.
LAUROCERASUS	:	Swelling of fingers which usually occurs in heart and lung diseases, medically called "clubbed fingers".
LEDUM PAL. 10M	:	This remedy relieves the pain from getting a foreign body under the fingers nails almost instantly.
NATRIUM MUR.	:	Fingers cannot hold things. Dryness and cracking about finger nails. Numbness and tingling in the fingers. Skin peels off partly at the root of the finger nail. Skin around nails dry and cracked.
PETROLEUM	:	Cracks at the tips of the fingers and on the back of hands.
PROPYLAMINUM Q	:	Tingling and numbness of fingers. Rheumatism, a needle held, feels too heavy. 10-15 drops in half a glass of water, a teaspoon full dose every two hours.
RHUS TOX.	:	Loss of power in forearms and fingers. Crawling sensation in the tips of fingers.
SARSAPARILLA	:	Burning on the sides of fingers and toes. Ulceration around ends of the fingers. Deep cracks in the fingers and toes.
SILICEA	:	Tip of the fingers are dry. The patient has to moisten them often by licking. Cracks at the ends.

THUJA OCC.   : Tip of the fingers toughened, feel
                               dead. Writer's cramps in fingers.

FISSURES

Fissure is a deep furrow, cleft, or slit.

ANTIMONIUM CRUD.,   : Fissures on the palms, hands and
LYCOPODIUM   heels.

CALCAREA FLUOR.   : Fissures or cracks on the palms.
                         Fissure of the arms.

GRAPHITES   : Fissures of anus, hands and fingers
                        in people who often have eczema
                        and severe constipation.

HEPAR SULPHURIS   : Chapped skin. Deep cracks on
                        hands and feet.

MALANDRINUM   : Fissures or chaps on hands and
                        feet in cold weather and from
                        washing.

MANGANUM ACET.   : Deep cracks in the bends of el-
                        bows or knees.

NITRICUM ACIDUM   : Fissures in the rectum. Constant
                        oozing of foul matter from fissures.
                        Fissures have clear cut edges as if
                        the cuts were made with a sharp
                        knife.

PETROLEUM   : Chaps and fissures which bleed
                        easily, worse in winter specially
                        on the tips of fingers.

PLATINUM MET.   : Crawling and itching in the anus.

RANUNCULUS BULB.   : Finger tips and palms chapped.
                        Blister like eruptions on the palms.

RATANHIA PERU.   : Sensation as if broken pieces of glass were in the anus. Anus burns for hours after stool. Fetid thin diarrhea. Hemorrhoids burn. Fissures in the anus, with great constriction, burning like fire; temporarily relieved by cold water.

SILICEA   : Fissures in finger tips and anus.

FISTULA

(ABNORMAL PASSAGE)

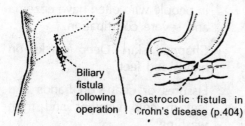

Biliary fistula following operation

Gastrocolic fistula in Crohn's disease (p.404)

Vesicovaginal fistula following radionecrosis in treatment of cancer of cervix

BACILLINUM 200   : It may be given when other well selected remedies fail to cure.

BERBERIS VULG. Q   : Fistula of anus. Increased bile. Sour eructations. Great itching of the anus.

CALENDULA OFF. Q   : Fistula not healing properly may yield to this when applied locally. 20 drops to an ounce of lukewarm water. An effective medicine for healing. The lotion may be used externally, always with other treatment.

CAUSTICUM 200	: Fistula and large piles.
GRAPHITES	: Fistula of anus. Discharge glutinous and fetid.
MYRISTICA SEB.	: Fistula of anus. Action similar to Silicea and Hepar sulphuris but it acts more powerfully than these two remedies.
NITRICUM ACIDUM 200	: There are one or two openings, internally or externally. Soreness and burning pain in the lower bowel. Constant oozing of thin, green, fetid matter from the fistula. It is the remedy of first importance.
PAEONIA OFF.	: Fistula ani. Hemorrhoids, fissures and ulceration of the anus covered with crusts. Burning, biting and itching in the anus.
SILICEA 1000	: Abscess fistula. It may be accompanied with piles. Give three doses in one day, cures in 1-3 weeks. Give Tuberculinum 1000 after cure.
SULPHUR	: Blind fistula, with cutting pains.

FLATTERY

PALLADIUM MET.	: Ladies of mild temperament with a lachrimose mood, who love to be appreciated for all their actions and reasonings. Likes to be told that they are beautiful or their dress is attractive. Likes flattery. Brownish yellowish spots on skin due to sun-rays or anemia.

FLATULENCY

(GAS OR WIND TROUBLE)

AGARICUS MUS. : Profuse fetid flatus. Gurgling in the abdomen. Flatulent distention of the stomach.

ALFALFA Q : Flatulence with distention of the abdomen. Shifting flatulent pain in the abdomen, several hours after meals.

ALOE SOC. : Copious flatus during passing stools.

ARGENTUM NIT. : Flatulence with painful swelling of stomach. Abdomen swollen with gas. Explosive belching.

ASAFOETIDA 3X : Pressure of wind is always upwards never downwards. Belching is loud.

CARBO VEG. : Wind bloats in upper parts of the abdomen. Eructation of wind by mouth with noise like hiccough, relieved by belching or passing wind. Pain in stomach on account of gas. Flatulent colic - pain extends to the chest.

CHINA OFF. : Wind bloats the whole abdomen. Patient says that everything eaten turns to gas. Passing of wind does not give relief.

COLCHICUM AUTUM.200: In dyspepsia when there is a burning or cold sensation in the stomach. Much gas in the stomach and abdomen. The smell of cooking food causes nausea. Distention of the abdomen with gas.

FUCUS VES. Q : Flatulence in fat persons. Digestion is furthered and flatulence diminished by the use of this remedy.

GRAPHITES : Very fetid gas preceded by colic.

KALIUM CARB. : Abdomen distended with wind immediately after eating. Excessive flatus. Everything he eats or drinks appears to be converted into gas, specially in aged and broken down patients.

LYCOPODIUM, LAC CAN. : Gas is emitted through the vagina.

LYCOPODIUM 200 : Immediately after a light meal, the abdomen bloats with gas. Sense of fermentation in the abdomen. Liver trouble. Wind in lower parts of abdomen. Passing of wind relieves.

MAGNESIUM PHOS. 6X : Bloating of abdomen with hot wind. Must loosen clothing, walk about, constantly passing flatus.

MYRICA C. : Constant discharge of flatus when walking. Urging to stool, with no other results than the passing of a great amount of flatus.

NUX MOSCH. : Dyspepsia. Everything eaten turns into gas and fills the stomach and abdomen to cause pressure on all the abdominal organs.

NUX VOM. : Flatus is due to indigestion and there is often pain in the stomach during its passage.

PSORINUM   : Flatus, which smells like rotten eggs.

RAPHANUS SAT.   : Wind formation around the navel. No emission for a long time.

RHUS G. 3X   : It disinfects the bowels so that the flatus and stools become free from odour.

SULPHUR   : Flatus smells like rotten eggs or sewage gas.

THUJA OCC. 200   : Flatulence in children. Abdomen distended. Loud rumbling in abdomen. Passing of wind does not give relief.

FOOD
(SEE ALSO ALLERGIES)

AETHUSA CYN.   : Nausea at the sight of food.

ARSENICUM ALB.   : Cannot bear the sight or smell of food. Allergic to preserved and cold foods and over ripe fruits.

BRYONIA ALBA   : Allergic to cabbage, vegetables, salad and chicken.

COLCHICUM AUTUM.   : The smell of food, especially fish causes nausea, even fainting.

FRAGARIA VESCA   : Strawberry causes urticaria.

SULPHUR   : Allergic to eggs.

THUJA OCC.   : Onions do not agree.

FOOD POISONING

ARSENICUM ALB.	: Bad effects of eating decayed vegetables and over ripe fruits.
CARBO VEG.	: Vomiting, nausea and diarrhea due to eating decayed meat.

FOREIGN BODIES

ACONITUM NAP.	: Profuse watering of eyes after removal of sand or other foreign bodies from them.
ANAGALLIS	: Favours expulsion of splinters, etc.
LEDUM PAL. 10M	: This remedy relieves the pain from getting a foreign body under the finger nail, almost instantly. It expels iron nails, etc.
SILICEA	: Promotes expulsion of foreign bodies from the tissues like fish bones, needles, bone splinters, etc.

FRACTURES

Bone

Fat embolism may occur in fracture of long bones due to entry of fat from the marrow cavity into the torn ends of veins.

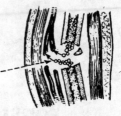

By sharp bone ends

Penetrating inuury from outside

Pathological fracture

A common condition is a secondary tumor growing in and destroying the bone.

Mixture of tumor and hematoma– healing inhibited.

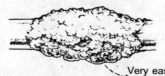

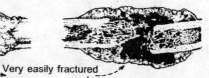

Very easily fractured

Factors influencing healing of fractures

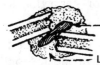 There may be interposition of soft tissue, e.g. muscle

Large irregular callus; slow repair, permanent deformity of bone.

 Small callus, qick repair.

  Callus formation inhibited

Fibrous union

In extreme cases, a rudimentary joint (pseudoarthrosis) may form.

 Small callus, good bone formation.

After the orthopedist has done his job, the following medicines will speed up the cure.

ARNICA MONT. 1000	: It should be given, four doses for one day only. It will remove bruises and pains.
CALCAREA PHOS. 6X	: Give four doses daily. It will help to unite the bones quickly.
RHUX TOX., BRYONIA ALBA	: These two remedies should be given alternately every two hours to remove pain, if any.
RHUS TOX., RUTA G.	: After the plaster has been removed by the surgeon, stiffness usually remains, sometimes for months. These medicines used alternately with a gap of two hours, will remove the stiffness in a few days.
RUTA G. Q, SYMPHYTUM OFF. Q	: From the second day, take 15-20 drops of the mixture of the two,

four times a day for 7 days.
Symphytum Q works as a glue, for
joining bones.

STICTA PULM. 200 : If the patient cannot sleep, due to
pain of fracture, give one dose and
if it fails to induce sleep, repeat
another dose after an hour. The
patient will go to sleep.

WIESBADEN : Stiffness remaining in old fractures
is benefited by its use.

FRECKLES
(LENTIGO)

Freckles are yellowish or brownish pigmentations on the
exposed parts of the skin, especially in persons of light complexion. The pigmentation increases in number on exposure to the
sun.

BADIAGA : Freckles on the skin, anywhere.

CAULOPHYLLUM : Discoloration of the facial skin in
women with menstrual and
uterine disorders.

CIMICIFUGA : Facial blemishes in young women.

KALIUM CARB. : Discoloration of facial skin specially after child birth or loss of
vital fluids.

LYCOPODIUM : Freckles, worse on the left side of
face and nose.

NATRIUM CARB. : Freckles. Yellow spots on the face.
Blue ring around the eyes.

NATRIUM HYPO SULPH. Q : Use locally and internally for removal of yellow and brown spots.

SEPIA 10M : Yellow blotches on the face. Yellow about the mouth. Saddle like brownish distribution on the nose and cheeks. Circumscribed discolored skin spots in young women.

THUJA OCC. : Dry skin. Circumscribed brown spots on the face and elsewhere, on the skin.

FRIGIDITY
(IMPOTENCE IN FEMALES)

This is an inability of the female to experience sexual pleasure and satisfaction. It can occur with certain diseases such as diabetes, pelvic disorders under an active thyroid, hypertension, etc. It can occur from over drugging specially with tranquilizers, etc. A poor technique of the male to arouse stimulation in the female partner also leads to it.

AGNUS CASTUS : Abhorrence of sexual intercourse. Mental depression. Relaxation of genitals, with leucorrhea.

BERBERIS VULG. : Painful intercourse with vaginal burning and soreness, in listless and apathetic women.

DAMIANA Q : Sexual weakness from nervous prostration and hence frigidity, it is an important remedy for its removal.

GRAPHITES	: Aversion to intercourse with a pale, thin, profuse vaginal discharge, in fat, chilly and timid women.
IGNATIA AMARA	: Total frigidity with great changes in moods. Sensitive and easily excited.
LYCOPODIUM	: A dry vaginal wall makes intercourse painful.
MUREX PURP.	: It produces violent sexual desire and the desire is easily aroused by touch of parts or by scratching the arm.
ONOSMODIUM	: Complete absence of sexual desire. The breasts ache, the nipples itch. The patient often suffers from migraine.
SEPIA	: Vagina painful during intercourse. Prolapse of the uterus. The women is sad and indifferent to the family.

FROSTBITE
(SEE CHILBLAINS)

Local tissue destruction resulting from exposure to extreme cold is known as frostbite.

FUNGUS DISEASES

| ALUMEN | : Whitish, ulceration patches on the vaginal membrane. |

ARSENICUM ALB. : Fungoid growth burns and itches specially at night, relieved by a warm water wash.

BORAX : Whitish ulceration on the mucous membrane of the mouth and on the hard palate, specially in young children. Lesions are sometimes formed beneath the tongue.

CALCAREA CARB. : Fungus infection of the vagina with an itchy and milky discharge, worse before menses.

LYCOPODIUM : Fungoid growth specially on palms of hands. Skin becomes dry, shrunken and fissured with violent itching.

MANCINELLA : Dermatitis. Oozing of a sticky substance from the crusts. Fungoid growths form heavy brown crusts, scales and fissures.

PHOSPHORUS . : Fungoid growths with blood like crusts and fissures which bleed easily.

SEPIA : Fungus infection of the vagina with a very offensive discharge.

THUJA OCC. : Fungus growth on any part of the body. Treatment should be started with 200 C potency of this remedy fails, any other indicated remedy may be given.

GALL BLADDER

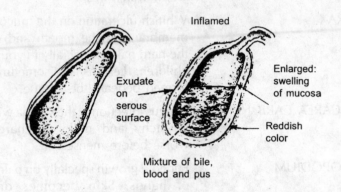

Inflamed

Exudate on serous surface

Enlarged: swelling of mucosa

Reddish color

Mixture of bile, blood and pus

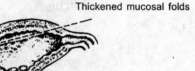

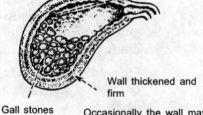

Thickened mucosal folds

Wall thickened and firm

Gall stones

Occasionally the wall may be calcified

ARSENICUM SULPH. RUB. 200	: Gall stone colic with fever.
BAPTISIA TINC.	: Soreness over the region of gall bladder with diarrhea. Stools very offensive.
BELLADONNA 200	: It is very valuable in gall stone colic. It can be repeated often, till the colic disappears.
BERBERIS VULG. Q	: Helps removal of gall stones and colic due to them.

CALCAREA CARB.	: Helps to remove colic due to gall or kidney stones. Should be repeated every 30 minutes.
CARDUUS MAR. Q	: Swelling of the gall bladder with tenderness and pain. Prevents further formation of gall stones.
CHELIDONIUM 200	: Gall stone colic and jaundice due to obstruction of the gall bladder by gall stones. Helps in the expulsion of gall stones and reduces pain, on this account.
CHINA OFF. 200	: It prevents formation of gall stones, and reduces pain, if occurring at night.
CHIONANTHUS Q	: A prominent remedy for prevention of formation of gall stones. Helps expulsion of the gall stones if already formed.
CHOLESTERINUM 3X	: It is almost a specific remedy in removing gall stone colic. Relieves pain at once.
FEL TAURI 2X OR 3X	: Increases the duodenal secretion, emulsifies fats and increases the action of intestines. Liquefies bile and removes the obstruction of gall ducts; helps expulsion of biliary calculi.
HYDRASTIS CAN.	: Gall stones with dragging in the right groin and right testicle. Jaundice and constipation.
MERCURIUS IOD.	: A lump on the gall bladder with enlargement of the liver. Urine smells like mustard oil. Great pain.
MERCURIUS SULPH.	: A lump on the gall bladder with inflammation of the liver. Stools black in color.

GANGRENE

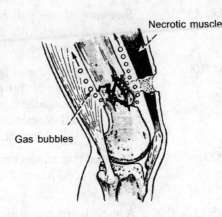

Necrotic muscle

Gas bubbles

Death of a tissue due to deficient blood supply or absence of blood supply. For healing, it is necessary that the dead matter is removed.

ACIDUM SULPH. : Blue and purple surroundings of the gangrene. Bleeding under the skin. Gangrene after an operation or after mechanical injuries.

ARSENICUM ALB. : Diabetic gangrene. Burning, fetid smell from the wound. Dry, specially of the uterus and lungs, better warmth.

BAPTISIA TINC. : Gangrene of the cheek. Symptoms like typhoid.

CARBO VEG. : Carbuncles and boils become gangrenous, wet, purple and icy cold.

CROTALUS H. : Wet gangrene emits a foul smell and oozes freely.

ECHINACEA Q : Gangrene, emitting a foul smell. Use 10 drops in an ounce of luke warm water locally as a cleaning and antiseptic wash and 5 drops in a little of water every two hours, internally.

KREOSOTUM : Specially of lungs and uterus, particularly in old age. Foul smell. Better warmth.

LACHESIS 200 : Bluish purple surroundings of the gangrene. Gangrene produced on account of injuries on septic wounds.

SECALE COR. : Dry gangrene of toes. Dusky blue tinge. Skin feels cold to touch yet covering is not tolerated.

TARENTULA CUB. : Painful and inflamed abscess with a tendency to gangrene.

GASTRIC TROUBLES

ABIES NIG. : A useful remedy for gastric ailments, specially of the aged. Constipation. Pain in the stomach after eating. Sensation of a hard boiled egg at the end of the stomach and as if food is lodged at the pit of the stomach.

ACONITUM NAP. : This remedy is very useful in acute gastritis. Burning from the stomach to the oesophagus. Intense thirst. Drinks and vomits.

ANTIMONIUM CRUD. : Gastric troubles caused by overloading of the stomach. Persistent nausea and occasional vomiting.

Eructations tasting of the ingesta. Heartburn. After nursing, child vomits the milk in curds and thereafter refuses to be nursed. Aversion to pastry and fatty foods. A thickly coated white tongue guides to the use of this remedy.

ARGENTUM NIT.   : Chronic duodenal ulcers with intolerable burning and pain in the stomach and duodenal region. Patients are usually thin and worried.

ARSENICUM ALB.   : For pain and cure of the ulcer, in the lower orifice of the stomach. Retching and vomiting after eating and drinking. Burning pain in the stomach. Long lasting eructations. Vomiting of blood mixed with green or dark brown mucus.

ATROPINUM·   : It is a very good remedy for subsiding the frightful pain of gastic ulcers.

BISMUTHUM   : A remedy for pure gastralgia.

CALCAREA CARB.   : Nausea with sour water in the mouth.

GRAPHITES 6   : Persistent scarring of the duodenal ulcers, this remedy will cure within 15 days.

HYDRASTIS CAN. Q   : In all the forms of stomatitis in children and ulceration of the stomach. A dose of 5 drops in water thrice a day, cures.

KREOSOTUM   : Nothing equals this remedy for the vomiting in gastric carcinoma.

NUX VOM.   : Gastric oppression after a good, heavy meal, and alcoholic drinks.

Feeling of nausea or diarrhea. Much flatulence. Gastric catarrh.

ORNITHOGALUM : Gastric induration and ulceration. Hemorrhage from stomach. Vomiting of coffee ground matter.

PHOSPHORUS ' : Excessive flatulence. In gastric problems, frequent palpitations, intermittent pulse with marked despondency and great thirst.

PULSATILLA NIG. : Heartburn is calmed down by its use. Heartburn after fried, fatty food.

ROBINIA : Gastric ulcers on account of hyper-acidity.

SULPHUR : It may cure 50% of chronic gastric ulcers. Rest may be cured with Carbo vegetabilis.

GIARDIASIS

It has symptoms similar to amoebiasis and stools under microscopic examination show the presence of giardia. Treatment is similar as in amoebiasis.

GIDDINESS
(SEE VERTIGO ALSO)

NUX VOM. : Giddiness, while eating.

FERRUM PHOS. 6X : Giddiness on seeing flowing water.

KALIUM PHOS. 6X   : Giddiness from exhaustion and
                        nervous weakness.

LACHESIS   : Giddiness, when closing eyes.

GLAUCOMA
(HARDENING OF THE EYE BALL)

GELSEMIUM   : Dilatation of pupils, disturbed
                        accomodation, pain in eyes, with
                        or without lachrymation.

SPIGELIA   : Pains sharp and stabbing through
                        the eye and head, worse on mo-
                        tion and at night.

COLOCYNTHIS   : Pain in the eye balls before glau-
                        coma has set in. Sensation as if the
                        eye balls would fall out. When the
                        pain travels to the head and is
                        better by pressure. It acts as a good
                        palliative.

COMOCLADIA DEN.   : Eyes feel large and protruded, spe-
                        cially at night. Feels as if pressed
                        outward. Sense of fullness. Eye
                        balls seem to be large.

CONIUM MAC.   : Sensation of pressure in the eyes
                        when reading, writing or doing
                        any fine work.

ESERINUM 6X   : Dilatation of pupils with harden-
                        ing of the eye balls.

PHOSPHORUS   : Thrombosis of retinal vessels and
                        degenerative changes in retinal
                        cells.

NOTE: This disease is better treated by an ophthalmologist because surgery is often needed in such cases.

GLEET

(THIN, MUCOID DISCHARGE FROM THE URETHRA)

KALIUM IOD.

: Emission of thin, watery, mucus from the urethra in chronic gonorrhea.

SEPIA

: Emission of thick, yellowish green mucus from the urethra of males or females. Micturition is slow and takes a long time to complete.

GOITRE

(ENLARGEMENT OF THE THYROID GLAND)

Commence with SPONGIA, followed by SULPHUR and later IODIUM. In severe cases, BROMIUM followed by CALCAREA CARBONICA, LYCOPODIUM and CAUSTICUM in the same order will cure most cases of goitre.

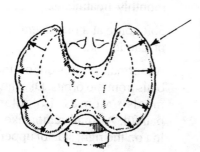

Gland is diffusely enlarged; pale pink in color

BELLADONNA	: Exophthalmic goitre. Marked protusion of eyeballs, increased heart action, enlargement of the thyroid gland, weight loss and nervousness.
BROMIUM CM	: If Iodium fails, this remedy may be needed for six months, one dose a month. Hard goitre.
CALCAREA CARB. 200	: A simple goitre with the symptoms of this remedy and fatness. Perspiration on the head and neck. Two doses daily.
CALCAREA FLUOR. 200	: For painful hard goitre.
CALCAREA IOD. 3X	: Goitre about the time of puberty.
FUCUS VES. Q	: It is a remedy for non-toxic goitre and exophthalmic goitre. Obstinate constipation and obesity. 20 drop doses thrice daily.
HYDRASTIS CAN. Q	: Goitre at puberty and pregnancy.
IODIUM CM	: Patient is always hungry. Eats well and yet emaciates. Enlargement of the thyroid gland. Always feels better by eating. When these symptoms are present with goitre, a dose every night for four days, after the full moon is waning will clear the symptoms with three-four monthly treatments.
LAPIS ALBUS.	: Soft goitre at a pre-ulcerative stage of carcinoma.
LYCOPODIUM 1M	: Abnormal protrusion of the eye balls from the orbits. Diarrhea after meals. Menses irregular and painful. A small tumor like swelling on the right side of upper neck.

NATRIUM MUR. 200	: Goitre with great emaciation, palpitation and sleeplessness. It is very useful for finishing and fixing the cure.
SPONGIA TOS.	: Thyroid gland is swollen. Throat is dry and burns.
THYROIDINUM 3X	: When there is a great craving for sugar and a tendency to obesity in this disease. This remedy may be given every two hours for a long time.
THUJA OCC. 200	: It is indicated when the veins are very prominent on the goitre. A dose every fifth day.

NOTE: Goitres are more prevalent in fresh water and lake countries and less so on the sea coast, due to the lack of iodine in fresh water. Iodine and iodized salts are used as remedies and preventives.

GONORRHEA

AGNUS CASTUS	: History of repeated gonorrhea. Suicidal thoughts due to the disease.
ARGENTUM NIT.	: Burning in the urethra. Frequent desire to pass urine. Sensation as if a few drops remained behind, after urination.
COPAIVA OFF.	: Burning pressure. Painful micturition by drops. Retention of urine. Urine has a bad smell. Discharge is of a greenish, turbid color with a pungent odour. Testicles swol-

len. In females, violent itching of vulva with a bloody discharge.

KREOSOTUM : Discharge is very fetid. Gonorrhea in females with itching of the vaginal canal and vulva.

MERCURIUS COR. : It is always indicated in one stage or the other. The stream of urine is thin, feeble and takes a longer time to finish urination. Discharge is yellowish green both in men and women.

NATRIUM SULPH. : Inflammation of the prepuce. Itching of glans and penis. Discharge is yellowish and greenish.

SILICEA 200 : The discharge of gonorrhea from the urethra is thick, foul and bloody. Two doses may be given daily, morning and evening.

THUJA OCC. 200 : Treatment should be started with this remedy in recent or long standing cases. No medicine should be given on the day when this remedy is given. Discharge is thin and greenish. Painful urination.

GOUT (RHEUMATISM)

ACTAEA SPIC. 3X : Rheumatism of small joints of the fingers and wrists.

AMMONIUM PHOS. : Chronic gout with nodosities in the finger joints and back of the hands. Rheumatic pain in the shoulder joints.

ARNICA MONT.	: Rheumatic or other pains due to an injury, such as a fall or a severe wrench. Burning pain and the part affected is sore to touch. The patient desires to be alone and is better by gentle movements for a short moment, worse by prolonged movement, heat, rest and light pressure.
ARSENICUM ALB.	: Rheumatic pain in the forearm worse during night. Burning pain, relieved by warmth.
AURUM MUR.	: Old cases of rheumatism and gout. Tearing, drawing, pressing and stitching pains, better by heat and worse by cold.
AZADIRACHTA	: Rheumatic pain in the sternum, ribs, shoulders and extremities.
BENZOICUM ACIDUM	: Rheumatic and gouty pains in patients suffering from urinary troubles. Urine contains several deposits, is of high color and smells like the urine of a horse. Pain often changes position. In such conditions, it relieves the pain.
BERBERIS VULG.	: Rheumatic pain in shoulders, arms, hands, fingers, legs and feet. Neuralgia under finger nails with swelling of finger joints. Pain in heels as if standing on a nail. Pain in the balls of heels on standing.
BRYONIA ALBA 200	: The pains are gouty, aggravated on motion; better by rest, pressure and warmth. The joints are red, hot and swollen.

CALCAREA CARB., LEDUM PAL., LYCOPODIUM	:	Deposits of chalk stones in the finger joints, wrists and toes.
CALCAREA CARB.	:	Rheumatic pains are sharp and stitching as if wrenched, after an exposure to wet weather. Rheumatism on account of defective bony growths.
CALCAREA PHOS.	:	Rheumatism, worse during winter and better in summer. Stiffness and pain with a cold and numb feeling. Buttocks, back and limbs go to sleep.
CAMPHORA 200	:	Rheumatic affections in cold climate.
CARBONEUM SULPH.	:	Chronic rheumatism and gout. Flying pains return regularly for a long time. Lightening like pain with cramps.
CASCARA SAG.	:	Its use proves useful in rheumatism of muscles and joints, also when there is obstinate constipation.
CAULOPHYLLUM	:	Rheumatic pain in small joints like fingers, toes, ankles, etc. Aching in the wrists. Cutting pain on closing hands. Erratic pains, changing place every few minutes.
CAUSTICUM	:	Manifests its action mainly in chronic rheumatism and arthritis. Deformities of joints. Restless at night due to pain. Cracking and tension in knees. Stiffness in the hollow of knees. Worse dry cold

winds, in clear fine weather and cold air. Better in damp, wet weather, and warmth specially heat of the bed.

CHAMOMILLA : Pains are violent, accompained with numbness. Patient is very sensitive to pain and often cries on this account, says that he would prefer death than pain. Very effective for pain with numbness. Ankles give way in the afternoon.

CHELIDONIUM : Rheumatism of feet and ankles, ususally accompanied by liver troubles.

CHINA OFF. : Chronic gout. Pain in the limbs and joints as if sprained, worse by the slightest touch. Joints swollen, pain in knees, worse by standing, and better by sitting.

CIMICIFUGA : Pain worse at night, in wet weather. Rheumatism of large muscles.

COLCHICUM AUTUM. : It has a specific power for relieving gouty attacks. The parts are red, hot and swollen. Tearing pains, worse in the evening, at night and from touch. Sharp pain down left arm. Gout of heels. Shifting rheumatism. Edematous swelling of legs and feet.

COLOCYNTHIS : Contraction of muscles. Cramp like pains in the hip. Pain from hip to knee. Pain in the left knee joint. The patient lies on the painful side as pressure and warmth relieve the pain.

DROSERA : Pain in ankles and feet with stiffness.

DULCAMARA : Symptoms similar to Rhus-t. Acts better when days are hot and nights are cold.

EUPATORIUM PERF. : Distressing pain in the bones of great toe, wrist, etc. accompanied with restlessness. Gouty soreness and inflammed nodosities of joints and headache. Aching in the back, arms and legs.

FLUORICUM ACIDUM : It works on any constitution, when heat aggravates the pain and the patient has the ability to withstand any amount of cold.

FORMICA RUFA : Rheumatism comes on with suddenness and restlessness. Sweat does not relieve. Relief after midnight and from rubbing.

FRAGARIA VESCA 200 : Prevents the attacks of gout.

GAULTHERIA OIL : Give in 20 drop doses, relieves much of the discomfort due to pain of gout, arthritis and rheumatism.

GINSENG Q : A useful remedy for treatment of rheumatium, lumbago and sciatica. Joints become stiff and contracted and there is an increase in urine.

GNAPHALIUM 200 : Chronic rheumatism, backache and pain in the neck. Sciatica. Numbness alternates with pain.

GUAIACUM OFF. Q : Rheumatic pain in hands, arms and shoulders. Sciatica and lumbago. Gouty pains, tearing and lancinating; worse from motion, heat, cold wet weather, touch and pressure, from 6 P.M. to 4 A.M. Better by external pressure. Nodosities of joints and contraction of muscles.

KALIUM BROM.

: Chronic gout of nodular form. Hands become hard. Fingers and muscles, jerk and twitch.

KALIUM CARB.

: Pain in knees and it may extend from hip to knee. Pain in the limbs and arms, from shoulders to wrist. Worse by pressure but better by moving about and warmth. Pains are sharp and cutting.

KALIUM IOD.

: Old gouty patients. Must keep in constant motion, as it gives relief.

KALMIA LAT.

: Rheumatic pains travel from above downwards with numbness. Rheumatic pain of the scapula and shoulder muscles, specially right side.

LEDUM PAL.

: Pain travels from below upwards. Patient feels chilly, yet he does not like to be covered as his pains are better by cold. In chronic cases, chalk stone oozes from the finger joints.

LYCOPERSICUM ESCU.

: Dull pain in the lumbar region. Sharp pain in right deltoid and breast muscles. Pain in the right elbow, wrist, in both hands and legs.

LYCOPODIUM	: Chronic gout with chalky deposits in joints. Numbness, drawing and tearing in limbs.
MAGNESIUM CARB.	: Tearing in shoulders, as if dislocated. Right shoulder painful. The patient is unable to raise it. Swelling in the bend of knees.
MEDORRHINUM 1M	: Rheumatism originated from gonorrhea, worse during the day.
MERCURIUS SOL.	: Lacerating pain in joints. Cold fetid sweat on the legs at night. Dropsical swelling of feet and legs.
MIMOSA P.	: Rheumatism of back and limbs.
NATRIUM PHOS.	: Rheumatic arthritis. Crackling of joints. Pain in the wrist and finger joints.
NATRIUM SULPH.	: Rheumatism of persons living in basements or damp houses. They are worse by bathing and in rainy weather. Edema of feet. Piercing pain between scapulae. Crackling of joints.
NUX VOM.	: Crackling in knee joints when walking. Drags feet, when walking. Sensation of sudden loss of power in arms and legs in the morning.
OXALICUM ACIDUM	: Pains through the lower lobe of left lung; pain under the scapula and between the shoulders to the lower back.
PROPYLAMINUM Q	: Palliates fever and pain in a day or two in acute rheumatism. Rheu-

matic pains change their place, specially in heart lesions. Pain in the wrists and ankles, worse by slightest motion. Fingers cannot hold things, even a needle held in the hand appears too heavy. Tingling and numbness of fingers. 10-15 drops in a glass full of water; teaspoonful doses every 2 hours.

PULSATILLA NIG. : Pain in the joints shift from place to place. It is generally due to changes associated with the menstrual cycle. The patient has a tendency to be emotional and tearful. She desires sympathy and consolation. Is worse in the evening, at night and by lying on the painful side.

RADIUM BROM. : It is a very useful remedy in chronic rheumatic arthritis. Severe pain in all the limbs and joints. Knees, ankles, shoulders, arms, hands, fingers, toes, calves, hip joints, etc., all have pain, which is worse at night, in open air, on touch, from cold air and movements.

RANUNCULUS BULB. : Rheumatic and muscular pains along the lower margin of shoulder blade. Pain like pleurodynia in chest. Worse in spring.

RHAMNUS CAL. Q : A positive remedy for muscular pains and rheumatism. 10 drops a dose, four times a day. It is indicated when there is constipation also.

RHODODENDRON CH.	:	Pains are wandering, now in this joint and then in that joint. Arthritic nodes. Pains are worse before thunderstorms and in the hot season. Gout of toe joints.
RHUS TOX. 200	:	Gout, worse in damp and rainy weather. Pain increases on rising from a sitting position or on first motion and becomes better by walking for sometime but increases again after a long walk. Rheumatism due to suppression of perspiration.
RUTA G.	:	Pain in the tendons, appearing after an injury. Pain due to a bruise on the lining of bones. Pain is better by movement and worse in damp, cold weather and during rest.
STELLARIA M. Q, AURUM MUR. NAT. 3X, CARBONEUM SULPH.	:	Chronic rheumatic pains.
SYPHILINUM 1000	:	Rheumatism of shoulder joint, at the intersection of deltoid. Muscles become hard, knotty or lumpy and contracted to form knots.
TONGO 3X	:	Severe pains in hip joints , femur and knees, specially the left.
TUBERCULINUM 1M	:	When the origin is tubercular. Acute rheumatism of joints. Inflammation of joints. Worse motion, standing, dampness and early in the morning after sleep. Better open air.

GROIN
(INGUINAL REGION)

BELLIS P. : Sore and bruised feeling in the pelvic region. Bad effects of injuries to the pelvic organs and deeper tissues.

CALCAREA CARB. 200 : When Rhus-t. ceases to work and the pain is worse in cold damp weather and better by movements.

DULCAMARA. : Pain in the groins.

PODOPHYLLUM. : Pain in the right inguinal region shoots from inner thighs to knees, worse early morning.

RHUS TOX. : Tearing pain in groins due to exposure to damp, wet winds or due to lifting heavy weights. Swelling of inguinal glands.

GUILT
(SEE DEPRESSION)

THUJA OCC., ARSENICUM : Hidden feeling of guilt and depression, thereof.
ALB., NATRIUM SULPH.,
STAPHYSAGRIA

GUMS
GINGIVITIS (INFLAMMATION OF THE GUMS)

AMMONIUM CARB. : Gums recede from the teeth and the teeth become loose.

ARGENTUM NIT. : Tenderness and bleeding of the gums. Inflammation of the gums.

CARBO VEG. : Teeth separate from gums. Pain from hot or cold drinks and their application.

CAUSTICUM : Gums bleed easily.

HYPERICUM PERF. 3X : Pain in the gums from extraction of teeth.

KREOSOTUM : Spongy and bleeding gums.

MAGNESIUM CARB. : Bloody saliva with swelling of gums but teeth are intact.

MERCURIUS SOL. : Sensative to hot or cold. Gums swollen. Offensive breath and excessive saliva in the mouth. Fresh air and fasting relieves, bleeding.

NATRIUM MUR. : Gums bleed with a taste of pus in the mouth and are sensitive to both hot and cold. There may be ulcers on the gums and mouth.

PODOPHYLLUM : Pressing of the gums together in children, with diarrhea.

GUM BOIL
(ABSCESS OF THE GUMS)

ACONITUM NAP.   : Early stage of the gum boil, with throbbing pain.

BELLADONNA   : If three hourly four doses of Acon. do not relieve the pain, give this remedy. Inflammatory redness and swelling of the gums. It will often arrest an incipient gum boil.

BORAX 3X   : Painful gum boils.

CARBO ANIMALIS   : Bleeding, painful and burning gum boils.

HECLA LAVA 3X   : For painful gum boils and abscesses of the gums.

MERCURIUS SOL.   : Gum boil is bright red. Excessive fetid saliva. Inflammation of the gums.

SILICEA   : Gum boils with pus.

HAIR

ACIDUM FLUOR.	:	Falling of hair after typhoid fever.
ACIDUM PHOS.	:	Falling of hair after an exhausting disease. Hair falls from head, eye brows, eyelashes, etc.
CALCAREA PHOS.	:	Falling of hair in bunches on combing is cured by this remedy.
FERRUM PHOS.	:	Hair falls from the head due to anemia.
KALIUM CARB.	:	For falling of hair due to dryness of the scalp and dandruff.
NATRIUM MUR.	:	Falling of hair after child birth. Hair comes out in excess while combing.
NITRICUM ACIDUM	:	Falling of pubic hair due to syphilis or gonorrhea.
SELENIUM MET.	:	Useful for falling of pubic hair, if needed at all.
SEPIA, CARBO VEG.	:	Use of either remedy stops falling of hair during pregnancy, after child birth and during nursing of a child.
SULPHUR, LYCOPODIUM	:	These remedies are also useful for the falling of hair in nursing mothers. Lycopodium is also useful for greying hair at a young age.
THALLIUM	:	Falling of hair after an acute, exhausting disease. Alopecia with profuse perspiration on the head. Loss of hair as an after effect of an atom bomb explosion.

THUJA OCC.	: Use this remedy when the hair grows slowly and splits after growing. Use it as a general remedy for falling of hair.
VINCA MINOR	: Use of this remedy cures matting of hair together, after a head wash.
WIESBADEN 200	: By the use of this remedy, the hair will grow more rapidly than usual and becomes darker. New hair take place of the fallen hair rapidly.

HAIR - PREMATURE GREYING

Hair contains a black-brown pigment and a yellow-red pigment. The amount and distribution of the pigments determine the hair colour. When the secretion of the pigment is lessened, the shaft of the hair whitens. Normally hair gradually greys then whitens as people grow older and the quantity and distribution of the pigment decreases. This is determined by heredity. Stress or illness may also affect the formation of pigment. As how to stop it, is discussed below.

ACIDUM PHOS 1C	: Hair thins out, turns grey early and falls out.
NATRIUM MUR., PHOSPHORUS	: Use of either of these remedies when indicated or otherwise also stops further premature greying of hair, after diseases.
PILOCARPUS M. 1000	: If the hair are greying prematurely due to the dryness of the scalp, the use of this remedy stops it by stimulating natural secretion of the scalp.

THYROIDINUM 3X : It stops premature greying of hair due to thyroid diseases. It also helps to restore the natural color of hair, not turned completely grey.

LYCOPODIUM : It is specific for premature greying of hair.

HAIR UNWANTED
FACIAL HAIR

OLEUM JEC. 3X : Give this remedy 3 times a day after use of Thuja 1M.

THUJA OCC. 1M : Start the treatment with this. One dose a day and no medicine for 24 hours. Repeat after a month.

WAXING : The medication takes a long time to be effective. Along with it, the method of waxing may be adopted. Take liquid wax from a drug store. Spread a light layer of it on the skin and on the strong cloth cut equal to size of the space between the nose and upper lip where there is unwanted growth of hair in a woman. Apply it firmly on the space, after about 2-6 minutes take off the cloth steadily but firmly. All the hair will be pulled out. Employ the same method for the chin. After about a fortnight, the hair roots will be destroyed or become too weak to grow. Skin will become softer. A similar method, if needed can be applied to the growth of pubic hair. Medication can be employed, alongwith.

A TOTAL CARE HAIR OIL

PILOCARPUS M. Q,   : Mix 5 ml of each with 100 ml of
EMBELICA OFF. Q,   Arnica oil. Rubbing the scalp with
CEANOTHUS A. Q   this mixture will stop falling of the
                           hair, make them darker and cure
                           dandruff in many recent cases.
                           Also helpful in vertigo and head-
                           aches.

NOTE 1.: Normally each hair on the scalp grows continuously for 2 to 4 years and then stops growing for 2 to 4 months and then falls out. In its place new healthy hair begins to grow and the cycle is repeated. On an average, there are approximately 100000 hair follicles in the scalp. Normally upto 100 hair are shed daily.

NOTE 2. : Hair needs protection and care during winter months just as it does with the summer, sun and humidity. Colds, cold winds and excessive heat zap, moisture from the hair often leaving it dry and brittle. Keeping the head covered during extreme winters and warm days helps hair to feel soft and manageable.

HANDS

ACONITUM NAP.   : Hands hot and feet cold.
APIS MEL.   : Tip of the fingers and the hands
                           become swollen and numb.

BOVISTA	:	Clumsy with her hands, drops things from hands. Enlarged sensation of mind. Awkwardness; everything falls from hands.
CAUSTICUM	:	Dull tearing pain. Unsteadiness of the muscles of forearms and hands. Numbness and loss of sensation in hands.
COLCHICUM AUTUM.	:	Jerking of the right hand without any apparent reason.
MENYANTHES TRI.	:	Icy coldness of the hands.
NATRIUM CARB.	:	Soreness between fingers and hands are chapped.
PHOSPHORUS	:	Burning in hands.
SQUILLA MAR., CACTUS, CALENDULA OFF.	:	Icy coldness of hands.
SYPHILINUM	:	The patient is always seen washing his hands, without any reason.
TORULA CER.	:	Hands cold like ice and go to sleep easily.

HASTE AND HURRIED

ACIDUM SULPH.	:	Everything is done in a hurry. Wants to finish work quickly.
ACONITUM NAP.	:	Hurried. Wants things done at once. Hurried in movements and speech.
ANACARDIUM ORI.	:	Swallows foods and drinks hurriedly although he is not in a hurry for a purpose.

ARGENTUM NIT.	:	He wants to do things in a hurry.
AURUM MET.	:	Constant rapid questioning without waiting for a reply. Speaks fast. Thinks he cannot do things fast enough.
COCCULUS IND.	:	Speaks hastily.
LILIUM TIG.	:	Hurried manners. Walks fast without any purpose. Will reach the railway station or airport, hours before due departure.
LYCOPODIUM	:	Eats hurriedly without proper chewing as though in great haste.
MEDORRHINUM 1M	:	The patient is always in a hurry without any cause. For him time passes too slowly.
SULPHUR	:	Walks briskly without any urgent work. Hurried for stool and urine.

HAWKING

AESCULUS HIP.	:	Hawking with expulsion of ropy mucus, which tastes sweet.
ARGENTUM NIT.	:	Much thick mucus in the mouth, which causes hawking. Sensation of a splinter in the throat. Hawking in smokers.
ARUM TRIPH.	:	Constant hawking.
AURUM MET.	:	Stitches and pain in the throat, making the patient hawk.
CAUSTICUM	:	Hawks to expel mucus under the sternum as it is hard to expel.

EUPHRASIA	: Hawking up of offensive mucus with bland coryza.
GERANINUM 1X	: Constant hawking and spitting in elderly persons.
HEPAR SULPHURIS	: Hawks to expel mucus. Sensation of a splinter in the throat.
KALIUM BICH.	: Stringy and ropy mucus is expelled on hawking.
MERCURIUS BIN IOD.	: Constant desire to swallow and hawk.
PHYTOLACCA DEC.	: Hawking on account of a sensation of a lump in the throat. Greyish white, thick, tenacious yellowish mucus difficult to dislodge.
SELENIUM MET.	: Hawking and raising transparent lumps of mucus every morning.
SILICEA	: Hawks to remove sensation of a pricking pin in the tonsil.
SPONGIA	: Cleans throat, constantly. Tickling causes cough. Dryness of the throat.

HAY FEVER

It is an acute irritative inflammation of the eyes and upper respiratory passages accompanied by itching and profuse watery secretion, followed occasionally by bronchitis and asthma. The episodes recur annually at the same or nearly the same time of the year, in spring, summer, or late summer and autumn. It is caused by an allergic reaction to the pollen of trees, grasses, weeds, flowers, etc.

ALLIUM CEPA : Copious, watery and extremely acrid discharge from the nose. Feeling of a lump at the root of the nose. Fluent coryza with cough. Hoarseness and headache.

AMBROSIA ART. : Lachrymation and intolerable itching of the eyelids. Watery coryza. Sneezing. Stuffed up nose.

ARALIA R. : The least current of air causes sneezing with copious watery nasal discharge.

ARUNDO : Hay fever begins with burning and itching in the palate and conjunctivitis. Annoying itch in the nose and at the roof of the mouth.

NATRIUM MUR. : Violent fluent coryza. Discharge thin and watery, like the raw white of an egg. Cold commences with sneezing.

NAPHTHALINUM : Coryza with hay fever. Sneezing.

SABADILLA : Spasmodic sneezing with a running nose. Copious discharge of tough mucus. Frontal headache, redness and watering of eyes.

TONGO 2X : Coryza. Nose stopped up. Must breath through the mouth. Hay fever.

HEAD

AGARICUS MUS. : Confused head; vertigo, better by lying down. Vertigo from sunlight and on walking. Constant motion of the head.

ARSENICUM ALB. : Head remains in constant motion. Great itching of the scalp which is sensitive to brushing.

AURUM SULPH. : Constant nodding of the head.

BUFO RANA : Sensation of hot vapours rising in the head. Numbness of the head.

CALCAREA CARB. : Large head of an emaciated child. Sense of weight on the top of the head. Icy coldness in and on the head. Lots of perspiration, wets the pillow.

CANNABIS IND. : Sensation as if the head is closing and shutting.

CARBO VEG. : Hat on the head is intolerable. Hat seems to press upon the head like a heavy weight.

CICUTA VIR. : Head is turned or twisted to one side. Cervical muscles contracted.

CIMICIFUGA : Wild feeling in the head. Waving sensation or opening and shutting sensation in the brain.

COCCULUS IND. : Sensation as if, the head is closing and shutting. Sense of emptiness in the head, specially in the occiput.

GELSEMIUM : Heaviness of the head. Sensation of a band around the head.

HEPAR SULPHURIS, SILICEA : Wrapping of the head gives relief.

JUGLANS REG. : Head confused, feels as if head is floating in air.

LYCOPODIUM, CANNABIS IND.	:	Shakes head without any apparent cause.
NATRIUM MUR. 200	:	Head sweats, while eating.
OSTRYA VIRGIN.	:	Anemia of the head from malaria. Numbness.
PETROLEUM	:	Sensation of cold breeze blowing on the head.
SEPIA	:	Sensation as if something was rolling in the head.
SULPHUR	:	Constant heat on top of the head, worse washing.

HEADACHE

ACIDUM PHOS. 1C	:	Crushing headache with pressure on top of the head. Dull headache after coition or from eye strain.
AGARICUS MUS.	:	Dull headache due to prolonged desk work. Vertigo when looking at passing cars. Headache as if from a nail. Headache with epistaxis. Desire to cover the head.
AMBRA GRISEA	:	Senile headache with depression. Tearing pain in the upper half of the brain.
ANTIMONIUM CRUD.	:	Headache from river bathing, cold, alcoholism and eating pickles or acidic things.
ARGENTUM NIT.	:	It is useful in dull chronic headaches of literary and businessmen.
BARYTA MUR.	:	Headache in old people but without any acute crisis, heaviness

rather than pain. Headache due to hypertension.

BELLADONNA : Severe jerking headache extending from the eyes to the nape of the neck, worse light, noise, jar, lying down and in the afternoon. Throbbing and burning headache from suppressed catarrhs or colds. Headache from having a hair cut.

BELLIS P. : Headache from the occiput to the nape of the head. Forehead feels contracted, bruised and sore.

BRYONIA ALBA : Bursting, splitting headache as if everything would be pressed out, as if hit by a hammer from within. Frontal headache. Worse on any movement and on coughing.

CALCAREA CARB. : Headache before menses. Sense of weight on top of the head. Headache from overlifting and from mental exertion with nausea. Head feels heavy and hot with a pale face.

CALCAREA PHOS. 6X : Anemic girls suffer from headache after studies or after school hours and from eye strains. Headache due to abdominal flatulence.

CARBO VEG. : Headache from any indulgence.

CHINA OFF. : Headache alternating with pain in the abdomen and relieved by stooping. Headache due to strain on eyes. Headache with a feeling as if the head will burst and that the brain is moving to and fro. Throbbing in the head and temples. Pain worse in open air, by contact or

strong wind . Vertigo when walking. Better by hard pressure and
warmth. Periodicity is marked.

CHIONANTHUS Q : It cures many types of headaches,
neurasthenic, periodical, sick,
menstrual and bilious. 5 drops a
dose thrice daily breaks up the sick
headache habit.

CIMICIFUGA : Headache from worry, mental
strain, overstudy or loss of sleep.

COCCULUS IND. : Headache in the occiput and nape.
Sick headache from carriage riding.
Headache on reading, writing,
watching a film, talking, noises
and worries. Sensation of opening
and shutting of occiput.

CROTALUS H. : Dull heavy occipital pain on the
right side and right eye. Pain in the
heart, lying on left side. Worse
jarring.

CYCLAMEN : One sided headache with frequent
sneezing.

GELSEMIUM : Dull tired headache at the base of
the neck. The patient desires to lie
with the head raised upon a high
pillow and to be perfectly still.
Headache from mental labour,
smoking tobacco and in the heat
of the sun. Better by pressure.

GLONOINUM : Congestive headache during menopause or due to suppressed menses.
Headache due to sun stroke.
Severe throbbing headache due to
high blood pressure. Headache
increases or decreases with the
sun. Headache in place of menses.

GRAPHITES	:	Headache on one side of the head extending to the teeth and nose. Usually in the morning on rising.
IGNATIA AMARA 200	:	Headache from exertion of mind like listening to a lecture or paying close attention to an oreator.
IPECACUANHA	:	Headache with nausea.
JUGLANS REG.	:	Pain at the base of the head. Pains are sharp.
KALIUM BICH.	:	Pain in the head, in small spots due to suppressed catarrh. Frontal pain usually over one eye.
LACHESIS	:	Headache during menopause due to non appearance of blood at the proper time and better when flow appears. Headache due to heat of sun.
LOBELIA PURP.	:	Headache between the eye brows with dizziness and drowsiness. Cannot keep eyes open.
LUPULUS H.	:	Headache due to an eye strain, sex or debauch. Dull headache with dizziness.
LYCOPODIUM	:	Throbbing headache after every paroxysm of cough. Tearing pain in the occiput, better in the fresh air. Pain in the temples.
NATRIUM CARB.	:	Headache from slightest mental exertion, worse during change of weather and by working under gas light or sun.
NATRIUM MUR.	:	Throbbing, blinding headache comes periodically. Headache as if thousands of little hammers were

knocking on the brains. Worse in the morning on awakening. Anemic headache in school girls. Chronic headache from sunrise to sunset with a pale face. Headache from eye strain and during menstruation.

NATRIUM SULPH. : Headache, worse during menses. Headache of dwellers in basements and wet houses.

NUX VOM. : Headache in occiput or over the eyes with vertigo. Brain feels as if turning in a circle. Headache in the sunshine. Headache after . debauch. Frontal headache with a desire to press the head against something.

ONOSMODIUM : Headaches from eye strain and sexual weakness. Head appears confused, heavy and dizzy after sexual intercourse.

PAULLINIA SORB. : Sick headaches in persons who
(GUARANA)   have used tea and coffee in excess. Throbbing headache after the use of alcohol.

PICRICUM ACIDUM : Slightest exertion or mental efforts bring on headache. This headache is often found in students, over worked businessmen and people depressed by grief or other emotions.

PLATINUM MET. : Headache in women with numbness. Pain increases and decreases gradually. Tense pressing pain in a small spot.

PSORINUM	: Periodical headaches with putrid stools. Chronic headache, hungry during an attack with vertigo, worse during change of weather. Awakens at night with a feeling of pain, as if from a blow.
PULSATILLA NIG.	: Wandering pains in the head. Pain extends to the face and teeth. Better open air. Headache from overwork.
SANGUINARIA CAN.	: Headache during menopause. Chronic headache. Periodical sick headache. Pain begins in the occiput, spreads upwards and settles over the right eye. Headache every seventh day, worse right side.
SEPIA	: Terrible headache due to suppression of menses or due to scanty flow during menses or on account of constipation.
SILICEA	: Headache due to fasting. Pain begins in the occiput and settles over the eyes. Better by wrapping the head and worse in the morning. Profuse sweat on the head.
SPIGELIA	: Pain beneath frontal eminence and temples extending to the eyes. Pain as a band around the head. Headache starts from the nape of the neck and extends to the left eye. This is used in many types of headaches.
SPONGIA	: Bursting headache due to rush of blood to the head, worse forehead.
SUCCINUM 3X	: Headache every 7 days.

THEA SIN.	:	Sick headache due to drinking excessive tea is cured by this remedy.
TILIA EUR.	:	Neuralgic headache starting on the right side and shifting to the left with sensation of a gauze or veil before the eyes.
TUBERCULINUM 1M	:	Headache is so severe that the patient bangs the head against a door. Intense neuralgia, as if an iron hand was around the head. Symptoms keep on changing.
VIOLA ODORATA Q	:	Tendency for pain immediately above the eyebrows. Headache across the forehead due to uterine fibroids.

HEARING - IMPAIRED

Hearing loss is generally gradual and painless in many cases developing so slowly that it is barely noticeable. At any age, hearing can be damaged by :

1. Middle ear infection.

2. Exposure to loud or constant noise.

3. Hereditary.

4. Illness or birth defects.

5. Natural aging process.

6. Traumatic injury.

7. Tumors.

It is suggested that after the age of 50, a regular hearing test must be done. It should also be done whenever hearing becomes impaired. Treatment should be done on the basis of the disease. In most of cases (90%), it will be necessary to have a hearing aid which should be on the advise of an ear specialist. In the rest of 10% cases, the following medicines are suggested. Please refer to "Deafness".

AMBRA GRISEA : Dullness of hearing without any of the defects mentioned above.

ARNICA MONT. : Hearing impaired due to a blow or an injury to the external and middle ear.

BARYTA CARB. : Hardness of hearing. Crackling noise in the ears. Glands around the ears are painful and swollen. Reverberation on blowing the nose. Indicated in infancy and old age when the tonsils are swollen.

CHENOPODIUM AN. : Numbness of the auditory nerve. Hearing better for high pitched sounds. Comparative deafness to the sound of voice but great sensitiveness to the sounds of passing vehicles. Buzzing in the ears. Defect due to the enlargement of tonsils.

HEART

Mitral regurgitation

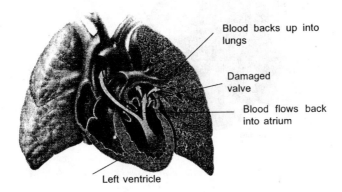

Blood backs up into lungs

Damaged valve

Blood flows back into atrium

Left ventricle

Myocardial infarction (heart attack)

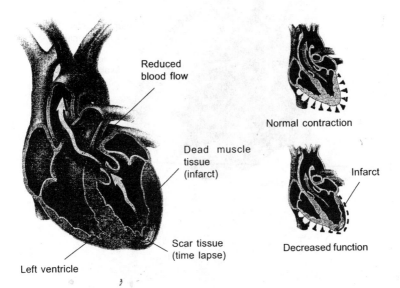

Reduced blood flow

Dead muscle tissue (infarct)

Scar tissue (time lapse)

Left ventricle

Normal contraction

Infarct

Decreased function

Dilated cardiomyopathy

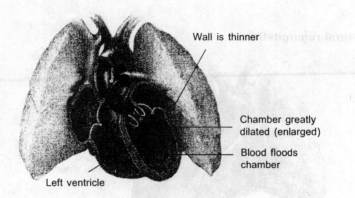

Wall is thinner

Chamber greatly
dilated (enlarged)

Blood floods
chamber

Left ventricle

Aortic stenosis

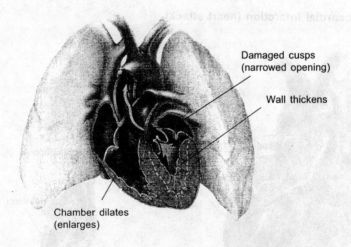

Damaged cusps
(narrowed opening)

Wall thickens

Chamber dilates
(enlarges)

Aortic regurgitation

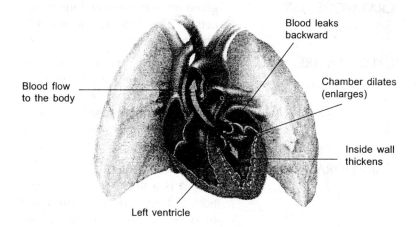

Blood leaks backward

Blood flow to the body

Chamber dilates (enlarges)

Inside wall thickens

Left ventricle

AGARICUS MUS.	:	In heart diseases when pain is prominent and the patient won't answer any question.
AMMONIUM CAUST. Q	:	This is a powerful cardiac stimulant and removes blood clots. May be given by inhalations in cases of fainting.
ARNICA MONT.	:	It is helpful in a tired heart which has become irregular in rate and volume whether as a result of a blood clot or not.
ARSENICUM IOD. 3X	:	Very specific in most of the heart diseases. Weakened heart, specially with a chronic lung condition. Breathlessness on going upstairs.
ARSENICUM ALB.	:	It is a very valuable remedy for the weak heart which is irritable on the slightest provocation.
BARYTA MUR.	:	Hardening and narrowing of cardiac orifice with pain.

CACTUS Q, : 10-15 drops mixed together and
CRATAEGUS OXY. given in water every four hours,
acts as a heart tonic and strength-
ens the heart.

CALCAREA ARS. : It is an excellent cardiac tonic
especially in dilatation and valve
mischief. It relieves pain, palpitation and dyspnea besides having a
marked influence over the dropsy,
always imminent in these cases.

CAMPHORA : As a heart stimulant for emergency
use, it is a most satisfactory remedy. 5 drops a dose on sugar (not
in water) every 5 minutes. Coldness of the body and extremities.

CARBO VEG. : Excessive flatulence pressing the
heart, causes a sinking sensation
and depression.

CHOLESTERINUM 20, 200: Insufficient function of the coronary blood vessels that supply
blood to the heart. Coronary pain
produced is usually dull and heavy
with a sensation as if the chest is
being squeezed.

CONVALLARIA MAJ. Q : Tobacco heart due to excessive
cigarette smoking. Palpitations on
the least exertion. Increases the
energy of the heart and renders it
more regular. 5 to 10 drops a dose
thrice daily. Palpitation and heart
failure of the aged from a sudden
loud noise or an explosion as of a
big cracker or a bomb. Feeling as
if the heart ceased beating and
then starts again suddenly. Angina
pectoris. Extremely rapid and irregular pulse.

CRATAEGUS OXY. Q : Increasing insomnia in cardiac affections. 5 drops in a teaspoon full of water every 3 hours. Common senile myocarditis with a previous history of hypertension, extreme weakness, irregular heart action. This remedy has no toxic effects. It can be given as a heart tonic for long periods of time for such senile hearts. Cardiac dropsy. Extreme dyspnea on least exertion. Cough. Angina pectoris.

DIGITALIS : It works wonders in heart block and bradycardia. Great weakness and sinking of strength, faintness, coldness of the skin and irregular respiration. Bluish face. In cardiac muscular failure, it increases the force of systole.

GLONOINUM : Heart beat is heard in the ears. Fluttering. Palpitation with dyspnea. Throbbing of the whole body. Any exertion brings a rush of blood to the heart.

MOSCHUS : Tightness of the chest. Patient takes a long breath. Hysterical palpitation. Trembling around the heart. Weak pulse and fainting.

NAJA TRI. : Heart cases without any symptoms. Sensation of weight on the heart. Anginal pain extends to the nape of the neck, left shoulder and arm. Fear of death. Pulse irregular. Threatened paralysis of the heart. Damaged heart after infectious diseases. Low blood pressure.

PITUITRINUM 30 : It has a valuable place in heart attacks of old people, when it is hard to pick a well indicated remedy. Attack may be due to coronary trouble or from chronic uremic conditions or from allergies. It relieves readily.

SECALE COR. : Anginal pain and hypertension. Numbness and coldness of the extremities. Pulse contracted and intermittent.

SELENIUM MET. : It is found in minute quantities in fish, meat, whole grain and dairy products. Selenium improves the oxygen supply to the heart. Use of these food articles or vegetables grown in selenium rich soil is useful for the oxygen starved heart, maintaining the elasticity of heart tissues.

SPIGELIA : Violent palpitations. Pain, worse motion. Foul odour from the mouth. Pulse weak and irregular; and dyspnea. Angina pectoris. Craving for hot water, which relieves. Pain extends to the arm or both arms.

STROPHANTHUS HISP. Q: Increases the power of cardiac muscles. Tones up the heart. Cures dropsical accumulations. It is safe for aged. Irritable heart of tobacco smokers. 5 drops, thrice daily.

SUGAR : Heart failure due to deficient heart muscles. One ounce of sugar morning and evening in combination with another indicated remedy.

SYPHILINUM 1000 : It prevents a recurrence of heart attacks.

TERMINALIA ARJUNA Q : Diseases of the heart, both organic and functional. Angina pectoris. Suffocation, palpitation, weakness and pain in the heart. It is a very good remedy for these disorders. In acute cases, give 10 drops half hourly and in chronic cases, 5 drops three hourly.

VERATRUM ALB. : A cold perspiration on the forehead, when indicated. Palpitation with anxiety and rapid audible respiration. Pulse irregular and feeble. Tobacco heart from chewing. Intermittent action of the heart in feeble persons with hepatic obstruction. One of the best heart stimulants.

VIPERA : Dropsy of the heart with swelling of veins, face, lips and tongue with a bursting sensation.

NOTE 1 : Exercise, diet, weight control, controlling blood pressure, stopping the use of drugs and smoking avoid the risk of heart diseases.

NOTE 2 : A team of scientists at the University of Pennsylvania confirmed, after a research, that the use of vitamin E gives protection against atherosclerosis characterized by fatty deposits in the arterial linings of the cardiovascular system, and protects against thickening, hardening, loss of the blood vessel walls and confers"Patient Protection" from heart disease.

HEELS

ACIDUM TART. 3X	: Pain in the soles and heels.
ALLIUM CEPA	: Ulcers on heels due to friction of the heels with shoes, etc. It is also useful for blisters on the feet.
AMMONIUM CARB.	: Pain in heels on standing with tenderness. Cramps in calf and soles. Big toe painful and swollen.
ANTIMONIUM CRUD., LYCOPODIUM	: Fissures on the heels.
ARANEA DIAD.	: Pain in the bones of heels. Sensation of swelling. Heels go to sleep.
ARISTOLOCHIA MIL.	: Stitching pain in the heels with itching.
ARSENICUM ALB.	: Ulcers on the heel with burning pain.
BERBERIS VULG. 200	: Pain in the heels relieved by putting the entire body weight on them. Pain in the heel as if ulcerated.
BORAX	: Pain in heels. Burning pain in great toe. Inflammation of the bulb of toes. Stitches in soles.
CALCAREA CAUST.	: Tearing pain in the left heel.
COLCHICUM AUTUM.	: Gout of the heel. Cannot bear to touch or move it.
CYCLAMEN	: Burning sore pain in heels, better by moving about, massage and warmth, worse sitting or standing and by a cold bath.
GRAPHITES	: Cracks in heels.

KALIUM CARB.	: Pain in the right heel.
LATHYRUS SAT.	: Heels do not touch the ground while walking. Walks on the front part of feet.
MALANDRINUM	: Fissures and chaps in the heels during winter and from washing.
PETROLEUM 200	: Stitching pain in the heels as if by splinters. Heels are rough with cracks and fissures. Worse in winter.
PHASEOLUS L.	: Gout of heels, accompanied with diabetes.
PHYTOLACCA DEC.	: Aching in the heels, relieved by elevating feet. Pain is like electric shocks.
PULSATILLA NIG.	: Pain in the heels like pricking of nails. Puts the feet outside the blanket to cool them as it has a pleasing effect on the pain.
RANUNCULUS BULB.	: Acute pain in the heels. Pulsative stitches in the left heel on standing.
SILICEA	: Tearing pain in the heels due to sprained ankles.
VALERIANA	: Stinging pain in heels while sitting.

HEMATEMESIS
(BLEEDING FROM THE STOMACH)

ACONITUM NAP.	: Hematemesis of newborn infants.
BRYONIA ALBA	: Vicarious hematemesis; vomiting

of bright red blood, followed by a dry, fatiguing cough.

CAUSTICUM : Nocturnal vomiting of dark blood.

CICUTA VIR. : Hematemesis in the aged.

FICUS IND. Q : A great anti hemorrhagic remedy, when blood is pure red.

HAMAMELIS Q : Blood is dark in color.

HYOSCYAMUS NIG. : Hematemesis in drunkards, with hiccough and bitter eructations, blood dark red or bloody mucus.

IPECACUANHA 1X : When the blood is bright red. Bleeding may be accompanied with continuous nausea.

MILLEFOLIUM : Active hemorrhage, bright blood in color.

OPIUM : Hematemesis in drunkards and old people.

PHOSPHORUS : Hematemesis after suppression of menses; coffee ground vomiting with oppression and burning in the stomach.

RHUS TOX. : Hematemesis from over exertion or lifting heavy weights.

STANNUM MET. : Hemorrhage from the stomach. Sensation of emptiness in the stomach. Smell of food causes vomiting.

VERATRUM ALB. : Hematemesis with continuous nausea, fainting, profuse cold sweat, prostration and collapse. Discharge of clotted blo.d from the bowels with crampy colic.

HEMATURIA
(BLOODY URINE)

APIS MEL.   : Stinging and burning in urethra while urinating. Urine is bloody.

ARNICA MONT.   : From mechanical injuries to any urinary part.

CANTHARIS Q   : Urine is voided in drops with burning in urethra. Urine is bloody.

FICUS REL. Q   : Frequent micturition with blood in it.

HAMAMELIS Q   : If Arnica fails give this remedy.

MILLEFOLIUM Q   : When the blood is suspected to come from the kidney and when there is pain in the region of the kidneys.

TEREBINTHINIAE 6   : Hemorrhage on account of inflammation of the kidneys. The blood is dark, passive and fetid. Urine is scanty or suppressed and has an odour.

VIPERA   : Hematuria due to ailments of the kidneys. This remedy exerts a special action on the kidneys when there is facial swelling and a bursting sensation in any part of the body.

HEMOGLOBIN
(SEE ANEMIA ALSO)

CALCAREA ARS. 3X   : Hemoglobin and R.B.C.'s are low,

specially suited to fat women and at menopause.

FERRUM PHOS. 3X   : Increases hemoglobin and makes up for the deficiency of iron.

LECITHINUM 12X   : Increases the amount of hemoglobin and red blood corpuscles.

NATRIUM CACODYL. 3X :   Increases the number of R.B.C.'s to double.

VANADIUM MET. 6   : Increases the amount of hemoglobin and W.B.C.'s. It also stimulates the action of W.B.C.'s.

NOTE: The amount of hemoglobin in blood, averages 12-16 gm/ 100 ml in females and 14-18 gm/100 ml in males. It is the iron containing pigment of the red blood cells and it functions to carry oxygen from the lungs to the tissues. 'Hemo' means iron containing pigment and 'globin' means a simple protein and their combination gives the name 'hemoglobin'.

HEMOPHILIA

In this disease, blood takes a long time to coagulate and, therefore, even the small wounds bleed profusely and for a long time. It is a hereditary disease and occurs almost exclusively in males. There is a deficiency of anti hemophilic factor in blood. In emergencies, transfusion of blood is required. The following remedies are used:

FICUS IND. Q   : It possesses great anti hemorrhagic properties and stops the bleeding quickly.

HAMAMELIS Q   : In every case, this remedy is applied on the wound and should be allowed to dry. It will make the blood coagulate. Distilled extract is better for local use and Q for oral use.

LACHESIS, CROTALUS H. : These may be used in 200 potency for a long time till cure - every week.

PHOSPHORUS   : Slightest wound bleeds too much.

SECALE COR.   : Slightest wound bleeds for weeks together. There is tingling in the limbs.

SYZYGIUM JAMB.   : This remedy is of a great help in hemophilia of diabetic patients. Use Jambalan Q, 10 drops every hour till the blood forms clots. May be used in 30C potency for cure.

NOTE: In the conventional method of treatment, anti hemo-philic factor is named factor 9. Such patients are treated with factor 9 taken from human blood or with protein taken from cell cultures, some of which are genetically engineered. Such blood is tested for H. I. V. infection, hepatitis and other blood diseases before such a use.

HEMOPTYSIS
(SPITTING OF BLOOD)

ACALYPHA IND. Q   : Cough with bloody expectoration. Pure red blood comes in the morning and dark lumps of clotted blood in the evening.

HAMAMELIS Q	:	It is considered as a specific remedy for the cure of this disease.
IPECACUANHA	:	Spitting of pure red blood with nausea or vomiting.
MILLEFOLIUM	:	Blood spitting originating from a disease.
NUX VOM.	:	Hemoptysis of bright red blood, usually in the mornings.
PHOSPHORUS	:	Blood spitting with dry, tight, fatiguing cough, intermixed with expectoration of mucus.
SEPIA	:	Hemoptysis in millers from inhaling flour-dust.
STANNUM MET.	:	Hemoptysis with a tendency to copious expectoration.

HEMORRHAGE

ACIDUM SULPH.	:	Hemorrhage into the skin, mucus membranes, internal organs and other tissues. The skin is red and darkens into purple.
AURUM MUR.	:	It is a very valuable remedy for hemorrhages from the womb, during menopause.
CHINA OFF.	:	Weakness on account of loss of blood. Faintness and ringing in the ears.
CINNAMOMUM Q	:	Hemorrhage after child birth, bleeding from the nose and bowels. A little strain on loins brings about a profuse flow of blood. Cancer with bleeding of an

offensive odour. Feeble patients with weak circulation of blood.

CROCUS SAT. : Blood is dark, slimy and stringy in all kinds of bleedings, even that of threatened abortion or of menses, when it contains clots with long strings.

CROTALUS H. : Hemorrhagic tendencies, blood is dark. Blood does not coagulate. Prolonged menses. Uterine hemorrhages.

ERIGERON Q : Cures epistaxis with congestion of the head, red face and fever. Hemorrhages from pelvic organs are marked with violent irritation of the rectum and bladder.

FERRUM PHOS. 1X-3X : It stops bleeding. The blood is bright red.

FICUS REL. Q, FICUS IND. : These are the best hemorrhage arresters. Bleeding piles, epistaxis, dysentery hemoptysis, hematemesis, hematuria, menorrhagia, etc. Hemorrhage from the mouth, throat or anywhere is arrested by these remedies provided the blood is red. Ficus indica has proved to be better than Ficus religiosa.

HAMAMELIS Q : Bleeding is very dark, clotted; venous blood from the nose, bowels, uterus, lungs or bladder.

IPECACUANHA 200 : Blood bright red and profuse with breathing difficulty and nausea. Bleeding may be from any orifice of the body, nose, stomach, uterus, lung, bladder, etc. provided nausea is present.

MANGIFERA IND. Q (MANGO TREE)	: One of the best remedies for passive hemorrhages, uterine, renal, gastric, pulmonary and intestinal.
MILLEFOLIUM Q	: A very good remedy for all types of hemorrhages when the blood is bright red.
PHOSPHORUS	: Persistent and profuse bleeding even from small wounds.
TRILLIUM PEND. Q	: It is a genuine anti hemorrhagic remedy. The blood is bright red whether of active or passive kind. Specially useful in the climacteric hemorrhages of the womb.

HEMORRHOIDS
(PILES)

CALCAREA FLUOR.	: Blind piles.
COLLINSONIA CAN.	: Sensation of sharp sticks in the rectum. Sense of constriction. Painful bleeding piles or blind piles. Hemorrhoids with most obstinate constipation. Constipation and piles during pregnancy, alternating with diarrhea.
FICUS REL. Q, FICUS IND. Q	: Either of the remedies may be tried if Mucuna fails. This will stop bleeding after about 4 doses of 5 drops each. Blood should be bright red.
HAMAMELIS	: Hemorrhoids after confinement Blood dark, profuse with soreness

in the rectum, great weakness after bleeding.

HYPERICUM PERF. 1X	:	Bleeding piles. It is a very specific remedy.
KALIUM CARB.	:	Piles relieved by hard pressure like sitting on horseback without a saddle.
MILLEFOLIUM	:	Bleeding hemorrhoids. Blood is bright red. Works better in tincture, 5 drops a dose thrice daily.
MIMOSA P. 1X	:	A single dose of 1X or 6X cures external piles. Its leaves made into a poultice with oil and tied on the anus, immediatly relieves the pain and causes receding of piles inside.
MUCUNA Q	:	One drop a dose is nearly the specific for bleeding piles. 4 doses will arrest the disease. If it does no good use the following.
PAEONIA OFF.	:	This is given for piles and fissure of anus occuring together. Burning in the anus.
STAPHYSAGRIA	:	Reappearance of piles after some time of their operation.
SULPHUR 30, NUX VOM., AESCULUS HIP.	:	A dose of Sulphur in the morning, a dose of Nux-v. at bed time and a dose of Aesculus at noon will cure piles, blind or bleeding in a short time.

HEPATITIS
(INFLAMMATION OF THE LIVER)

BAPTISIA TINC.	: Inflammation of the gall bladder.
BRYONIA ALBA	: From cold, sharp pain, worse on touch or on movement and better by lying on the painful side.
HEPAR SULPHURIS	: Due to an abscess on the liver.
IPECACUANHA	: Due to an abscess on the liver after dysentery. Nausea and vomiting.
MERCURIUS SOL.	: Tongue dirty, yellowish white, fetid breath, skin jaundiced. Liver region sore to touch and offensive perspiration. Pain better by lying on the painful side.
PHOSPHORUS	: Inflammation of the liver. Degeneration of the liver under anemic conditions.

HERNIA

Inguinal hernia

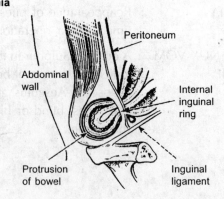

Peritoneum

Abdominal wall

Internal inguinal ring

Protrusion of bowel

Inguinal ligament

ACONITUM NAP.	:	Hernia of intestines which is a form of inguinal hernia in which the hernial sac lies between the layers of abdominal muscles. Pain in the strangulated bowel.
AESCULUS HIP. 3X	:	Hernia of the groin (inguinal) if on the left side with pain.
ASAFOETIDA 3X	:	Hernia of the stomach. Stomach protrudes upwards through the oesophagus. Hiatus hernia.
AURUM MET.	:	Hernia of the scrotum.
CALCAREA CARB. 200	:	Hernia occurring at the navel (umbilical), it is more frequent in children and women than in men. It works in all forms of hernia. Four doses per day.
CALCAREA PHOS.	:	Hernia of the navel, if the patient is thin.
GRANATUM	:	Hernia of the navel (umbilical hernia).
LYCOPODIUM 1000	:	Inguinal hernia of the right side with pain or no pain. A dose every 15th day. Strangulated hernia. Distention of the abdomen with rumbling of gas.
MAGNESIUM MUR.	:	Hernia, scrotal.
MAGNESIUM PHOS. 6X	:	Scrotal hernia which is inherited.
NUX VOM.	:	Right sided hernia with troubles of digestion. Give 200 potency every 5th day. Nux-v. IX reduces the pain in old hernias and in very recent cases. It cures umbilical hernia of infants.

PLUMBUM MET.	: When the hernia is strangulated and Acon., Bell. and Nux-v. have not worked properly.
SEPIA	: In vaginal hernia (i. e. hernia of the vagina).
STAPHYSAGRIA	: In cystic hernia, that is, hernia of the bladder.
WIESBADEN	: Hernia of the thigh bone or femur.

NOTE 1: In case of strangulation of hernia, when there is great pain, surgery is needed when the indicated remedies fail to reduce the pain and discomfort of the patient. Nux-v. IX - given every 10 minutes helps in case of threatened strangulation.

NOTE 2: In case where it is practicle, the patient should be made to lie down on the back with hips raised upto the level of shoulders. The hernia may be pushed back and a truss be applied. In case of scrotal and inguinal hernia, a loin cloth tied adequately helps.

HERPES

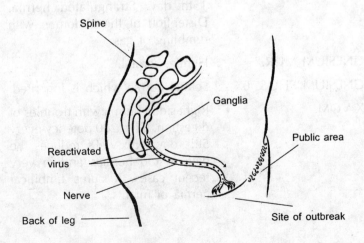

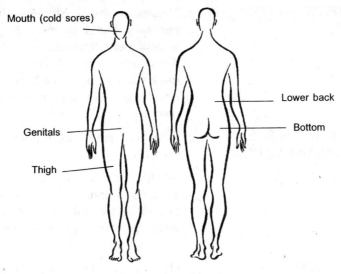

Common sites of herpes

ARSENICUM ALB. : Suppurating herpes with violent burning pains. Thirst for small quantities of water at short intervals. Clusters are dark and deep. It cures pain, etc. within 10 days

CALENDULA OFF. Q : After the vesicles and crusts have disappeared, 50 drops mixed with one ounce of vaseline may be applied on the affected parts to soothe the skin.

CANTHARIS : Herpes of the right side.

CISTUS CAN. : Herpes on the back.

GUNPOWDER 3X : Herpes of the face. Herpes facialis

HEPAR SULPHURIS 10M : Herpes very sensitive to touch. Ulcers on the prepuce, bleeds easily. Herpes circinatus. A single dose cures , such herpes when they appear again and again, after cure.

HYPERICUM PERF.	: Herpes zoster or shingles. It is generally found in men. Painful vesicular eruptions occuring along the course of spinal nerves in a unilateral way or on the face, nose and eyes. Herpes in circular patches.
MERCURIUS SOL., NITRICUM ACIDUM	: Herpes of the penis, prepuce or testicles.
MEZEREUM 200	: Intolerable itching. Chilliness. Vesicles shinning or fiery red. Ulceration forms thick scabs under which purulent matter exudes, in chronic cases.
NATRIUM MUR., CAPSICUM, RHUS TOX.	: Herpes of the vulva. Herpes genitalis and herpes labialis.
RANUNCULUS BULB.	: Herpes zoster. Shingles. Burning and intense itching. Bluish vesicles. Burning pains.
RHUS TOX.	: It is a routine remedy for this disease. Its use reduces pain. It is also used for herpes on lips.
SEPIA	: Herpes behind the ears on the nape of the neck. Herpes circinatus in isolated spots.

NOTE: **Genital herpes is mostly spread through sexual contact through the moist membranes of the penis, vagina, urinary opening, cervix, anus or mouth. Swellings, blisters and sores are caused when the body, immune system tries to fight the infection and actually this is the curative re-action of the nature to fight the disease. Many people with genital herpes experience repeat or recurrent out-breaks. This happens when the body's** immune system is low, for example, at times of stress, fatigue, after an illness or surgery. The patient should avoid sharing intimate articles like towels and razors used on the area of herpes and use safer sex methods.

HICCOUGH

ACIDUM SULPH.	: Persistent hiccough.
CHAMOMILLA	: Hiccough of infants.
CINNAMOMUM Q	: Three drops on sugar for hiccough.
CYCLAMEN	: In chronic cases and in pregnancy, it is given every 10 minutes.
GINSENG Q	: 5 drop doses every 15 minutes if the cause of hiccough is indigestion.
KALIUM BROM.	: Persistent hiccough and hiccough during pregnancy.
MAGNESIUM PHOS.12X	: It is a very good remedy for this disease. Repeat it every 10 minutes till relief.
MOSCHUS	: In hysterical cases give after every 10 minutes.
NUX VOM.	: Hiccough of infants or due to gastric trouble.
RANUNCULUS BULB. Q	: Hiccough after drinking alcohol.
STRAMONIUM 200	: Hiccough, convulsive and violent.

HIPS

AGARICUS MUS.	: Pain over both the hips.
BRYONIA ALBA	: Pain in the hips, worse on motion and better on rest and pressure.
CIMICIFUGA	: Muscular or rheumatic pain in the hips.
CONIUM MAC.	: Very severe pains in the hips.
HYPERICUM PERF.	: Severe nerve pains in the hip joints are relieved by this remedy.
KALIUM CARB.	: Sharp pain from hip to knee. Inflammation of the hip joints.
MERCURIUS IOD.	: Chronic inflammation and pain in hips is removed by the use of this remedy.
NATRIUM SULPH.	: Pain in the hip joints. Worse left side, stooping.
RHUS TOX.	: Pain in both the hip joints.
TONGO 2X	: Tearing pain in the hip joints, femur and knees, especially left side.

HOARSENESS

ANTIMONIUM CRUD.	: Hoarseness or loss of voice every time a person is exposed to heat.
ARUM TRIPH.	: Hoarseness of speakers, politicians, clergymen and lawyers who have to speak much, at a stretch.
BARYTA CARB.	: Chronic hoarseness.

BORAX   : A piece of borax, the size of a pea dissolved in the mouth acts magically in restoring the voice, in cases of sudden hoarseness brought about by cold and frequently for an hour or so, it renders the voice silvery and clear.

CAUSTICUM   : Simple hoarseness from catarrh of nose or throat or both. Hoarseness of singers, with pain in chest. Larynx sore.

COCA Q   : Loss of voice. Give 5-6 drops every half an hour for two hours, before expected demand of voice.

IODIUM 3X   : Hoarseness with general weakness.

NATRIUM SEL.   : Chronic laryngitis. Hoarseness of singers with frequent clearing of throat.

PHOSPHORUS   : Pain and burning in the larynx, Can't speak. Hawking, clears hoarseness temporarily.

POPULUS CAN. Q   : Acute hoarseness. Pharynx and larynx feel dry with rawness and soreness of the chest and throat. Restores voice quickly.

RHUS TOX.   : Hoarseness due to weakness of the vocal cords.

SELENIUM MET.   : Hoarseness of singers appearing, as soon as they begin to sing or after prolonged use of voice. Frequent necessity to clear the throat.

SPONGIA   : Hoarseness with cough. Cleans the throat constantly. Stitches in the throat, which is dry.

HOMESICKNESS

CAPSICUM 30 : Homesickness. The patient will travel miles to reach home in the evening after work. Office goers will rush home after office hours. They often contact their families on phone whenever they get a little time off, from work.

HOMOSEXUALITY

NATRIUM MUR. 1000 : A dose every 15 days for several years will remove the attraction of the persons to the same sex.

HORMONES

Secretions of the ductless glands are called hormones. These remedies are sometimes used to remove their deficiency in production by the respective gland.

ADRENALINUM : It is produced by the adrenal cortex which is situated one above each kidney. Adrenaline is used to stimulate the sympathetic nerve endings.

INSULINUM : It is secreted by the pancreas, which is situated behind the stomach and in front of L1 and L2 lumbar vertebrae. It converts sugar to blood sugar for production of heat and energy in the body.

OOPHORINUM : It is an extract of the ovaries. It is useful for treatment of menopausal symptoms and ovarian cysts. Oestrogen, another hormone present in the urine of pregnant women and mares is also widely used for similar purposes in the conventional treatment.

ORCHITINUM : It is an extract of the testes and is used for sexual weakness, senile decay of males and develops secondary sexual characteristics in males.

PITUITRINUM : It is secreted by the anterior portion of a small gland located at the base of the brain, called the pituitary gland. Pituitrinum influences growth, sexual development, skin pigmentation and thyroid functions. In homoeopathic doses, it is used for cerebral hemorrhage and for absorption of blood clots. The posterior part of pituitary, which is attached to the anterior part also produces pituitrine which aids the absorption of water by the kidneys and influences contractions of the uterus.

STEROID HORMONES : This is secreted by four small para thyroid glands situated near the thyroid. Steroid hormones also help in the secretion of thyroidine.

TESTOSTERONE : It is an androgen isolated from the testes of a number of animals including man. It is considered to be the principal testicular hormone produced by man. It is powerfully associated with masculinity. This is a steroid that gives man a hairy chest, deep voice and rippling muscles. Its use in small doses fuels sexual desires and protects against bone loss during and after menopause.

THYROIDINUM : It is secreted by a butterfly like gland situated in the interior portion of the neck, in the throat. Thyroidinum is used indirectly in growth and nutrition. In homoeopathic doses, its effects are striking in thetreatment of myxedema and cretinism.

NOTE 1: Recent studies have shown that adding hormones to the body does not cause hormone levels to rise. Instead the body compensates by producing less hormone.

NOTE 2 : Graphites is the most positive remedy for female diseases due to the diminishing hormonal activity. It makes up for the deficiency of female hormones.

HYDROCELE
(DROPSY OF SCROTUM OR TESTICLES)

ABROTANUM : Hydrocele of boys.

ARNICA MONT. : Hydrocele as a result of an injury or blow.

AURUM MET. : Chronic hydrocele and enlargement of testes. It cures the condition after using it for several months.

BRYONIA ALBA : Hereditary hydrocele.

GRAPHITES : Aids in absorption of fluid from the testicles and scrotum.

PULSATILLA NIG. : Hydrocele is painful. Pains wander from scrotum to testicles and vice-a-versa.

RHODODENDRON CH. : Left sided hydrocele. Testicles swollen.

SILICEA : Hydrocele of chilly patients with burning and soreness of genitals.

HYDROCEPHALUS
(COLLECTION OF WATER IN THE HEAD)

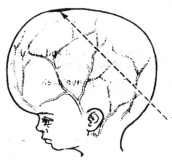

There is great enlargement of the head with prominent scalp veins and forehead overhanging the eyes. The fontanelle remains open. Clinically mental deficiency is common.

APOCYNUM CAN. 3X : Acute hydrocephalus. A diminished frequency of pulse is the prime indication. It is one of the most efficient remedies for all kinds of dropsies.

APIS MEL.	: It is a good remedy when the whole brain feels tired. Extreme sensitiveness to touch. Face swollen.
CALCAREA CARB.	: Lot of perspiration on the head with hydrocephalus. Patient is fat and flabby.
CALCAREA PHOS.	: This is given for lean children.
HEDERA HELIX Q	: Chronic hydrocephalus. 1 drop per dose only. Next morning, a clear flow of fluid through the nose appears and generally only one dose is sufficent to cure. Repeat, if recurrence is threatened.
HELLEBORUS NIG.	: When numbness predominates. Child asks for nothing but drinks greedily when given water. Urine is suppressed.
TUBERCULINUM 200	: May be used intercurrently.

HYDROPHOBIA
(RABIES)

BELLADONNA 200	: Actions violent. Jumps, strikes and bites like a mad dog.
LYSSINUM 200	: Convulsions brought at the sight of running water. Hypersensitiveness of all senses. Start the treatment with this remedy.
STRAMONIUM 200	: Madness of a person on seeing running water or even by drinking water.

XANTHIUM SPIN. 200   : It is said to be specific remedy for hydrophobia.

HYPERACTIVITY
(SEE ALSO CHILD ABNORMAL)

AGARICUS MUS.   : It is suited to impatient people who are clumsy in appearance, have a clumsy handwriting and whose clothes are generally stained. They cannot concentrate and forget everything immediately.

ARGENTUM NIT.   : The patient is always hurried and impatient. He likes to finish before he has even begun. He does not live in the present and constantly asks, what is next. Children crave for sugar and candy though it makes them ill.

ARSENICUM ALB.   : An Arsenicum patient has an immense liking for cleanliness. She is well dressed and well groomed. Always likes all the articles to be placed in the right place and in the right order. She is over sensitive to her troubles and sometimes thinks that it is useless to take medicine. She is miserly, selfish and very sensitive to disorder and confusion. She is actually not overactive but despair drives her from place to place.

BARYTA CARB.   : Child is very shy, averse to meet strangers. Hides on seeing a stranger.

CHAMOMILLA	:	The patient is always moving, is impatient and angry. Never stays in one place. They are often unbearable. Want a thing they do not have, but will reject it when offered. They do not like to be spoken to or even looked at. Children are better when carried. They sleep poorly and are oversensitive to pain. Specially suits children and ladies.
CYPRIPEDIUM PUB.	:	Child wakes up at night and begins to play. He smiles and laughs.
KALIUM BROM.	:	The patient cannot keep his hands still. Touches everything. Bites nails. Forgets what to write, while writing. He has a poor memory and fails to concentrate. Sleeps poorly and grinds teeth during sleep. Nocturnal tremors.
MAGNESIUM CARB.	:	Child is very sensitive to touch. It causes startling. His whole body smells sour.
TARENTULA HIS.	:	Cannot stay still for even a moment to read or write. They eat while standing or sitting, but always move their legs. They are however calmed by music and film songs.
ZINCUM MET.	:	Cannot keep his legs still.

HYPEROPIA
(FAR SIGHTEDNESS)

Use of properly and accurately selected lenses (spectacles) is the only remedy.

HYPOGLYCEMIA
(LOW BLOOD SUGAR)

ALUMINA SIL.

: Level of blood sugar becomes very low sometimes due to excessive intake of insulin. It causes irritability, confusion and possible coma i. e. unconsciousness. In such cases, give sugar in any form and when the patient regains consciousness, give Alum-sil. 200 one dose weekly.

HYSTERIA

AGARICUS MUS.

: Hysterical fits and faintness after sexual intercourse.

AMMONIUM CARB. 200 : Patient weeps incessantly during the fit. Depressed and weak. Dyspnea.

AQUILEGIA VUL.

: Globus hystericus. Severe headache.

ASAFOETIDA 3X

: Globus hystericus. Nausea. Offensive diarrhea with flatulence.

CAMPHORA Q	: It acts like magic in paroxysms of hysteria. 5 drops can be given on a lump of sugar every 5 minutes.
CICUTA VIR.	: Jerking of arms, fingers and legs during fits.
CIMICIFUGA 200	: Hysterical shivering. Irregularity of menses or uterine problems give rise to hysteria.
CINNAMOMUM Q	: Hysterical hiccough. Give three drops on a lump of sugar and repeat as desired.
CONIUM MAC.	: Hysteria due to suppressed sexual desires.
CROCUS SAT.	: Sudden changes in moods. Spasmodic twitching of muscles.
HYOSCYAMUS NIG.	: Feeble hysterical fits, mostly pretended. Laughing and weeping alternately.
IGNATIA AMARA Q	: Hysteria due to grief. Crying and laughing alternately. Does foolish things. During the attack, give it mixed with Pothos Q-5 drops each, half hourly. For cure, use 200th potency.
KALIUM PHOS.	: Nervousness, anxiety and great irritability. Night terrors. Any work seems like an effort.
KREOSOTUM	: Vomiting during hysterical fits.
MOSCHUS Q	: The odour of this remedy is liable to bring the patient to work. It readily does away the hysterical attack and unconsciousness or uncontrollable laughter and extreme coldness.

NATRIUM MUR. 1M : It is the chronic of Ignatia amara and has the same symptoms. Should be used, when Ignatia amara fails.

PLATINUM MET. : Hysteria of over sexy women. Hysteria due to over excitement of sexual desire.

POTHOS Q : 10 drops in water is very effective to relieve the patient from distress.

TARENTULA HIS. : Patient pretends a hysterical fit. Uncontrollable laughter. Sings and dances. Destructive impulses. Pulls hair and tears clothes.

THYROIDINUM 200 : Hysteria during pregnancy. It can be repeated as it bears repetition well.

VALERIANA Q : When well chosen remedies fail. Hysterical flatulence. Sensation of a thread in the throat.

VIOLA ODORATA : Difficulty in breathing, anxiety and palpitation.

ZINCUM VAL. : The hysterical patients cannot sit still. Must move about or keep the ' legs in constant motion.

ILL EFFECTS

ABROTANUM : Ill effects of suppressed diseases, specially gout.

ACETICUM ACIDUM : Ill effects of acid thrown on the face and of inhaling carbon monoxide gas.

ACIDUM PHOS.	: Ill effects of excessive loss of semen or blood, grief, mental shock and eating sour food or drinks.
AMMONIUM CARB.	: Ill effects of inhaling charcoal fumes.
ANTIMONIUM CURD.	: Ill effects of swimming, falling into a river and very cold bathing.
ANTHRACINUM Q	: Ill effects of inhaling foul odours.
ARNICA MONT. 1M	: Ill effects of realization of financial losses. Grief or remorse. Ill effects of over exertion.
ARSENICUM ALB.	: Bad effects of eating ice cream or decayed food. Ill effects of excessive alcoholism.
BELLADONNA	: Ill effects of cold weather and hair cut.
BELLIS P.	: Ill effects of cold winds, complaints due to cold wind or cold drinks when the body is heated. Ill effects of masturbation.
BRYONIA ALBA 200	: Ill effects of inoculation for typhoid fever.
CALCAREA CARB.	: Ill effects of working in water.
CAMPHORA	: Ill effects of shock.
CARBO VEG., KALIUM CARB.	: Ill effects of drinking too cold or icy water or soft drinks.
CARCINOSINUM 200	: It is worthy of consideration in cases of ill effects of severe fright, prolonged fear of unhappiness.
CAUSTICUM	: Ailments from long lasting grief and sudden happiness or grief. Thinking of complaints aggravates.

Emaciation due to worry, etc. Ill effects from burns like pain, etc.

CHAMOMILLA : Bad effects of inhaling chloroform. It cures nausea and vomiting.

CHEIRANTHUS C. : Ill effects, like deafness, otorrhea, nose stopped up at night due to irritation of cutting wisdom tooth.

CHININUM ARS. : Eating eggs causes diarrhea.

COCA Q : Ill effects of mountaineering such as palpitation, breathlessness and insomnia.

COCCULUS IND. : Ill effects of night watching, loss of sleep or overwork.

COFFEA CRUDA : Ill effects of sudden emotions, surprises, sudden bad news or sudden joy.

COLCHICUM AUTUM. : Ill effects of suppressed sweat, night watching and hard studies.

COLOCYNTHIS : Colic or other complaints arising as a result of anger.

CONIUM MAC. : Ill effects of suppressed sexual desire.

DULCAMARA : Ill effects of taking a very cold bath.

FERRUM PHOS. 6X : Ill effects from the heat of sun and sun stroke.

GELSEMIUM : Bad effects from fright, fear and exciting news.

GINGER (ZINGIBER) : Ill effects of eating water melons and impure water.

GUNPOWDER 3X : Bad effects from extraction of an abscessed tooth. Ill effects of taking bad food or drinking bad water.

HELLEBORUS NIG.	:	Ill effects of head injury.
HELONIAS	:	Patient is worn out due to hard work. He feels tired and sleepless, his muscles ache. He feels better, when he is busy and engaged.
HEPAR SULPHURIS	:	Ill effects of dry cold winds.
IGNATIA AMARA	:	Ill effects of grief and worry make her sad, sighing and sobbing. It is a remedy for sudden shocks, grief and disappointments, which may lead to semi-unconsciousness.
KALIUM HYPO PHOS.	:	Ill effects of excessive tea drinking.
KALIUM PHOS.	:	Ill effects of worry like mental and physical depression, overwork, excitement are wonderfully removed by this remedy. For insomnia use 200X potency and for other ill effects use 6X potency.
MAGNESIUM MUR.	:	Ill effects of sea bathing.
MALANDRINUM, SILICEA,:		Ill effects of vaccination.
THUJA OCC.		
MERCURIUS CYAN. 200	:	Ill effects of inoculation for diphtheria.
NATRIUM SULPH.	:	Ill effects of head injury and mental troubles, there from.
NATRIUM CARB.	:	Ill effects of drinking cold water when overheated.
NATRIUM MUR.	:	Ill effects of grief, fright, anger, quinine, etc. which are of long standing. It is an excellent remedy for the ill effects of sun strokes.

	Give alternately with Ferr- p. every half hourly.
OPIUM 200	: Ill effects from fright and fear of long standing, are antidoted by this remedy.
PHOSPHORUS	: Ill effects following the iodine and excessive use of salt.
PHOSPHORUS, STRONTIUM CARB.	: Ill effects following the explosion of an atom bomb.
PHYTOLACCA DEC.	: Ill effects of getting wet in rain, exposure to damp and cold weather are removed by the use of this remedy.
PULSATILLA NIG. 200	: Ill effects of inoculation for whooping cough.
PYROGENIUM 200	: Bad effects of miscarriage or poisoning by sewer gas.
RHUS TOX.	: Ill effects of getting wet, when perspiring.
RHUS TOX., FORMICA RUFA, MILLEFOLIUM	: Ill effects of over lifting or fall from heights.
SELENIUM MET.	: Antidotes the bad effects of X-rays and radiations.
STAPHYSAGRIA	: Ill effects of insults and anger.
STRAMONIUM	: Ill effects of suppressed eruptions, like scarlatina.
THLASPI BURSA 6	: Ill effects of suppressed uterine diseases.
TRIBULUS TER. Q	: It corrects the ill effects of masturbation like spermatorrhea, partial impotence and too early an ejaculation in coitus.
TUBERCULINUM 200	: Ill effects of hair dyes.

IMMUNE SYSTEM

ECHINACEA Q   : It is an immune system stimulant.
                                 5 drops a dose thrice daily till
                                 required.

IODIUM   : It increases the defensive system of
                                 the body by assembling the white
                                 blood corpuscles to fight and
                                 destroy the injurious, invading
                                 bacteria.

IMPOTENCY

According to Dr. Alain Jardin, a french urologist, about 26 million European men have regular problems in getting an erection. About one in ten Europeans, over the age of 18 have difficulty in achieving erection at least once out of every two times they attempt to have sex. A 1994 survey conducted in France, found that only about one in five men with erection problems ever consulted a physician about their condition even though several types of treatment are available.

Impotency is stressful for both partners. Fatigue, increased stress, job loss, illness or depression may cause rapid onset of impotence. If a man is suffering from a low sex drive, he may well experience difficulty in attaining or maintaining an erection firm and lasting enough for satisfactory sex. The following treatment may be given alongwith some soothing advice. Also, please read the Chapter "Erections".

ACIDUM PHOS.   : Impotency due to the sexual
                                 excesses. Testicles tender and swol-
                                 len. Parts relax during an embrace.
                                 Edema of the prepuce.

AGNUS CASTUS	: Simple impotence. Yellow discharge from the urethra. No erections. Parts cold and relaxed. Desire gone. Scanty emission without ejaculation. Testicles swollen, cold, hard and painful.
ARNICA MONT. 200, HYPERICUM PERF. 12X	: Impotence due to a fall or blow on the sexual parts. Give Arnica 200, one dose daily in the morning and Hypericum 12X twice daily at an interval of 3-4 hours.
BUFO RANA	: Impotency as a result of masturbation. Involuntary emissions. Discharge, too quick.
CALADIUM SEG.	: Impotence due to masturbation. The violent sexual desire fails to bring about an erection. Impotency of the advancing age, persons who indulged too much during the ripe days. No emission and no orgasm on sexual intercourse. Erections while half asleep they cease when fully awake. Penis relaxes on attempting to sex.
CONIUM MAC.	: Desire increased, power decreased. Very feeble erection. Impotency due to suppressed sexual appetite. Testicles large and hard.
DAMIANA Q	: 10 drops thrice daily are very good in curing impotency. Use it for a month or so.
GINSENG	: It improves the blood supply to sexual organs and improves the erectile functions in impotency.
GRAPHITES	: Want of thrill and emission of semen in coition.

KALIUM BROM.	: Debility and impotency due to sexual excesses.
KALIUM BROM., KALIUM IOD.	: Impotence due to wasting away of testicles or due to syphilis.
LECITHINUM 3X	: Increases the sexual desire in both sexes and also increases the strength of penile erections in males by supplying more blood to it.
LYCOPODIUM 1000	: Long standing impotency. No erec tile power. Premature emission.
MOSCHUS, CUPRUM MET.	: Impotent due to diabetes.
NATRIUM MUR.	: Emissions even after coition and ejaculation. Retarded and very late ejaculation in coitus due to impotency.
NUPHAR LUT. Q	: Absence of erection and desire. It tones up the sexual system.
NUX VOM.	: Impotency accompanied by general nervous depression and irritability, digestive disorders and constipation.
SABAL SER.	: Impotent due to urinary troubles. Parts cold. Penis and testicles shrunken.
SALIX NIGRA	: Impotency with excessive desire for intercourse. Erections painful, painful movements of the testicles.
SAPONINUM	: It is a steroid and is stated to cure impotency. Its long use should be avoided.
SELENIUM MET.	: Impotency due to dribbling and wastage of semen during sleep. Increased desire and decreased

ability. Semen thin and colorless. On attempting coition, penis relaxes.

STAPHYSAGRIA : Impotent due to masturbation. Patient remains gloomy on this account.

SULPHUR : Complete absence of erections and sexual desire. Involuntary emission during stool or while urinating.

THUJA OCC. : Loss of confidence. Seminal emissions without dreams. Does not want to marry due to fear of inability to perform.

TRIBULUS TER. Q : Partial impotency due to over indulgence in advancing age or when accompanied by urinary problems, spermatorrhea or prostrate gland enlargement. It is considered as one of the best remedies for spermatorrhea. Dose, 15 drops thrice daily.

YOHIMBINUM Q : An excellent remedy for impotency. Excites sexual organs. 10 drops four times a day for a month or so. During the period of treatment, restrict the sexual activities.

INDIGESTION
(SEE ALSO DYSPEPSIA)

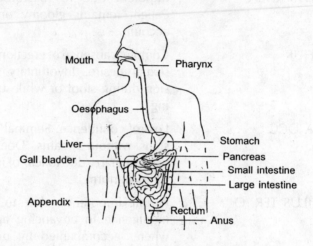

Mouth — Pharynx

Oesophagus

Liver — Stomach
Gall bladder — Pancreas
Small intestine
Large intestine
Appendix
Rectum
Anus

The passageway between
the mouth and stomach

Improves clearance re-
lieves HEARTBURN

SPHINCTER: The open/close
barrier that prevents food from
coming back up

Improves stomach emptying:
relieves DISCOMFORT
Bloating
Too full to finish a meal Fullness after meals Burping

Improvies sphincter pressure:
relieves REGURGITATION

ABIES NIG.   : Indigestion with a feeling of
                              constriction in the oesophagus.
                              It is very useful in dyspepsia of the

aged with functional heart systems, pain in the stomach always after eating. Offensive breath and eructations.

ANACARDIUM ORI.   : Indigestion after taking cold drinks or stress. Such patients are always relieved by eating. There is a sensation of a plug, anywhere in the alimentary canal. Heartburn, after 2-3 hours of eating.

ARGENTUM NIT.   : After taking too much sweet or due to constipation. Loud belching.

ARSENICUM ALB.   : Indigestion caused by taking preserved food.

CARBO VEG.   : Indigestion with excessive flatulence. It may result from over eating, eating rich fatty foods or eating too late in the evening and sleeping soon, thereafter. Burning in the chest and headache often result. Simplest food disagrees.

COLOCYNTHIS   : Indigestion after anger.

GRAPHITES   : Pain in the pit of the stomach, after about 2 hours of eating. Constant desire to retch or swallow.

HEPAR SULPHURIS   : Even after eating a small meal, there is heaviness and bloating in the stomach.

IPECACUANHA   : Indicated in constant nausea; not relieved by vomiting, when the tongue is clear.

KALIUM BICH.   : Pain, heartburn and weight in the stomach immediately after eating.

NATRIUM MUR.   : Indigestion due to drinking excessive coffee.

NUX VOM.	: Indigestion with painful retching; may be as a result of loss of sleep, stress or anxiety. There is burning in the chest, after about 30-60 minutes of eating. The patient is better by warmth and sleep or when left alone. He craves alcohol and spicy food. Indigestion after over eating.
ORNITHOGALUM Q	: Useful in chronic gastric and alimentary canal ailments. Gastric ulceration even bleeding and vomiting of coffee ground matter.
PEPSINUM 1X	: It digests the contents of the stomach and acts upon the secretory tissues of the stomach. Diarrhea, due to indigestion. Dose 3-4 grains, thrice daily. Alcohol and carbonated drinks should not be taken during this treatment.
PULSATILLA NIG.	: Indigestion with nausea and vomiting, begins after about 2 hours of eating and is worse in the evening. Taste may be bad. It may also be as a result of rich fatty foods, stress, emotions or may be associated with menstruation or pregnancy.
THUJA OCC.	: Indigestion due to drinking excessive tea.

INFANT DISEASES

AETHUSA CYN.	: Milk is not digested and vomited out. Indigestion. Troubles, worse

in hot weather. Ill effects of over feeding babies.

ALOE SOC. : Involuntary stools. Child cries soon after feeding, as it feels uneasy and has pain in the liver region.

CALCAREA ARS. : Enlarged liver and spleen, specially if the child had malaria.

CALCAREA PHOS. : Infant wants to nurse all the time and vomits easily. Complaints during teething. Diarrhea, stool green, slimy, hot and spluttering, undigested with foul smelling gas.

CHAMOMILLA : Diarrhea. Stools green, watery, slimy and fetid, and contain yellow mucus. Soreness of the anus. Colic and restlessness.

CINA : Stool contains pieces like popcorn. Colic before passing stool. Child touch his anus frequently, as it itches. He is restless and wants to be rocked.

PULSATILLA NIG. : Ill effects of eating rich, fatty, non-vegetarian food, chocolates, etc.

SAMBUCUS NIG. : Cold. Cannot breathe easily. Nose blocked. Loose cough which can choke.

SENNA : Lot of wind. Child appears full of wind. Enlarged liver. Constipation with colic. Loss of appetite.

SULPHUR 6, CALCAREA PHOS. 6X : If a woman repeatedly gives birth to babies who die soon after birth or in early infancy, give these medicines, one dose each, daily during the last two months of pregnancy. The child should be given Alfalfa Q-5 drops, three times a day for several months before 10 minutes of each feeding.

INFERTILITY

(FOR ORAL HOMOEOPATHIC TREATMENT SEE STERILITY)

When a lady is unable to have a child even after a prolonged medical treatment. Many couples employ high technical treatment and enjoy the joys of parenthood. Any of the following six procedures can be employed, only under the supervision of a competent surgeon who specialized in this kind of treatment.

(I) Intracytoplasmic sperm injection (I. C. S. I): The sperm is injected directly into the egg under a microscope. The embryo is then implanted in the female's womb.

(II) Ovulation induction: A women who is unable to produce eggs, is treated to produce a lot of eggs. The intercourse is timed at an optimal period during the woman's cycle to create pregnancy.

(III) Intra - uterine insemination (I. U. I.): The husbands sperms are collected and placed directly in the wife's uterus. This type of insemination helps, if the man has a low sperm count or they are slow in movement, which hampers their journey to the egg.

(IV) Invitro fertilisation: Some of the eggs are combined with the sperms in a test tube. If fertilization takes place, the embryo is transferred into the woman's uterus.

(V) Gametic intra fallopian transfer : An egg and sperm are directly transferred into the fallopian tubes and on fertilization, it travels to the uterus.

(VI)   Another woman's egg or another man's sperm is employed to produce the   embryo which is then planted in the uterus of the barren woman.

NOTE 1: It is said that for obtaining a male child, the women should take Nat-m. 6X one dose daily and for obtaining a female child, she should take Puls. 6X one dose daily from the 3rd to 6th month of pregnancy.

NOTE 2: Aur-m. CM one dose given at the commencement of pregnancy, usually results in the birth of a male child.

NOTE 3: Doctors at the genetics and I. V. F. Institute, Fairfax, Va are researching that a baby of choice- male or female can be produced. The only difference between male producing Y chromosome sperm and female producing X chromosome sperm is that Y chromosome sperms have about 2. 8 percent less genetic material.

INFLUENZA

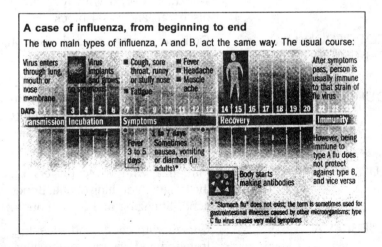

A case of influenza, from beginning to end

AMMONIUM CARB. 200, : For cough remaining after influ-
BRYONIA ALBA 200,   enza.
MEPHITIS 200

ARSENICUM ALB.	: It is the best remedy to be prescribed in routine on its symptoms of thirst for small quantities of water at short intervals, restlessness, sneezing and a running nose. It cures many cases.
BRYONIA ALBA	: Indigestion remaining after influenza. Intense nausea, worse by motion better from eructations and hot drinks or when the influenza is accompanied with pain in the chest.
CARBO VEG. 200	: After effects of influenza, like debility or cough. Give a dose daily.
CARBOLICUM ACIDUM 3X	: Cures most of the cases of influenzal attacks. Also removes debility left after the cure when used in 30 potency.
CAUSTICUM	: High fever without chill. Great weakness. Coryza with free watery discharge and nasal blockage.
COTYLEDON UM., BAPTISIA TINC.	: Delirium during severe influenza with a sensation as if the body is separated into parts.
DULCAMARA	: Influenza during rainy season, in cold weather or when the nights are cold and days are comparatively hot. Sore throat with cough.
EUPATORIUM PERF. 3X	: Influenza with white blisters on the tongue. Vomiting of bile. Bones ache. Sneezing and loose cough.
EUPHRASIA	: Coryza with cough and sneezing. Irritation and watering of the eyes.
GELSEMIUM 1X	: Its use can be considered in the early stage, when chills and sneez-

ing are present. Nasal irritation, watery discharge from the nose. No thirst. Severe headache and muscle ache.

INFLUENZINUM 200 : It is given as a preventive for safety against this disease to those not effected by it, when influenza has come into the family. Treatment can also be started with it, when so, it cuts short the disease.

KALIUM BICH. : Persistent, ropy discharge with a sense of obstruction in the nose. Symptoms are aggravated in cold damp weather and are better by the warmth of bed.

KALIUM IOD. 6X : It is a prophylactic against colds and influenza.

LYCOPERSICUM ESCU. : Influenza with severe aching pains all over the body. Pains left after influenza. Symptoms, worse open air.

LYCOPODIUM : Pains left after influenza.

MEDORRHINUM 200 : A good antidote to the ill effects of influenza.

NATRIUM SAL. 3X : One of the best remedies for the prostrating after effects of influenza.

NATRIUM SULPH. 6X : A good remedy for influenza when it is in epidemic form. Influenza during rainy or wet season. Thick, yellow discharge and salty mucus. Cough with bursting pain in the head and flow of tears. Weakness left due to flu.

NUX VOM.	:	If given early at the onset of the disease, averts influenza.
PHYTOLACCA DEC.	:	Influenza with a sore throat and toothache.
PICRICUM ACIDUM, PHOSPHORUS, COCCULUS IND.	:	Mental weakness remaining after influenza. The patient shows his inability to do any mental work.
PYROGENIUM	:	It works wonderfully and cures the influenza.
RHUS TOX.	:	Hard tickling cough. Great chilliness. Pain in the legs. Restlessness. Dry tongue with a triangular tip and temperature.
SARCOLACTICUM ACIDUM	:	Influenza with nausea and uncontrollable vomiting with extreme weakness.
SULPHUR 200	:	If by the use of other indicated remedies, the temperature does not subside, a dose of Sulphur will have the desired effect.
THALLIUM	:	Specially suitable in cases of chronic influenza with violent pains and trembling of the limbs. The temperature is low.
TUBERCULINUM 1M	:	Recurrent influenza with a long, continuous teasing cough.

INJURIES

ARNICA MONT.	:	This is the remedy of first importance in all kinds of injuries, traumatic or bruised. It is mostly suited to cases, when any injury,

however remote seems to have caused the present trouble. Higher potencies are as effective as lower.

BELLIS P. : Injuries to deeper tissues and nerves.

CALENDULA OFF. Q : A lotion of it, 20 drops to an ounce of water may be used in all kinds of injuries and wounds. Internally, it is most effective in healing. It is a great antiseptic.

CAUSTICUM : Healed wounds and scars re-open. Affects of old injuries come back.

ECHINACEA Q : Ulcers or wounds with a foul smell and with a tendency to gangrene. 10 drops in an ounce of luke warm water may be used locally for cleaning and as an antiseptic wash. 5 drops in a little water may be used internally, every two hours till the curative effects appear.

HELLEBORUS NIG. : 200, 1M or 10M potency of this remedy, is very special for the after effects of head injuries.

HYPERICUM PERF. 12X : Injuries to nerves in the soft parts of the body like finger tips. It is useful in the injuries of coccyx and spine. Injuries of long standing duration.

LEDUM PAL. : Injuries caused by piercing of nails "punctured wounds", insect bites, etc.

NATRIUM SULPH. : Injuries to the head and mental troubles, thereafter.

RUTA G. : Bruises caused by blows and from blunt weapons, when there is

	bleeding under the skin, giving it a blue black appearance.
SILICEA	: Corneal abscess after traumatic injury.
STAPHYSAGRIA	: Injuries caused by sharp instruments, like knife and sword.
SULPHUR	: Use it when every little injury suppurates.
SYMPHYTUM OFF.	: Injuries of the bones, eye balls, tendons and ligaments.

INSANITY
(MANIA)
(SEE ALSO SCHIZOPHRENIA)

It is a mental disorder characterized by the patient's inability to distinguish between right and wrong. He has impulses which he cannot resist and which become a menace to others. This chapter may be read with the chapter 'Schizophrenia'.

ACIDUM FLUOR.	: The patient sits in a corner of the room. He does not talk or answer any questions.
AGARICUS MUS. 1M	: Destroys things which are otherwise required. The patient sings and whistles, when it is not required. Seems foolish and acts like a fool. He is fearless and threatens others.
ANACARDIUM ORI.	: Excessive anger at the slightest offense. Insanity with loss of memory. Dual personality.
ARGENTUM NIT.	: Progressive paralysis in the insane.

ARSENICUM ALB.	:	Great anguish and restlessness. Changes places continuously due to despair. Fear of death. Fear of being left alone. Cold sweats. Malicious and selfish. Immense liking for cleanliness.
AURUM ARS.	:	Insanity of fanatics, drunkards and religious persons. Extreme irritability on hearing any adverse remark about his religion. Obstinate and hard to convince.
AURUM MET.	:	Great inclination to commit suicide, but is afraid of death. Depressed, dejected and low spirited. Has no guts, cannot face difficulties and considers, that he is unfit to live in this world.
BARYTA MUR.	:	Many kinds of manias are cured with this remedy, when there is a maddening, excessive sexual desire. He will catch hold of the opposite sex even in a public place like bazaar or street.
BELLADONNA	:	The patient is violent, will kick and cry. There is rush of blood towards the brain and eyes. Eyes become blood shot when he is furious. Actions midway between Hyoscyamus and Stramonium.
CALCAREA CARB.	:	Religious mania.
CANNABIS IND. Q	:	Dual nature state. Hallucinations and imaginations. Extremely happy and contended. Talkative. Time seems too long, seconds seem years. Has a great soothing influence in many nervous disorders,

like mania, dementia and delirium. Anxiety and depression. Must move constantly. Forgetful. Uncontrollable laughter. Insomnia. Constant fear of becoming insane. Sensation, as if the top of the head is opening and shutting. Clairvoyance. Rapid change of moods.

CIMICIFUGA : Mania following disappearance of neuralgia.

COCCULUS IND., PULSATILLA NIG. : Mania due to suppression of menses.

CROCUS SAT. : Anger with violence followed by repentance. Laughing mania. Drowsiness and lassitude. Laughter followed by weeping.

HELLEBORUS NIG. : Mania of the melancholic type, sensation of depression and sinking.

HEPAR SULPHURIS, CAUSTICUM : Threatens to kill his family and to burn the house. Insanity due to suppression of skin problems.

HYOSCYAMUS NIG. : Face is red and the gaze wild. Tears everything, he can lay hands upon. Talkative, restless and quarrelsome. Will tear his clothes to uncover. Sometimes sad and at other times laughs. Dangerous, can stab and murder. Some end their life by drowning. She is hurried in manners and is intensely jealous. Makes motions as if brushing hair or face. Stupid. Wants to be naked.

IODIUM : Chronic mania in scrofulous patients. Mania after acute affections of the respiratory organs. Unconcerned about the future. Depression. Sudden impulses to run and to become violent. Suicidal tendencies. Talkative, can talk for hours with enthusiasm and over confidence.

KALIUM BROM. : Violent only on seeing a particular person or a particular thing.

LACHESIS : Suspicious. If sees people whispering, thinks they are talking about her. Religious mania. Cruel to everybody and to the pets. Jealous and hates others. Mania during or after menopause.

LILIUM TIG. : Profound depression of spirits. Constant inclination to weep. Fears some organic and incurable disease. Swears and curses. Aimless hurried manners.

LYCOPODIUM 200 : Patient is always ordering and dictating. Envious. Easily aroused to anger with violence.

MANCINELLA, HYDROPHOBINUM, CANNABIS IND. : Fear of becoming insane. Mentally depressed states at puberty and menopause, with raised sexuality.

MELILOTUS OFF. : Unable to fix mind. Treacherous stupor, wants to run away and hide. Thinks everyone is looking at her. Fear to talk. Threatens to kill the physician or parents, approaching him. Insomnia.

MERCURIUS SOL. : Frequent spitting. Spreads the saliva out with her feet and licks some of it again. Licks mud of ponds and eats cow dung. Generally does not harm any one.

Manical, catches the strangers passing by.

NUX VOM. 200 : Mania caused by sleeplessness, prostration and excitement. Very irritable, sensitive to all impressions, malicious. Cannot bear noises, odours, light, etc. Fault finding. Scolds and insults others. Loquaciousness.

RAUWOLFIA Q : Insanity due to high blood pressure and an irritative condition of the central nervous system. Violent maniacal condition. 10 drops a dose, four times a day and more often, when needed.

SEPIA : Mania, during or after menopause with dyspepsia and constipation. Mania due to profuse menses.

SILICEA : Insanity after influenza.

STAPHYSAGRIA, PHOSPHORUS : Insanity due to excessive masturbation.

STRAMONIUM : Sees and hears imaginary things and persons. Talkative, sad and desires light. Refuses food and water saying that they are poisoned, will ask the person serving, to taste them in his presence. Violent with a tendency to commit murder. Religious mania. Claps hands. Wants to pray all the time. Mania from childhood. Talkativeness. May have involuntary stools and urine. Insanity during pregnancy.

SULPHUR : Mania following child birth. Does not feed her baby. Walks briskly.

Wants to remain quite. Does nothing else except praying.

TARENTULA HIS. : Sudden alteration of the mood. Destructive impulses. Breaks and throws away costly things without any reason. Mania with increased sexual desire. Sensitive to music. Must keep legs in constant motion, though walking aggravates. Wants the scalp rubbed.

USTILAGO MAY. : Mania of always taking a bath. Impulses to commit suicide by drowning.

VERATRUM ALB. : Sadness with stupor and mania. Mania after giving birth to a child. Unsocial. Unwilling to talk. Insanity after a major operation. Cold sweat on the forehead with a pale face. Aimless wandering away from home. Cursing and howling at night. Mania during heart diseases. Cuts and tears things. Religious mania and mania of a destructive nature. Always busy praying. Covers many types of insanity.

INSOMNIA
(SLEEPLESSNESS)

ACIDUM PHOS. : Sleeplessness after depressing events, sorrow or loss and death of a friend and a relative.

ACONITUM NAP. 200 : In badly shocked cases, give Acon. 200 every 15 minutes to induce sleep. Sleeplessness is caused by fear, over excitement or shock. Restlessness.

ALFALFA Q : Sleeps better in the morning. It induces a quite, peaceful and refreshing sleep.

AMBRA GRISEA : Sleeplessness due to worries or business problems.

APIUM GRAVE. : Patient of insomnia is not fatigued from loss of sleep. Awake from 1 to 3 A.M. Unrefreshed.

ARGENTUM NIT. : Sleeplessness from worry about an event the next day, such as an interview or an examination.

ARNICA MONT. : Sleeplessness caused by over exertion, mental or physical. Bed appears too hard. Tosses about to find a soft portion of bed.

ARSENICUM ALB. : Inability to fall asleep or waking up at about 2 A.M. due to an anxiety. Great restlessness with a great need to get up and walk about in the room. Sleepy yet unable to sleep. Child tosses and kicks the clothes.

AVENA SAT. Q : Sleeplessness in alcoholics and those with morphine habits.

BELLADONNA : Sleeplessness after midnight from anxiety and restlessness. Gets up and walks. Insomnia during pregnancy.

BELLIS P. : Wakes up early in the morning and cannot get to sleep again, specially after 1-2 A.M. at night.

BRYONIA ALBA	:	Insomnia due to business worries.
CANNABIS IND. Q	:	Very sleepy, but unable to do so. Obstinate and severe forms of insomnia. Give 10 drops a dose.
CAUSTICUM	:	Cannot sleep due to heat, specially dry heating of houses with natural gas.
CHAMOMILLA	:	Sleeplessness and restlessness during the first part of night. Gets up and walks.
CHININUM ARS. 6, ACIDUM MUR.	:	They produce sleep after taking one dose only. Sleepy but unable to sleep. Tosses about with restlessness.
CHLORALUM 200	:	It is a powerful sleep producing remedy for patients with mental diseases, asthma, hallucinations and night terrors.
CIMICIFUGA	:	Sleeplessness in children during the period of dentition.
COCCULUS IND.	:	Constant drowsiness and spasmodic yawning after loss of sleep. Vertigo.
COFFEA CRUDA	:	Insomnia after happy news, pleasant surprises and overwork. The problems of the day seem to go round and round, in the mind. It can happen even with bad news. Cannot sleep during the early hours of night. Insomnia during pregnancy and after child birth.
COLCHICUM AUTUM.	:	Great prostration as a result of loss of sleep, due to hard study or night watching. There is a feeling of internal coldness.

CONIUM MAC.	: Sleeplessness due to neuralgic pains.
CUPRUM MET. 12X	: Sleeplessness due to cramps in the body.
CYPRIPEDIUM PUB.	: Insomnia of children. Child wakes up at night and starts playing.
HELONIAS	: Sleeplessness on account of tiring, hard labour with aching of muscles.
IGNATIA AMARA	: Sleeplessness due to grief and an event like death. There is continuous yawning and a fear that she can never sleep again.
KALIUM CARB.	: Drowsy after eating. Wakes up around 2 A.M. and cannot sleep again.
KALIUM PHOS. 200X	: A great remedy for sleeplessness. The patient is weak nervously. Sleeplessness due to business worries and due to mental disturbances.
LYCOPODIUM	: Wakes up at about 4 A.M. and then cannot go back to sleep due to an overactive mind.
MAGESIUM PHOS.	: Sleeplessness on account of indigestion.
NATRIUM MUR. 200	: Sleeplessness due to grief and unpleasant events of the past.
NUX VOM.	: Sleeplessness is due to over excitement, exhaustion and stress. He is very irritable. Falls asleep but wakes up between 3 to 4 A.M., remains awake for a few hours and then again falls asleep till the usual time of getting up. Criticises others. Sleeplessness due to alcohol, drug habits, abuse or coffee.

OPIUM	:	Sleeplessness and restlessness during the time of sleeping but is sound asleep when it is time to get up. Feels chilly when uncovered and hot when covered.
PASSIFLORA Q	:	Sleeplessness due to insanity and worries. Give 15 drops a dose after 30 minutes at bed time till asleep. It produces a normal sleep.
PHOSPHORUS	:	Insomnia of old people.
PISCIDIA Q	:	Insomnia due to worry, nervous excitement, dysmenorrhea, cough and pain. Give 30-40 drops a dose near bed time. Generally, one dose is sufficient to produce a long and undisturbed sleep.
PLANTAGO	:	Insomnia of smokers.
PULSATILLA NIG.	:	Falls asleep but cannot sleep. Bed feels hot. Moves about in vain in the bed to find a cool spot. Even the ticking of a clock disturbs. Sleeplessness on account of eating very late at night.
SECALE COR.	:	Insomnia in drug and liquor habituals.
SENECIO AUR.	:	Sleeplessness during menopause, prolapse of uterus or urinary disturbances. Great drowsiness with unpleasant dreams.
STICTA PULM.	:	Insomnia due to a fracture or wound.
TABACUM	:	Insomnia due to nervous breakdown.

NOTE: Some sleep disorders are caused by physical problems, the treatment of which can make sleeplessness disappear. Some are caused by medications and can be resolved by a change of prescription. Still others are caused by poor sleep habits, such as too much napping which can be broken with education and efforts.

Below are some helpful hints for getting a good night's rest:

1. Maintain a regular sleep schedule.

2. Keep the bed room for sleeping. Do not read, watch TV or eat in bed.

3. If you do not fall asleep within 20 minutes of going to bed, get up and read or listen to some quite music, until you get sleepy.

4. Limit daytime naps.

5. Take a 20 to 30 minutes warm bath before going to bed.

6. Drink a glass of milk just before going to bed (warm or cold).

7. Avoid caffeinated beverages and chocalate in the afternoon and evening.

8. Don't drink alcohol before going to bed. It can cause sleeplessness at night.

9. Exercise during the day but not before going to bed.

IRITIS

ACIDUM NITRIC. 200	: Iritis in syphilitic patients.
COLOCYNTHIS	: A useful palliative in the pain of iritis, the pain extends to the head and is better from pressure.
HEPAR SULPHURIS	: Iritis after an exposure to cold dry

winds. Profuse discharge with pus in the anterior chamber of the eye.

MERCURIUS SOL. : Iritis after an exposure to the glare of fire usually found in foundrymen and workers of the steel rolling mills. Pus may have been formed in the interior of the eye. Iritis in patients with venereal diseases.

RHUS TOX. : Iritis after an exposure to cold and dampness. Increased lachrymation.

SYMPHYTUM OFF. : Iritis due to an injury to the eyeballs.

ITCH

AGARICUS MUS. : Itching without eruptions, changing place, sometimes here and sometimes there.

ALOE SOC. : Great burning and itching in the anus and around it. The patient bores his finger in the anus and rotates it to calm the itching. Such people are inclined towards anal intercourse.

AMBRA GRISEA : Great itching in the female organs and labia, during menses. Itching is so great that sometimes virgin girls have to bore their fingers inside the vagina and thus they rupture the hymen.

ANAGALLIS : Itching and tingling, everywhere. Itching of the palms. Skin is dry with bran like eruptions specially on hands, fingers and palms.

ANTIMONIUM CRUD.	:	Measle like eruptions. Skin dry and burns. Itching is worse at night in bed.
ARUM TRIPH.	:	There is constant picking at nose. It is so much that the patient may scratch it till it bleeding.
BELLADONNA	:	Itching with eruptions like scarlatina. Burning and redness of the skin.
CROTON TIG.	:	Itching around eyes, genitals , penis and scrotum.
DOLICHOS 6	:	Itching without eruptions. Diabetic itching. Itching is worse on the hairy parts, across the shoulders and about the elbows and knees.
GELSEMIUM	:	Itching. Measle like eruptions. Skin is hot and dry.
GRANATUM	:	Itching of palms.
HEPAR SULPHURIS, MERCURIUS SOL.	:	Pimple like eruptions on the skin, itching violently. Scratching causes ulcers.
HYDRASTIS CAN.	:	Eczema with eruptions like small pox, discharging a yellow fluid on scratching.
JUGLANS REG.	:	Itchy small red pustules. Itching more violent at night.
KALIUM ARS.	:	Intolerable itching, worse while undressing. Dry scaly acne. Itching worse from warmth, walking and undressing.
MEDORRHINUM 200	:	Intense and constant itching, worse at night and when thinking of it.

MERCURIUS SOL.	: Itching, worse from warmth of the bed at night. Vesicular and pustular eruptions. Skin is always moist.
NATRIUM SULPH.	: Itching while undressing. Wart like red lumps all over the body.
PETROLEUM	: Itching, worse in winter. Itching at night. Skin dry. Slightest scratch makes the skin suppurate. Burning.
PSORINUM	: Skin has a dirty and clingy look. Intolerable itching. Itch, worse on the scalp, bends of joints and by the warmth of bed. Skin is oily. Itching returns every winter. Scratches until the skin bleeds. Itching between fingers.
RANUNCULUS BULB.	: Burning and itching vesicles of a bluish color. Barber's itch.
RHUS TOX.	: Red, swollen skin with intense itching. Burning. Barber's itch. Urticaria like eruptions..
RUMEX CRIS.	: Intense itching of the skin specially of the lower extremities, worse on exposure to cold air and when undressing.
SELENIUM MET.	: Itching of the palms. Dry scaly eruptions on palms. Itching about the ankles and in the folds of skin, between the fingers. Skin oily. Itching of the ear.
SULPHUR	: Itching causes burning. Skin is dry and unhealthy. Itching, worse from washing. Itching, worse in the folds of skin, from warmth of the bed, in

the evening and it often recurs at spring time and in damp weather. Pruritis.

SULPHURICUM IOD. 3X : Obstinate skin affections, barber's itch and acne. Itching in the ears, nose and urethra. Papular eruptions on the face.

SULPHURICUM ACIDUM : Very useful in removing. the tendency to terrible itching.

SYPHILINUM 200 : Itching, worse at night. Hot bath relieves.

THUJA OCC. : Itching and eruptions on the covered parts only. Worse after scratching and very sensitive to touch.

THYROIDINUM : Skin dry. Itching without eruptions, worse at night.

JAUNDICE

ACONITUM NAP. : It is a good remedy in jaundice of infants, when used in the very early stages.

AESCULUS HIP. : Dull pain in the liver region radiating to the navel.

ARSENICUM ALB. : Chronic jaundice with fever. Thirst for small quantities of water at short intervals. Jaundice after abuse of quinine.

CARDUUS MAR. : Jaundice and pain in the liver region are corrected by the use of this remedy, specially in alcoholics and beer drinkers.

CARICA PAPAYA Q	: Eyes yellow. Loss of appetite. Nausea and vomiting. Pain in the right hypochondrium.
CHAMOMILLA	: Jaundice in a new born baby. Baby cries a lot.
CHELIDONIUM 6	: Pain in the right shoulder blade. Eyes are yellow and the face is also yellow. Taste is bitter. Urine is deep yellow or brown red. Stools are clay colored. This remedy is usually required in most of the cases. It is to be used for a long time.
CHINA OFF.	: This remedy will commonly ward off the development of a commencing attack of jaundice. Liver is hard and painful. Yellowish skin and eyes. White colored stools. Flatulant abdomen.
CHIONANTHUS	: A prominent liver remedy. Aching in the umbilical region. Liver sore and enlarged. Constipation. Clay colored stools or soft, yellow colored stools. No appetite.
HYDRASTIS CAN.	: There are imprints of teeth on the tongue. Nausea, vomiting and constipation may be present. Its action is marked on the liver. Liver torpid and tender. Pain in the right groin.
MERCURIUS SOL.	: It is a very specific remedy for a great number of jaundice cases. Whitish grey stools. Boring pain in the right groin, liver enlarged, sore to touch. Bile secreted deficiently.

| MYRICA C. | : | Persistent sleeplessness with jaundice. Complete loss of appetite. Bitter taste. Dull pain in the liver region. |

NATRIUM PHOS. 1X : Skin yellow. Feet icy cold during day time and burn at night. This may be given in alternation with any other remedy, especially Nat-s.

NATRIUM SULPH. 6X : Liver sore to touch with sharp stitching pains. Great size of the stools.

NUX VOM. : Throbbing pain in the region of liver. Appetite scanty. Alcoholic patient.

PLUMBUM MET. : Jaundice with a very pale skin.

PODOPHYLLUM : Liver region is sore, better by lying on the abdomen. Most suited to children. Liver region is painful, better by rubbing the part. Constipation alternating with diarrhea.

SULPHUR : In all the cases of jaundice, the treatment may be started and ended with this remedy.

THYROIDINUM 3X : In desperate cases of jaundice in new born babies, this remedy will bring back the patient, almost from the jaws of death.

JAW

ACIDUM FLUOR. : Necrosis of the upper jaw, specially right side.

ACONITUM NAP., HELLEBORUS NIG.	:	Constantly moves the lower jaw, as if chewing.
CALCAREA FLUOR., SILICEA	:	Given alternately cures necrosis of jaws.
HECLA LAVA	:	Tumor of the jaw with swelling of the jaw after tooth extraction.
LAC CAN.	:	Cracking in the jaw while eating.
PHOSPHORUS	:	Necrosis (mortification-death of) of the bones of the lower jaw.
RHUS TOX., LAC CAN.	:	Cracking in the joints of jaw, while eating or yawning.

JEALOUSY

HYOSCYAMUS NIG.	:	A suspicious person is jealous of others doing good things. He feels jealous on the property holdings of others.
LACHESIS	:	A Lachesis patient is full of love for their spouse and children. Feels very jealous on seeing them talking to others. The jealousy is on account of suspicion.
NATRIUM MUR. 1M	:	Psychic causes for jealousy. Irritable, depressed and becomes violent on little suspicions or trifles.
PLATINUM MET.	:	The jealousy in such patients is on account of their sense of pride. They like flattery particularly women and if they see somebody praising others, they feel jealous.

JOINTS

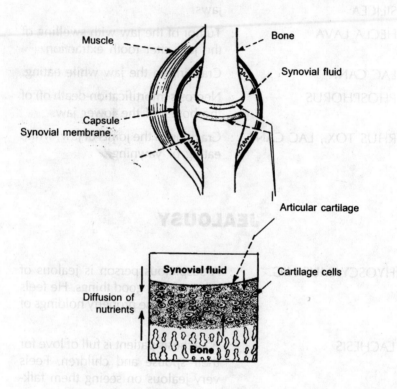

ACONITUM NAP.	:	Painless crackling in all joints of extremities.
APIS MEL., ARSENICUM ALB., CAUSTICUM, RHUS TOX., SULPHUR	:	Burning in the joints.
ARISTOLOCHIA MIL.	:	Pain in the ball and socket joints.
CALCAREA CARB., LEDUM PAL., RUTA G.	:	Nodosities (calcareous deposits on the joints).

CAUSTICUM : Rheumatic pain with tearing and drawing in the joints make him restless at night. Deformities about the joints. Pain, worse at night and better by warmth, especially heat of bed.

CROCUS SAT. : Crackling in hip joints and knees.

GINSENG Q : Crackling in joints, stiffness and contraction of the joints.

GUAIACUM OFF. Q : Rheumatic pains in the joints of arms and shoulders. Stiffness of joints with contractions. Lameness. Pressure cannot be tolerated. Pain is worse from 6 P.M. to 4 A.M., from motion and cold wet weather.

HYPERICUM PERF. : Severe nerve pains in the joints of the hips are relieved by the use of this remedy.

KALIUM BICH. : Crackling in all joints of extremities.

MAGNESIUM CARB. : Swelling in the bend of knees.

NATRIUM PHOS. : Crackling in all joints.

NATRIUM SULPH., : Crackling in knee joints.
NUX VOM.

RHODODENDRON CH. : Pain and inflammation of the great toe.

THUJA OCC. : Crackling in the joints of lower extremities.

TONGO 3X : Tearing pain in hip joints, femur and knee specially, the left.

KELOID

Scar formation in the skin following an injury or a surgical incision. The point of skin is raised with a scar on it. It takes some months to cure.

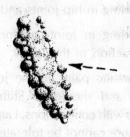

The formation of excess collagen in the form of thick interlacing bundles which causes marked swelling at the site of the wound is known as a KELOID. The essential cause is unkown but it may be due to deficent polymerisation of fibrin (factor XIII deficiency): the condition is more common among negroes.

ACIDUM FLUOR. : It acts specially on the scar tissue and is indicated in deep, destructive, processed ulcers.

GRAPHITES 200 : In the early stages of keloid. The keloid may ooze out a thin, sticky discharge.

SILICEA 200 : Keloid growth may be on the spot vaccinated or anywhere. Fistulous burrowing under process of suppuration. More suited to patients who are chilly.

THIOSINAMINUM 1X : It is a great resolvent externally and internally for dissolving scar tissues. Give three doses per day.

TUBERCULINUM : May be given once or twice during the treatment. It fastens cure.

KIDNEYS

INFLAMMATION (NEPHRITIS)

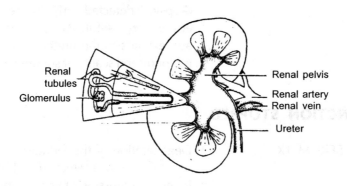

APIS MEL.	:	Burning in urine. Rash on skin. Puffiness and paleness of face. Pain in the head, back and limbs. Urine contains casts.
ARSENICUM ALB.	:	Tubular nephritis. Urine contains albumin and other casts. Dropsy. Thirst for cold water in small quantities and at smaller intervals. Restlessness and anxiety.
CANTHARIS	:	Inflammation of the kidneys. Urine is passed in drops with burning. Acute pain in the lumbar region. Urine may or may not be bloody.
FERRUM MET.	:	Pale, bloated face. Chilly. Vomiting of food or passing stools containing undigested food particles.
FERRUM PHOS. 6X	:	Fever, headache. Irritation of the bladder and a frequent desire to urinate.

MERCURIUS COR.   : For albumin in urine and inflam-
                            mation of the kidneys in pregnant
                            women.

TEREBINTHINIAE   : When congestion is prominent with
                            dropsy. If detected early, this rem-
                            edy is very useful. Pain is severe
                            and extends to the urethra. Urine
                            is bloody and scanty or suppressed.

FUNCTION STOPPED

EEL SERUM 1X   : Degeneration of the kidneys. He-
                            moglobinuria. Hematuria. Pro-
                            longed suppression of urine. Albu-
                            minuria. It puts an end to renal
                            obstruction and produces abun-
                            dant urine flow.

KIDNEY STONES
(RENAL CALCULI)

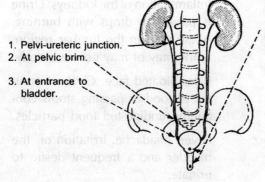

1. Pelvi-ureteric junction.
2. At pelvic brim.

3. At entrance to
   bladder.

Bilateral obstruction: in
or around bladder or ure-
thra. The ureters are also
affected and become di-
lated and become dilared
and tortuous.

Surface is rough; color brown, probably due to old blood pigment.

1. Calcium oxalate

Smooth light brown color.

Flaking surface, greyish white.

2. Uric acid and urates

3. Phosphate (calcium apatite)

BERBERIS VULG. Q	: This is the head remedy for renal stones. There is an acute pain in the region of kidneys and urethra, with a frequent desire to pass urine. Very useful for pain, when the stone is in the left kidney. Give 10 drops every hour.
CALCAREA CARB. 30	: When there is difficulty in passing urine and an attack of pain on passing the stone. Give a dose every 15 minutes.
EEL SERUM	: In affections of the kidney when there is diminished urine or when it is completely suppressed due to renal failure, this remedy produces abundant urine, cures albuminuria and removes the infection.
HYDRANGEA Q	: A remedy for gravel and for breaking stones enabling their easy passage. Can be mixed with Berberis vulgaris Q and Pareira brava Q.
LYCOPODIUM 1M	: When the pain is due to calculi in

the right kidney. It expels it.

OCIMUM CAN. : Renal calculus, specially, in the right kidney with pain on the right side. Urine smells like musk and when allowed to stand for a while, brick dust red or yellow sediment settles at the bottom. Urine contains uric acid.

PAREIRA BRAVA Q : When the renal stone has been present for a long time and is difficult to expel, give 5 drops a dose every hour. It can be given mixed with Berb. Q.

URTICA URENS Q : Its use in expulsion of renal stones is very old. It acts as a cleaning agent of the kidneys and eliminates gravel from them.

KNIFE (HOMOEOPATHIC)

MYRISTICA SEB. : Hastens suppuration and shortens, its duration. Acts more powerfully than Hepar and Silicea 3X, opens up carbuncles, fistula, abscess, etc. and does away the operation. It is often the "homoeopathic knife".

LABOR PAINS

The following symptoms will differentiate true labor pains and false labor pains :

TRUE LABOR PAINS	FALSE LABOR PAINS
1. Pains come and go, at regular intervals.	1. Pain is constant and does not go away.
2. Pains press downwards to expel the baby.	2. Pain is colic like and radiates in all the directions of the abdomen.
3. Pains arise from the uterus to produce dilatation in the uterus.	3. Pains are in the abdomen. They have no associated dilatation of the mouth of womb.
4. Each spell of pain is accompanied by a little watery discharge to dilate the os.	4. Not accompanied by any discharge and are usually due to the regions of colic and on account of gas or indigestion.

ACONITUM NAP., SULPHUR	: When lochia is suppressed or insufficient.
AGARICUS MUS.	: This remedy covers most of the complaints after the delivery of a baby.
ANTIMONIUM TART.	: The new born cannot breathe or there is difficulty in breathing although there are pulsating movements of the cord. Two small globules, dry on the tongue remove the problem.
ARNICA MONT.	: Soothes the muscles of vagina and uterus, gives a great sense of relief and comfort after delivery. The child is born after some difficulty and seems to be doing well. However within a few days, it may seem that an arm or a leg is rather limp and is not used properly. The face seems somewhat unsymmetrical or there is some difficulty in sucking. On investigation, some hemorrhages within the skull are

seen. Arnica will absorb the blood and induce maximum recovery of the damaged nerve tissue.

BELLADONNA : Retention of placenta with profuse hot blood.

CANTHARIS : Retention of placenta with painful urination.

CARBO VEG., : Falling of hair after delivery.
NATRIUM MUR., SEPIA

CAULOPHYLLUM : Extraordinary rigidity of os. Spasmodic and severe pains fly in all directions. Shivering without progress, false pains. Revives labor pains and furthers progress of labor. Caul. 200, two doses induces child birth.

CAUSTICUM : Retention of urine after delivery. Absence or weakness of uterine contractions in labor.

CIMICIFUGA : Pain shoots across the abdomen and the patient doubles up with pain. It may be given 3 to 4 months before the expected day of delivery. It ensures, safe and virtually painless delivery. It should be discontinued a week before delivery. It checks labor pains and ensures, live birth. It is very helpful when a woman habitually gives birth to dead babies.

HAMAMELIS : Hemorrhoids after confinement. Anus feels sore and raw. Black, dark and profuse blood in bleeding piles.

KALIUM CARB. : One of the best remedies after

labor and following weakness or hemorrhage, which occurs after about a week of delivery.

KALIUM PHOS. 6X : Delayed labor. Labor pains are feeble and ineffectual.

LILIUM TIG., LYCOPODIUM : Constipation after delivering a child.

PITUITRINUM 1X : Os fully dilated but labor does not takes place.

PODOPHYLLUM : Pendulous abdomen after confinement.

PSORINUM : Patient has never felt well, after delivery.

PULSATILLA NIG. 1M : Insufficient labor pains. Hemorrhage after delivery. Pains after delayed and strenuous delivery. It corrects the position of the child in the womb. Avoids false labor pains and ensures safe delivery in due time. Three doses, only at the time of delivery at an interval of 15 minutes each, before the membranes are ruptured. It avoids many complaints of labor.

STAPHYSAGRIA : For any difficulty when the child is born after Cesarean section.

SULPHUR 6, CALCAREA PHOS. 6X : If a woman habitually gives birth to dead babies or when the babies die soon after birth, give one dose each of Sulphur 6 in the morning and Calc-p. 6X in the evening during the last two months of pregnancy.

TRILLIUM PEND. : Dribbling of urine after labor.

VIBURNUM OP.	: Great uterine tonic. Cures false labor pains, which may occur prematurely, a week or a month before the actual date of delivery. Removes uterine displacement.
VISCUM ALB.	: For placental retention.

LACTATION

ACETICUM ACIDUM, CALCAREA PHOS.	: Child rejects milk because it is faulty - sour.
ACONITUM NAP., BRYONIA ALBA, PULSATILLA NIG.	: Milk is suppressed.
ACONITUM NAP., BELLADONNA	: For milk fever.
AETHUSA CYN.	: Milk and milk products cannot be digested and are vomited in large curds, as soon as taken, causing weakness and drowsiness.
AGARICUS MUS.	: Complaints from suppression of milk.
AGNUS CASTUS, ASAFOETIDA, PULSATILLA NIG.	: Absence of milk or scanty milk coming down slowly on lactating the child.
ARNICA MONT., BELLIS P.:	Inflammation of breasts, because the head of the child violently strikes against the breast while nursing.
ASAFOETIDA	: Milk appears late after labor or diminishes in quantity.
BORAX	: Milk too thick and tastes bad. Child does not want to take breast

	feed on this account. Pain in the opposite breast while nursing one breast.
BRYONIA ALBA	: Inflammation of the breasts due to accumulation of milk.
BRYONIA ALBA PULSATILLA NIG.	: Ill effects of weaning.
BUFO RANA	: Milk is bloody.
CALCAREA CARB.	: For increasing the milk supply. Menses during nursing.
CALCAREA CARB., PULSATILLA NIG.	: Milk is too profuse. To dry up milk during weaning.
CALCAREA PHOS.	: Milk tastes salty. Child refuses breast feed. Sexual excitement during nursing.
CARBO ANIMALIS	: Weakness of nursing woman.
CAUSTICUM	: Suppression of milk due to any cause which cannot be determined.
CHAMOMILLA	: Suppression of milk due to anger.
CHINA OFF., KALIUM CARB.	: Weakness during lactation.
CHIONANTHUS	: For stopping milk supply in woman who cannot nurse the baby.
CINA 200	: Child refuses to take breast feed within the first few hours of delivery. One dose sets. him right. If it fails, give Merc. 200.
COD LIVER OIL (OLEUM JEC.)	: Mix a few drops of this oil in the milk for children who cannot take milk. A few days of forced treatment will cure.
CROTON TIG.	: Pain from nipples to the back while nursing. Nipples are very sore.

GALEGA OFF. Q	:	Increases the quantity and quality of milk. It corrects anemia and impaired nutrition of nursing women.
GRAPHITES, SEPIA	:	Nipples fissured from nursing.
LAC VACCINUM DEF., LAC CAN.	:	For reducing the milk supply. Lac-c. 200 helps to dry up milk in women who cannot nurse the baby.
LACTUCA VIR.	:	For increasing milk supply.
LECITHINUM 12X, RICINUS COM. Q, ALFALFA Q	:	Excellent remedies to increase the quantity and quality of milk in nursing women.
LYCOPODIUM, BUFO RANA	:	Milk mixed with blood, as the child sucks the nipples. The child vomits blood.
MAGNESIUM MUR, NATRIUM CARB.	:	Milk disagrees.
MILLEFOLIUM Q	:	Milk does not come after labor.
NATRIUM MUR.	:	Pubic hair falls out during nursing.
PHYTOLACCA DEC.	:	Excessive secretion of milk in nursing women. Breasts hard and lumpy. Sucking and nursing causes pain in the nipples and the pain radiates to other parts of the body.
PODOPHYLLUM	:	Prolapes of uterus during nursing.
PULSATILLA NIG., SILICEA	:	Pain in the nipples and all over the body, while nursing.
PULSATILLA NIG., CALCAREA CARB., CIMICIFUGA	:	Suppression of milk flow due to sudden emotions.
RHEUM	:	Milk ceases to flow after starting.

RICINUS COM.	: To produce milk supply in nursing mothers, even in virgins.
SABAL SER.	: For producing milk supply when suppressed.
SALVIA OFF.	: Excessive flow of milk from the breasts (galactorrhea).
SECALE COR.	: Nursing women do not get sufficient milk in their breasts or there is suppression or non appearance of milk after delivery and the breasts do not fill adequately.
SEPIA	: Drinking milk makes the patient worse. Milk just does not agree.
SILICEA	: Discharge from the vagina while nursing.
STICTA PULM.	: Scanty milk. It increases the quantity of milk and removes suppression.
URTICA URENS	: Diminished secretion of milk to arrest its flow after weaning.
YOHIMBINUM Q	: Stimulates the function of lactational glands.

NOTE : Breast fed babies have a much lower chance of infection than babies fed on formula milk or milk from other animals. Breast feeding boosts the immune system of infants.

LAMENESS

BELLIS P.	: Lameness as if, sprained.
DULCAMARA	: Lameness after getting wet and cold.

LARYNGITIS
(INFLAMMATION OF THE LARYNX)

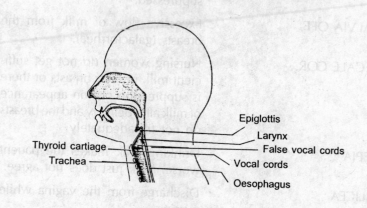

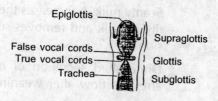

Detail of larynx

ACONITUM NAP.   : Recent laryngitis with irritating, hacking cough. Restlessness, anxiety and fever. If there is no improvement within 6 hours, select another remedy.

ANTIMONIUM CRUD.   : Laryngitis of singers. Loss of voice, improves by heat or wrapping a warm cloth around the neck.

ARGENTUM NIT.   : Loss of voice from too much singing or shouting. Hoarseness. He is better in fresh air. Raising the voice causes cough.

ARSENICUM ALB.	:	Dry, hoarse cough with burning pains.
BELLADONNA	:	Acute laryngitis. Deep red throat, painful on talking.
CALCAREA CARB.	:	Suits chronic laryngitis in fat persons.
CAUSTICUM	:	Dry, raw throat with violent cough; which may cause leakage of urine, involuntarily. Mucus drops at the back of the nose and is so copious that it becomes difficult to speak. Occasionally, loss of voice may be quite painless.
HEPAR SULPHURIS	:	When cough becomes loose and there is still hoarseness. Pain extends from ear to ear.
KALIUM BICH.	:	Cough with sticky, yellow mucus and hoarseness. Chronic laryngitis.
MENTHOLUM	:	It is curative for laryngitis.
NATRIUM SEL.	:	Chronic laryngitis and laryngeal phthisis. Hoarseness of singers. Expectorates small lumps of mucus with frequent clearing of throat.
PHOSPHORUS	:	Larynx very painful. Hoarseness, worse in the evening. Violent tickling in the larynx while speaking. Laryngitis with dry, tickly cough and hoarseness. Talking hurts.
SPONGIA	:	Barking cough and hoarseness. Burning and tickling in the larynx.

LAUGHTER

CROCUS SAT.	: Laughing and crying alternately, in cases of mental troubles.
MANGANUM ACET.	: Involuntary laughing and weeping; walking backwards.
MOSCHUS	: Uncontrollable laughter in hysterical patients.
PHOSPHORUS	: Uncontrollable laughter followed by sadness.
ZINCUM SULPH.	: Stupid laughter. The patient repeats everything said.

LAXATIVE

A glass of cold water on rising in the morning with a teaspoon full of common salt makes an excellent laxative.

CASCARA SAG. Q	: 15 drops in half a cup of water, restores the normal function of intestines and is a palliative for constipation.

LEGS

AGARICUS MUS.	: Numbness after crossing the legs.
ALUMINA	: Legs feel asleep, when sitting with legs crossed.

AMYLENUM NIT.	: Must stretch legs for hours together. Feels relieved on doing so.
ARNICA MONT.	: Soreness of the thighs.
BELLADONNA	: Jerking of the limbs during sleep.
BELLIS P.	: Pain down the front part of thighs.
CARBOLICUM ACIDUM	: Painful contraction of calves when walking.
CAUSTICUM	: Crackling and tension in the knees. Stiffness in the hollow of the knee.
CHAMOMILLA, PLATINUM MET.	: Sleeps with legs apart.
CINA	: Must lie on hands and knees.
CANNABIS IND.	: Feeling of shortness in the left leg.
COBALTUM	: Weakness of legs after emissions.
CONIUM MAC. 200	: Difficult gait, trembling, sudden loss of strength while walking, painful stiffness of the legs. Better by lying down or by putting feet on a chair.
CROCUS SAT.	: Weakness of the legs and knees.
ILLICIUM	: Pain in the thighs.
KALIUM CARB.	: Uneasiness, heaviness and tearing in the limbs with jerking. Legs and back jerk out and go to sleep easily. Constant pain in the lumbar region and legs with weakness. The patient cannot move.
LATHYRUS SAT.	: Cannot cross or extend legs while sitting. Legs feel asleep when sitting with legs crossed.
LYCOPODIUM	: Limbs go to sleep, jerk and twitch at night, in bed.

MEDORRHINUM 200	:	Legs feel heavy, ache all night. Cannot keep them still despite the of pain.
MERCURIUS SOL.	:	Weakness and trembling of the legs. Dropsical swelling of the legs and feet.
NATRIUM CARB.	:	The hollow of knee is painful on motion.
PAREIRA BRAVA	:	Pain in the upper part of the sides of thighs.
PHYTOLACCA DEC.	:	Pain in the legs. The patient is afraid to get up and stand. Pain like electric shocks in the thighs and legs.
PICRICUM ACIDUM	:	Great heaviness in legs, can hardly lift them from the ground. Tired feeling and aching in the back.
RHODODENDRON CH.	:	Must lie with legs crossed.
RUTA G.	:	Pain when straightening the limbs.
SEPIA	:	Legs, lame and stiff. Legs appear, too short. Likes to sit with legs crossed. Likes energetic exercise. Coldness.
SILICEA	:	Loss of power in the legs. Legs tremble while walking.
STANNUM MET.	:	Must lie with one leg drawn up and the other stretched out.
STAPHYSAGRIA	:	Muscles of the calves feel bruised. Extremities feel beaten up. Pain in the upper part of thigh, on its inner side. Pain in buttocks and back.
TARENTULA HIS.	:	Weakness and numbness of legs,

with twitching. Must move them constantly even though walking aggravates his troubles.

TEUCRIUM MAR. 3X	: Legs go to sleep with a tingling sensation while sitting.
THUJA OCC. 200	: Legs feel heavy, as if made of wood or glass.
VIPERA	: Patient likes to keep the legs elevated. Hanging down of legs causes an aggravation in pain and gives a feeling as if they would burst.
ZINCUM MET.	: Lameness, weakness, trembling and twitching of legs. Cannot keep them still.
ZINCUM VAL.	: Must move about. Cannot keep the legs still.

LEUCODERMA
(VITILIGO)

ARSENICUM SULPH. FLAV.	: This remedy can be given in 3X potency, thrice daily; when the improvement is retarded, give 30 potency and if it fails to cure completely, give 200 potency weekly.
BORAX	: White skin with red patches.
HYDROCOTYLE A. Q	: 5 drops thrice daily if Ars-s-f. fails to cure.
NITRICUM ACIDUM.	: Discolored zigzag patches on the

skin.The base looks like raw flesh.

PSORALEA CORYL. 3X : 5 drops thrice daily is an excellent remedy for leucoderma. It is used externally, in the form of an oil. After applying the oil, exposure to sun rays must be avoided.

PSORINUM 200 : It may be required at some stage of the disease Hair on eye brows and even eye lashes may become grey. A dose of this remedy given every week can restore the original color of hair affected by the disease.

TUBERCULINUM 200 : A dose should be given at the start of treatment.It should be repeated every month.

NOTE: Avoid milk products and citrus fruits.

LEUCORRHEA

ABROMA AUG. : Leucorrhea in diabetic ladies. Thick, whitish discharge. Dysmenorrhea.

ACIDUM FLUOR. : Acrid and profuse discharge.

ACIDUM PHOS. Q : Leucorrhea in nursing women who nurse the child longer than a year. Discharge is yellow with itching of the parts.

AESCULUS HIP. 3X : Chronic cases. Discharge dark yellow, thick and sticky. Pain in the hips and back.

AGARICUS MUS. : Discharge profuse, dark and bloody.

AGNUS CASTUS	: Discharge stains the underwear yellow or is transparent.
ALUMINA	: Discharge transparent, profuse, ropy, acrid and runs down to the legs and feet. Burning leucorrhea.
ARISTOLOCHIA CLEM.6X	: Leucorrhea of all kinds.
ARSENICUM ALB.	: Leucorrhea acrid, burning, offensive and thin.
BORAX	: Leucorrhea like white of an egg, with a sensation as if warm water is flowing. Leucorrhea and backache. Sensation as if the spine is broken and tied together.
CALCAREA CARB.	: Milky discharge. Leucorrhea in children.
CALCAREA PHOS.	: Leucorrhea like white of an egg, worse morning.Menses every two weeks and prolonged for a week or more. Backache.
AMBRA GRISEA	: Profuse, bluish leucorrhea.
CARBOLICUM ACIDUM	: Offensive leucorrhea in children.
CHELIDONIUM	: White leucorrhea that leaves yellow stains on clothes.
CHINA OFF.	: Leucorrhea before menses, fetid or bloody.
EUPIONUM	: Gushing discharge.
GRAPHITES	: Constipated patients. Discharge white, causing irritation and itching of the parts.
IODIUM	: Chronic leucorrhea, which is abundant and also corrosive as to eat holes in the underwear.

MERCURIUS SOL.	:	Discharge burns and itches, worse at night.
NATRIUM MUR.	:	Leucorrhea acrid and watery with constipation.
OVA TOSTA 3X	:	Leucorrhea and backache. Sensation that the spine is broken and tied together.
PHOSPHORUS	:	Discharge profuse, smarting and corrosive. Leucorrhea instead of menses.
PULSATILLA NIG.	:	Leucorrhea acrid, burning and creamy. Also in children.
SARACA IND. Q	:	Leucorrhea in small girls who become weak and emaciated, despite good food and regular nourishment.
SEPIA	:	Leucorrhea yellow, greenish with much itching.
SYPHILINUM 200 (LUETICUM)	:	Leucorrhea profuse, thin, watery, acrid with sharp knife like pains in the ovaries. The discharge is so profuse that it runs down to the feet. Very useful for those having a history of syphilis in the family.
THLASPI BURSA Q	:	Leucorrhea before and after menses, bloody, dark, offensive and stains the underwear. Stains do not go on washing.

LEUKEMIA

Circulatory system*

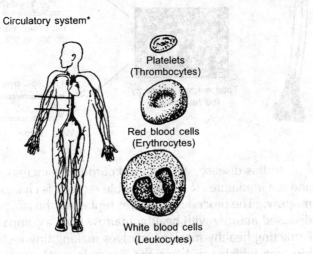

Platelets
(Thrombocytes)

Red blood cells
(Erythrocytes)

White blood cells
(Leukocytes)

*Cells not shown in actual proortion to one another.

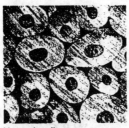

Normal cells

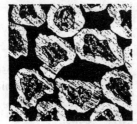

Cancer cells

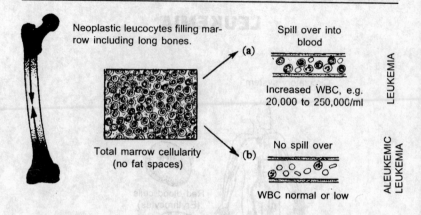

Neoplastic leucocytes filling marrow including long bones.

Total marrow cellularity (no fat spaces)

(a) Spill over into blood

Increased WBC, e.g. 20,000 to 250,000/ml

LEUKEMIA

(b) No spill over

WBC normal or low

ALEUKEMIC LEUKEMIA

In this disease, white blood corpuscles increase in number and are immature. The only reliable remedy is changing of bone marrow. The procedure involves replacing the afflicted person's diseased marrow with healthy marrow from a compatible donor. Extracting healthy marrow involves making tiny incisions in the hip area which can leave the donor in a minor discomfort for a short time. The following remedies may be used according to the symptoms :

BARYTA MUR. 3X : Vertigo, increased tension of pulse and high systolic pressure with comparatively low diastolic pressure. Cardiac symptoms are usually present.

BENZINUM 30 : Decrease in R.B.C. and increase in W.B.C.

CEANOTHUS A. Q : Splenomegaly, pain in the spleen and violent dyspnea are guiding symptoms.

CHININUM SULPH. : A rapid decrease in red blood cells and hemoglobin with a tendency to polynucleate and irregular white cells.

FERRUM PIC. 3X : Symptoms like leukemia i.e. pseudoleukemia.

MERCURIUS SOL. 1000, : High count of white blood cor-
CALCAREA CARB. 200, puscles.
BARYTA MUR.

PSORINUM : Phagocytes are defective. Patient is chilly, weak and very hungry always.

RADIUM BROM. : This remedy may prove useful when there is a marked increase in the white blood cells, having more than one nucleus.

THIOSINAMINUM : It is a remedy for wasting of spinal marrow and should prove useful in this disease.

VANADIUM MET. 6 : It is a carrier of oxygen. Increases the amount of hemoglobin and stimulates the function of white blood corpuscles (phagocytes).

NOTE: Research is required for treatment of this disease homoeopathically. Dr. Raymond Warell, a leukemia specialist at Memorial Sloan Kettering Cancer Centre, New York (USA), found low doses of Arsenicum extremely effective in the treatment of·leukemia without any side effects.

LIARS

CONIUM MAC.200 : A person is accustomed to tell lies by habit though, it may or may not benefit him. A dose or two will bring him on the right path.

LICE

Life cycle of the head louse

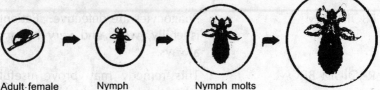

Adult female glues the nit to the hair with a cement bond, close to the scalp.

Nymph resembling miniature adult hatches in 7 to 10 days.

Nymph molts or sheds skin 3 times to reach adult stage in 10 to 14 days.

Adult life span on head about 20 days.

LYCOPODIUM 200 : It is a specific remedy for lice on the skin. 1 dose a week.

PSORINUM 200 : For lice on the hair of head, 1 dose a week.

STAPHYSAGRIA : Lice on pubic hair.

NOTE: Lice can also be picked by hand in strong light. A magnifying glass can be used if needed. Lice thus picked should be destroyed by burning. The entire head should be checked. A person suffering from this disease should not share his comb, head gear or clothes with a healthy person. His clothes should be washed separately with hot water and detergent powder.

An external lotion prepared with 50 drops of Camphora Q in 30 ml of mustard oil kills 90% of the lice with one application. The lotion should be applied on the hair, rubbing gently. The hair should be combed after about 10 minutes after placing a cloth beneath and watch dead or half dead lice and nits (eggs) falling on it. These should be destroyed by burning. This lotion should not be allowed to fall into the eyes. Then wash with soap and water after 30 minutes. Another application, if needed, should be done after a week.

LIGHT
(PHOTOPHOBIA)

BELLADONNA : General photophobia. Likes to wear sun glasses always. Aversion to light in eye troubles.

CALCAREA CARB. : Sensitive to light, which causes lachrymation. Sun light cannot be tolerated.

CROTALUS H. : Very sensitive to light specially, lamp light.

ELAPS COR. : Aversion to light. Letters run together while reading.

GRAPHITES : Intolerance of artificial light as that of electricity, lamps and candles.

MERCURIUS SOL. : The light of fire is intolerable. It dazzles the eyes. Also dislikes day light. Foundry light is not tolerated.

NUX VOM. : Photophobia, worse in the morning. Must blink eyes several times to become accustomed to light.

RHUS TOX. : General dread of light. Eyes cannot be opened for sometime in light.

SILICEA : Aversion to light specially, day light. It produces dazzling.

LIMPING

ARNICA MONT.	: When limping is due to an injury or bruise.
CALCAREA CARB.	: If lameness and limping remains after reunion of bones, after a fracture, this remedy will cure it. It also cures stiffness, which is very usual even after several months of the union of fracture.
SULPHUR	: If limping is due to weakness of the legs.

LINGUAL DELIRIUM

AILANTHUS G.	: Semi conscious. Delirious muttering and speaking unintelligently, while asleep.
KALIUM PHOS.	: Semi conscious walking in sleep.

LIPS

ALOE SOC.	: Marked redness of the lips. Lips cracked.
AMMONIUM CARB.	: Middle of the lower lip parched.
APIS MEL.	: Lips swollen specially, the lower.
ARSENICUM ALB.	: Ulceration of the lips with a burning sensation, which is relieved by taking tea or other hot drinks.

Tumor of the lips. Accumulation of dry skin debris on the lips. Cancer of the lips.

ARUM TRIPH. : Constant picking of the lips until they bleed.

BRYONIA ALBA : Lips dry and parched with excessive thirst for large quantities of water. Burning in the lower lip of old smokers.

CAPSICUM : Eczema of the lips. Give 30C orally and a drop of the mother tincture on the affected part.

CANNABIS IND., HELONIAS : Lips stick together.

CONDURANGO Q : Painful cracks, cancer on the lips.

CONIUM MAC.1M, HYDRASTIS CAN. Q : Cancer of the lips, a very important remedies in cancer.

HEPAR SULPHURIS : Middle of the lower lip is cracked.

MAGNESIUM MUR. : Blisters on the lips.

MANCINELLA : Lower lip hanging down.

MERCURIUS SOL. : Inflammation of the lips.

NATRIUM CARB., SEPIA : Swelling of the upper lip.

NATRIUM MUR. : Deep crack in the middle of the lower lip. Lips and corners of the mouth dry, ulcerated and cracked. Blisters on the lips.

NUX MOSCH. : Extreme dryness of the lips and tongue with no desire for water.

PETROLEUM : Painful cracks at the corners of the mouth.

PULSATILLA NIG. : Frequent licking of lips.

SILICEA : Cracks in the skin of lips, worse

washing.

SULPHUR   : Lips dry and burn. Bright red.

TARENTULA CUB.   : Swelling of the lower lip with dryness.

LIVER

Anatomy

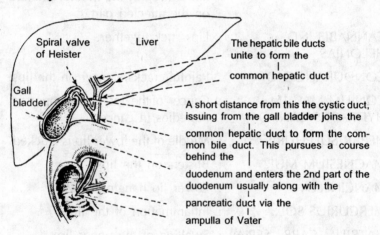

Spiral valve of Heister

Liver

Gall bladder

The hepatic bile ducts unite to form the
|
common hepatic duct

A short distance from this the cystic duct, issuing from the gall bladder joins the
|
common hepatic duct to form the common bile duct. This pursues a course behind the |

duodenum and enters the 2nd part of the duodenum usually along with the
|
pancreatic duct via the
|
ampulla of Vater

ENLARGEMENT

ACETICUM ACIDUM   : Enlargement of the liver and spleen, with emaciation.

ANTIMONIUM TART.   : Enlargement of the liver with respiratory troubles.

CALCAREA ARS. 200   : Enlargement of the liver in infants.

CHINA OFF.	: Hard and an enlarged liver. White stools.
CHIONANTHUS Q	: Enlargement with soreness of the liver and yellow urine. Pain in the liver and back.
CHOLESTERINUM 3X	: Obstinate distention and congestion of the liver. Burning pain on the right side, on walking holds the hands on sides, as it hurts.
MERCURIUS SOL.	: Constipation. No appetite. Depression or deficient bile secretion.
NATRIUM SULPH. 6	: Chronic enlargement of the liver. Soreness and tenderness in the liver region. Urine is yellow, foamy and scanty.
PHOSPHORUS	: Enlargement in anemic people.
PODOPHYLLUM	: Diarrhea due to liver problems.

INFLAMMATION

CHELIDONIUM 6	: Removes enlargement, inflammation, etc. of the liver. A long use is required. 3-4 doses a day.
NATRIUM MUR.	: Liver region is sore with gastric troubles.
PHOSPHORUS	: Inflammation of the liver in anemic subjects. Enlargement.
VIPERA	: Enlargement of the liver with severe pain, jaundice and fever. Pain extends to the hips and shoulders.

DROPSY

ARGENTUM NIT.	:	Dropsy in first stage, when the emaciation and marasmus starts on account of liver problem.
CARDUUS MAR. Q	:	Chronic cases of liver troubles with dropsy.
LYCOPODIUM	:	Hardness of the liver with dropsy. Inherited liver affections.

CONSTIPATION

CHIONANTHUS Q	:	5 drops in water thrice daily for constipation and other conditions of the liver.
MAGNESIUM MUR.	:	Patient has no desire for stool for days together with liver problems.
NASTURTIUM AQUA.	:	Dropsy of the liver with degenerative changes in its cell; resistance to the flow of blood through the liver.

SWELLING

ACETICUM ACIDUM	:	Swelling of feet and legs with emaciation.
PTELEA TRI.	:	Swelling of feet and legs. Strenuous breathing.

HEADACHE

MYRICA C.	:	Headache, worse in the morning. Color of the skin, eyes, tongue and urine is yellow.

FEVER

FERRUM ARS. 6
: Fever due to enlargement and inflammation of the liver is cured by this remedy.

EMACIATION

ACETICUM ACIDUM
: Emaciation produced due to liver defects. Unquenchable thirst and diarrhea. Enlargement of the liver and spleen.

LIVER ABSCESS

HEPAR SULPHURIS
: This is given in liver abscesses and suppurative conditions of the liver.

PTELEA TRI.
: Aching and heaviness in the liver region, which is greatly aggravated by lying on the left side.

LIVER SPOTS

There may be light yellow to black spots on the skin. These may be due to indigestion, or due to syphilis or cancer and in pregnancy and some other uterine conditions. These conditions must be found out and cured. Liver spots will disappear automatically.

Liver spots of pregnancy disappear after the birth of the baby. The following medicines are usually indicated:

CURARE	: Spots of yellow brown color.
LYCOPODIUM	: Spots on the face and especially on the abdomen.
MEZEREUM	: This is indicated when the color of the spots is dark brown, blue or black. Spots may be on the chest and arms.
NATRIUM HYPO SULPH. Q	: Use for liver spots - locally and internally. 5 drops in water thrice daily.
PLUMBUM MET.	: Liver spots during the period of menopause. They disappear after menopause.

LOCHIA

Discharges from the vagina consist of mucus, blood and tissue debris following child birth.

CIMICIFUGA	: Suppression of lochia, due to anxiety or emotional disturbances.
CROCUS SAT.	: If the quantity of discharge is profuse and contines too long.
PULSATILLA NIG.	: Sudden suppression of lochia.
KREOSOTUM	: Acrid, offensive and intermittent lochia.

LUMBAGO
(PAIN IN MID AND LOWER BACK)

ACONITUM NAP.

: Lumbago, after exposure to draught. Pain sharp, as if sprained.

AESCULUS HIP. 3X

: Very difficult to rise from a sitting position. Dull pain in the back with hemorrhoids. Backache during pregnancy.

ANTIMONIUM TART.

: Backache from fatigue, worse while sitting. Sensation of weight on the coccyx. Slightest effort to move cause retching.

ARNICA MONT.

: Lumbago from an injury.

BRYONIA ALBA

: Pain excited by every motion. Muscles sensitive to touch.

CALCAREA FLUOR.

: If Rhus-t. fails, try this remedy.

CIMICIFUGA

: Muscular pain with restlessness.

GINSENG Q

: When no other remedy is well indicated, use this remedy. Stiffness and feeling of contraction in the back.

GNAPHALIUM Q

: Chronic lumbago. Backache, worse from movement. Feeling of stiffness and contraction in the back. Pressure cannot be tolerated. Pain worse from 6 P.M. to 4 A.M. and cold weather.

PHYTOLACCA DEC.

: Pain in the lumbar and sacral region. Worse in the morning and damp weather.

RHUS TOX.

: Bruised or burning pains. Stiffness of the back. Lumbago on exposure to cold and long standing.

LUNGS

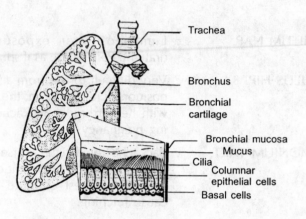

ANTIMONIUM ARS.   : Useful in destruction of lung passages causing breathing difficulties.

ANTIMONIUM TART.   : Rapid, short, difficult breathing, seems as if he would suffocate. Better by lying on the right side. Emphysema of the aged.

APOCYNUM CAN. 1X   : Congestion of the lungs in dropsy. Gasping respiration. Water is swallowed the wrong way into the wind pipe, which is a very dangerous condition.

ARSENICUM ALB.   : Breathing is oppressed. Respiration, wheezing on account of lung troubles.

ASPIDOSPERMA Q   : It is a lung tonic. Removes temporary obstruction to the oxidation of blood by stimulating respiratory centres, increasing oxidation and excretion of carbolic acid. Thrombosis of the pulmonary artery. 5 drops a dose every 2 hours till required. A great lung tonic.

COCA Q

: Emphysema. Want of breath, short breath.

QUEBRACHO Q

: Emphysema. Want of breath during exercise.

SENEGA

: Chronic emphysema. Portion of lungs is destroyed. Old asthmatics with congestive attacks.

TRIBULUS TER. Q

: This remedy is given in lung cancer. 10 drops a dose four times a day.

LUPUS

(ULCERATING SKIN DISEASE)

APIS MEL.

: Lupus with characteristic effects of bee stings with rosy swelling, stinging pains, and intolerance of heat and slightest touch.

CISTUS CAN.

: Lupus with hard and indurated glands. Skin hard, dry, fissured with deep cracks. Itching all over. Can be used locally in tincture form, 5 drops in one ounce of water to wash and arrest the fetid discharge.

GUAREA T. Q

: Lupus with red, yellow or brown pigmentation of skin.

HYDROCOTYLE A. Q

: Dry eruptions with great thickening of the epidermoid layer and exfoliation of scales. Lupus non-exudens.

KALIUM BICH. : Papular or vesicular eruptions resembling small pox with itching and burning.

RADIUM BROM. : Inflammation and swelling of the skin with ulceration and redness. Burning and itching of skin. A good remedy under these circumstances for lupus.

THUJA OCC. 1000 : Treatment may be started with this remedy. Next indicated remedy should be given 24 hours after its use. In some cases, the use of this remedy alone in 30C potency for a very long period may cure the disease.

NOTE: **In 1851, the french dermatologist Cazenave employed the latin term 'LUPUS' (meaning wolf) to describe the skin rash that spread over the bridge of nose and cheeks in a characteristic butterfly shape. Why he named it so, is unclear. The disease affects women 8 to 10 times more than men. It usually appears in women between the ages of 20-40 years, although it can occur at any age. Nausea, vomiting and abdominal pain may accompany. It is an ulcerating skin disease and requires a prolonged treatment.**

MARASMUS

Marasmus is general weight loss or wasting, especially is young children, primarily due to prolonged dietary deficiency of protein and calories.

ABROTANUM
: A very useful remedy in marasmus, especially of lower extremities with a good appetite.

BARYTA CARB.
: Child is weak and sluggish with tonsillitis. Abdomen is large.

FERRUM PHOS. 6X.,
CALCAREA PHOS. 6X,
NATRIUM MUR. 6X
: Two tablets of each and all the three mixed, should be given once early in the morning along with other indicated remedeis at an interval of three hours.

IODIUM 200
: It may be noted that this remedy in lower potencies reduces weight and in higher potencies 200-1000 increases weight. There is extreme hunger, the child eats well and yet emaciates rapidly. The skin appears yellow and there is a problem with the thyroid gland.

PEPSINUM
: Marasmus of children fed on artificial food.

PLUMBUM MET.
: Emaciation due to anemia.

SYPHILINUM 1M
: A dose of Syph. should be given after Tuberculinum. Follows it advantageously but it should be given, only if, there is a history of syphilis in the family.

TUBERCULINUM 1M
: Treatment should be started with this remedy and no other remedy should be given for the next 24 hours.

MASTURBATION

BELLIS P.
: Ill effects of masturbation are remedied by the use of this medicine.

CALADIUM SEG.
: Women have excessive sexual desire. May also be due to pruritus of vulva and vagina. Desire is more during pregnancy. If they cannot get a partner, they masturbate.

CONIUM MAC.
: A man who is unable to penetrate the woman due to deficient erections of the penis, masturbates to satisfy his lust. This remedy improves his sexual powers and thus eradicates this habit.

GRATIOLA OFF.
: It is specific for removing the bad habit of masturbation, in ladies.

ORIGANUM MAJ. 3X
: Women who have unexplained nervous disorders. Irritation in the sexual system causes an irresistible desire for sexual intercourse and when it cannot be had for some reasons, they masturbate. These lascivious impulses are cured by this remedy.

PLATINUM MET.
: Sexual excitement, both physical and mental in young boys. It is useful to subdue the excitement and helps boys to stop masturbation. Such boys are inclined to sodomy i. e. anal sex with other boys due to excessive sexual excitement. This remedy is useful in such cases.

STAPHYSAGRIA : Masturbation in children of both sexes for the sake of thrill only. This remedy cures this habit and its bad effects.

MEASLES

It is an acute disease, characterized by a catarrhal inflammation of the respiratory mucous membranes with fever and a generalized eruption of a dusky red color, on the skin.

ACONITUM NAP. : In the beginning, on appearance of the catarrhal symptoms, the patient demands water at night though he has seldom done so in the past. He is chilly and restless.

BELLADONNA : If Acon. in four doses does not help and there is a sore throat, headache, cough and swollen face, give this remedy.

BRYONIA ALBA : It is a very useful remedy when the patient is quite and does not want to be disturbed.

CAMPHORA 1X : If the eruptions do not appear or are deficient in appearance, give 2 or 3 drops a dose on a lump of sugar, till the reaction sets in.

CUPRUM ACET. : When there are convulsions during the disease.

HYDRASTIS CAN. : For weakness remaining after measles.

KALIUM BICH. : Measles complicated with respiratory troubles.

MERCURIUS SOL., SILICEA	: If after the fever, cough remains use either of these remedies according to the indications.
MORBILLINUM 200	: It should be given at the commencement of the disease. As a prophylactic, one dose daily for three days. It will prevent the disease from attacking them.
NATRIUM MUR.	: Blisters remaining in the mouth after measles are cured by this remedy.
PULSATILLA NIG.	: Pulsatilla 1M, one dose every night for three days acts as a prophylactic in this disease. When the disease has taken hold and there is marked digestive catarrh with diarrhea and the patient does not want to be covered though he has fever, give this remedy in 30 potency, thrice daily.
RHUS TOX.	: Soreness all over the body. Restlessness and pain.

MEMORY

ACONITUM NAP.	: Does not remember dates and recent events.
AETHUSA CYN.	: No interest in remembering things.
AGARICUS MUS.	: Suited to children who forget their lessons. Stupid children.
AGNUS CASTUS, ACIDUM PHOS.,	: Loss of memory due to sexual excesses and masturbation. Take

STAPHYSAGRIA	other symptoms of the remedy into account.
AILANTHUS G.	: Words spoken a little while ago, are forgotten.
AMBRA GRISEA	: An old man or a man who has grown old before time cannot remember the simplest words to express himself. Changes irrelevantly from one subject to another.
ANACARDIUM ORI.	: Loss or weak memory after small pox and chicken pox. Remembers a thing now and a moment after forgets it. Irresistible desire to curse. The patient is depressed and irritable.
ARGENTUM NIT.	: The patient is absent minded and has a poor memory.
AURUM MET.	: Absent mindedness. The patient is apathetic and listless.
BARYTA CARB.	: Absent mindedness in old people. Age has impaired all the functions including memory.
CAMPHORA	: Loss of memory after hysterical attacks.
CANNABIS IND.	: Very forgetful. Starts to speak but forgets, what he has to say.
COCCULUS IND.	: Mind distracted. Easily worried.
CONIUM MAC.	: Absent mindedness, debility and hypochondria. Poor memory, accompanied by disorders of urinary tract and sexual weakness.
DIGITALIS	: Thinking difficult. Forgets everything.
GLONOINUM	: He forgets the name of his own street and the number or location

of his own house, where he has been staying for a long time.

KALIUM BROM.	: Absent mindedness. Impaired co-ordination. Numbness and tingling in the limbs.
LAC CAN.	: Makes purchases and goes home without picking them up. Goes to post a letter and comes back with the letter in his pocket. Cannot concentrate while studying or in anything.
LYCOPODIUM	: Weakness of memory after an attack of influenza. Uses wrong words and cannot express himself properly. Commits mistakes in spelling, writing and is averse to any mental work. Suitable for old people.
MANCINELLA	: Wandering thoughts. Sudden vanishing of thoughts.
MERCURIUS SOL.	: Absent mindedness with loss of will power and a weak memory.
RHODODENDRON CH.	: Sudden disappearance of thoughts. Omits words while writing.
RHUS TOX.	: Incapable of a continuous thought. Writes incorrect figures. If he has to write 31, he writes only 3 or 1.
SCUTELLARIA LAT.	: Loss of memory or weakness of memory in nervous persons.
STRAMONIUM	: Uses incorrect words while talking or delivering a speech because he has no memory of the correct words.
SULPHUR	: Does not remember names and words.

THYROIDINUM 3X	: Improves memory of patients with thyroid problems.
VANADIUM MET.	: It helps to increase memory.
ZINCUM PHOS.	: Weakness of memory due to mental weakness. Cannot keep his legs still.

MENINGITIS

It is an inflammation of the membranes covering the brain or spinal cord.

ACONITUM NAP. ·	: It is the first remedy to be thought of in this disease. Nocturnal furious delirium. Fullness of head. Heavy, pulsating, hot and bursting pressure in the head. Sensation as if the brain was floating in boiling water.
APIS MEL.	: It is very useful in spinal and cerebral meningitis. Heat, throbbing and distensive pains, better by pressure and worse by motion.
ANACARDIUM ORI.	: Brain confused with total loss of memory.
BELLADONNA	: High fever. Face is red and hot but lower extremities are cold. Violent delirium is usually present.
CICUTA VIR.	: When there are convulsions.
CUPRUM MET.	: It is useful when there are convulsion resembling epilepsy.
GLONOINUM	: Indicated during pulsations in the temples, fever and vomiting.

NATRIUM SULPH.   : It is a very good remedy for spinal meningitis, specially if the patient is living in a damp house or basement. The patient dislikes speaking or to be spoken to. Any sound, even the ringing of a telephone is unbearable.

ZINCUM MET.   : Useful in children suffering from this disease. Child is awakened by fear. Rolls his head and cries in his sleep.

MENOPAUSE
(CHANGE OF LIFE)

In women, it occurs between 35-55 years of life. Menses may stop suddenly or there may be a decreased flow each month until there is a final cessation or the periods may be lengthened until complete cessation is accomplished. Surgical menopause occurs in almost 50% of women aged 50-64 years. It is surgically induced·by removal of ovaries irrespective of age, characterizing the end of child bearing years.

In men, it is generally between the age of 50-60 years when some changes in his behaviour may be noticed. When menses in a woman halts,the estrogen level begins to drop. Fatigue, insomnia, headache, irritability, depression, loss of the memory and concentration are a series of conditions associated with climacteric. All these symptoms have been dealt with under the appropriate heads and may be consulted in case of need. Calc-p. and Symphytum (tincture) will be found useful. Weight bearing exercise, calcium supplement and soyabean foods are helpful during this difficult period of change in life.

ALOE SOC.	: Given in frequent doses cures protracted, exhausting and obstinate hemorrhage from the uterus which occurs in women of nervous, relaxed and phlegmatic habits during this difficult period of change of life.
AMYLENUM NIT. 3X	: Climacteric headache and flashes of heat with anxiety and palpitation. It may accompany facial flushing.
AURUM MUR.	: Hemorrhage from the womb during menopause.
CALCAREA ARS.	: Slightest exertion causes palpitations of the heart. It suits specially to women, especially those who are fleshy.
CALCAREA CARB.	: Diseases of fat women around climacteric. Pituitary and thyroid dysfunction.
CAMPHORA	: Flushes of heat and sweat in a warm room. Feels hot when covered and cold, when uncovered. Feet and limbs feel cold.
CIMICIFUGA	: Rheumatic pains. Headache. Menses, when they appear, are clotted, painful and profuse. Amenorrhea.
CONIUM MAC.	: Problems of women, specially old maids during and after menopause. Great debility in the morning in bed.
FICUS REL. Q, FICUS IND. Q	: 5 drops of either in a little water given four times a day arrests the unusual bleeding during meno-

pause.

FRAXINUS A. : Mental disorders at the time of menopause. Cold creeping and hot flushes.

GELSEMIUM : Otalgia during menopause. It is a sure remedy.

GINKGO BILOBA Q : It helps mood disorders and memory problems during the climacteric period.

GUNPOWDER 3X, HECLA LAVA 3X : Osteoporosis. Inflammation of the bones during menopause.

HELONIAS : Debility and menorrhagia, during menopause.

HYPERICUM PERF. : It eases depression during menopause.

LACHESIS : Flooding at climacteric and in precancerous flowing. Palpitations, hot flushes, headache and hemorrhage. Mental troubles.

MANCINELLA : Mental depression at menopause.

OOPHORINUM 3X : Nervous climacteric disturbances generally - whether menopause is natural or is produced surgically by the removal of ovaries. Skin disorders, acne rosacea.

PLATINUM MET. : Suits arrogant and proud ladies, who are prone to localized numbness and coldness. Ovaritis with excessive bleeding.

PULSATILLA NIG. : Menses suppressed, appear too late and are scanty. Suits ladies who are sad, mild, gentle and yeilding with a weeping disposition. Likes open air even if she feels chilly.

SANGUINARIA CAN. : Burning sensation as from hot water. Bearing down with leucorrhea smelling like fish or old cheese. Headache during menopause. Climateric disorders with sensation of burning in various parts, face, palms, soles, stomach, etc. Hot flushes.

SENECIO AUR. : Insomnia during the menopausal stage. Great drowsiness with unpleasant dreams.

SEPIA : Unusual bleeding during menopause. Hot flushes at menopause with weakness and perspiration. Aversion to coitus.

VALERIANA Q : Sleep disturbances. Sleepless with nocturnal itching and muscular spasms.

NOTE1: Hot flushes are felt by women 2-4 years before menopause (pre-menopause) and after the post-menopausal period. This usually occurs when the hormones are low. Hot flushes are highest when the hormonal levels are lowest. The flushes involve a sensation of heat spreading up from the abdomen to the neck. The exact cause of this remains a mystery.

NOTE 2: Post menopausal period can also be a difficult time for some women. It can be a time for emotional distress,anxiety, depression with physical symptoms like hot flushes,intermittent bleeding, palpitations,weight gain, insomnia and headaches. In homoeopathy, the diagnosis and the consequent treatment of pre or post menopausal difficulties is specific to the patient individually as it reflects her unique experience of the disease.

MENORRHAGIA

(MENOSTAXIS)

Excessively prolonged or profuse menses.

ALOF SOC. : Too early ,too profuse, too long lasting periods.

AMBRA GRISEA, BOVISTA: Discharge of blood between periods.

ARSENICUM ALB. : Chronic menorrhagia with thin, corrosive and burning leucorrhea.

BELLADONNA : Bright red, hot flow with head symptoms.

CALCAREA CARB. : Too early, too profuse, especially in pale subjects with cold and damp feet; marked tendency to gain weight.

CHAMOMILLA : Periods prolonged due to disturbing emotions. Great irritability.

CHINA OFF. 1X : Black lumps in' blood.

CROCUS SAT. : Blood clotted, with long strings; worse from least movement.

CYCLAMEN : Profuse, black, membranous, clotted blood, too early, with labor like pains from back to pubes.

ERIGERON : Menorrhagia with bright red flow of blood. Continuous profuse bleeding during menses.

FERRUM MET. : Simple increase in normal flow.

HAMAMELIS Q : Dark blood accompanied with ovarian irritation caused by a fall.

HELONIAS : Too early, too profuse,too long lasting periods with bearing down, prolapsed and rectal urging. Menses protracted, exhausting and obstinate.

IPECACUANHA : In severest form of prolonged menses, which otherwise is simple. Bright red discharge with or without nausea.

KREOSOTUM : Menses too early, prolonged. Menstrual flow intermits, ceases on sitting or walking; reappears on lying down.

MILLEFOLIUM : Menses early, profuse, protracted (prolonged). Hemorrhage from the uterus; bright red fluid.

NITRICUM ACIDUM : Coming on too soon and again returning, soon after. Violent cramps with irritable, green leucorrhea. Urine smells like horse's urine. Restless after midnight.

NUX VOM. : Menses before time. Copious and lasts a few days longer. Blood black.

SABINA : Bright red flow with bearing down in the abdomen.

SARACA IND. Q (ASHOKA) : Profuse menses black in color, painful foul smelling, and various uterine troubles.

SECALE COR. : Menses irregular, copious, dark; continuous oozing of watery blood until next period.

SEPIA : Heavy menstruation with faintness and tearfulness. Pain in the uterus is severe enough to cause fainting.

THLASPI BURSA Q : Increased, copious flow with clots

and debility which remains even between periods.

TRILLIUM PEND.   : Menses every two weeks lasting a week or longer.

USTILAGO MAY.   : Menorrhagia at climaxis; oozing of dark blood, clotted forming long strings.

MENTAL DEVELOPMENT

AGARICUS MUS.   : Children are slow in learning due to slow development of brain. He makes mistakes and does not remember lessons. The patient is sluggish in habit and appears foolish. Late in learning, talking and walking.

CALCAREA CARB.   : Child is late in learning to walk.

NATRIUM MUR.   : Child is late in learning to talk.

METRORRHAGIA

BOVISTA   : Bleeding between periods and profuse, bloody leucorrhea. Inter menstrual bleeding.

ERIGERON   : Metrorrhagia with violent irritation of rectum and bladder, prolapsus uteri. Bright red flow.

FERRUM PHOS.   : Menses every three weeks, with a bearing down sensation and pain

	on top of the head. Vagina dry and hot.
NITRICUM ACIDUM	: Bleeding between periods with pain in the back and legs. This may happen due to over exertion or lifting heavy weights.
PHOSPHORUS	: Slight hemorrhage from uterus between periods. Menses too early, scanty and last too long. Weeps before menses.
SABINA	: Discharge of blood between periods, with sexual excitement. Hemorrhage from the uterus with partly clotted blood, worse from least motion.
SECALE COR.	: Continuous oozing of thin watery blood between periods and until the start of next period.
THLASPI BURSA Q	: Too frequent and copious menses. Hardly recovers from one period when another starts.
TRILLIUM PEND. Q	: Menses every two weeks, long lasting for a week or over and leucorrhea between the periods of bleeding.

MIGRAINE

A throbbing, one sided severe pain in the head often with nausea, vomiting and photophobia. Neck stiffness and depression may accompany.

BELLADONNA	: Throbbing the pain with fullness, especially in the forehead, also

occiput, and temples. Pain worse light, noise, and semi-erect posture. Headache worse on right side.

BROMIUM : Migraine, chiefly of the left side worse stooping, after drinking milk and at the sight of running water.

CANNABIS IND. : It is one of the most useful remedies in cases of migraine. Its use decreases the pain and distress. Sensation as if the top of the head was opening and shutting. Flatulence. Throbbing in the occiput, attacks after unusual excitement. Worse from coffee, liquor and smoking and better by rest.

CARBOLICUM ACIDUM : Migraine in children. Tight feeling on the head as if compressed by a rubber band, worse over the right eye, better by smoking and drinking tea.

CHIONANTHUS Q : 5 drops of this medicine every two hours, relieves the immediate distress. Thereafter, it should be given in 30 potency. Also Damiana Q should be given every two hours during the attacks, if they occur at all. This treatment usually cures migraine.

CIMICIFUGA : In migraine, pains are like electric shocks, worse during menses. More the flow more the suffering. Pain is better by warmth and eating. Sensation of opening and shutting in the brain.

COCA	: Migraine with fatigue and worry, accompanied with vertigo.
COFFEA CRUDA	: A good remedy for patients who suffer from sleeplessness. Migraine caused by excitement.
CYCLAMEN	: Migraine is accompanied by sparkling before the eyes.
DAMIANA Q (TURNERA)	: Give 15-20 drops in a dose every 30 minutes during the attack. It usually puts the patient to sleep after two doses and gives relief. Rest in a quite, darkened room during the attack gives relief to all the symptoms.
IPECACUANHA	: Migraine accompanied with constant nausea and vomiting. Pain may extend to the face, teeth and tongue. Vomiting does not relieve. It is better with eyes closed, rest and pressure. The cause may be stress or indigestion.
IRIS VERS.	: Migraine with acidity due to indigestion and sour vomiting. Right temple is especially affected. It is worse while resting.
LAC CAN. 200	: If pain changes sides, first on the right side of the head, then on the left side and so on. This remedy will cure it.
MELILOTUS OFF.	: Headache with retching, vomiting, sense of pressure over orbits and black spots before eyes; sick headache. Neuralgia around and over the right side of head and neck.

NATRIUM MUR. : It cures chronic severe migraine, with throbbing, as if a thousand little hammers striking the brain. The patient is anemic. Vomiting generally accompanies. It suits school girls with this disease. Pain is worse on rising in the morning and gradually subsides as the day advances. Terrible, severe headache accompanied with high blood pressure and during menstruation.

NUX VOM. : Heavy pressive headache with giddiness, flushed face, gastric derangement after overeating, drinking or smoking. Better in fresh air and cold applications.

ONOSMODIUM : A remedy for migraine. Pain in the morning on walking, chiefly left sided. Headaches from eyestrain and sexual excesses.

PSORINUM : Headache relieved by keeping a hot water bottle on the head. Pain is worse at night and is like that of a blow on the head. During the attack, patient feels hungry.

PULSATILLA NIG. : Migraine due to emotions, hormonal changes specially in women, with weeping tendencies. It is better by cold, cold drinks, fresh air and sympathy and is worse towards the evening and in a warm room.

SANGUINARIA CAN. : Headache usually starts in the morning at the back of the head and gradually spreads upwards to the right eye where it settles down.

Pain may spread to the right shoulder. Sun headaches, worse right side and at climacteric. Headache every seventh day.

SAPONARIA OFF.   : Pain in the left temple and left eye, photophobia, hot sticks in the eyes, severe pain before menstrual flow and worse left side. Severe sore throat and sneezing may be present along with the headache.

SCUTELLARIA LAT. Q   : Sick headache appearing after excitement and over exertion. 5-10 drops a dose.

SENECIO AUR.   : Sharp pain over the left eye and through the left temple. Dull, stupefying headache. Some problem of the female organs or urinary organs is generally present.

SEPIA   : Periodic, weekly headaches. Sensation as if the head would burst and the eye would come out. Better by rest, closing eyes, in open air and lying on the painful side. Throbbing, sticking pain with nausea and vomiting. Headache at climacteric and menses with scanty flow.

SILICEA   : Migraine with a strong desire to cover the head. Pain starts at the back of the head and settles over one eye. Pain is relieved by pressure and urinating. It is worse in cold windy weather.

SPIGELIA   : Headache starts from the nape of the neck and extends to the left

eye. Pain as if a band was around
the head.

TONGO Q   : Neuralgic headaches with throbbing and heat.

NOTE : Here are some ways of minimising the headache:

1.   Get up and go to bed at the same time, each day.

2.   Always eat at the same time during the day.

3.   Stretch neck and shoulders regularly.

4.   Take a few deep breaths, each day.

MILK

Milk is one of the most precious gifts of nature. For a few
months of its life, a child takes only milk as food. It contains all
the nourishment required for growth like vitamin A, B, C and D
in adequate quantities for the needs of the growing child. Breast
milk contains antibodies which are present in mother's blood,
a number of enzymes, proteins, etc. and this makes it, perfect
food. It is digested easily and is an essential diet for all young
and old. If it causes disorders, the following remedies can be
used to remove the disorders. See chapter "Lactation" also.

AETHUSA CYN.   : Intolerance of milk, which is vomited out in large curds soon after
swallowing.

BORAX   : Milk is too thick and tastes bad;
the child does not take; breast
feed. This remedy when given to
the mother will remove this defect.
The other way is to change the
milk.

CALCAREA PHOS. 6X   : Milk tastes salty. If so, change the
milk. In other cases, give this

remedy both to the child and the mother.

CINA : Vomiting and diarrhea, immediately after taking milk.

MAGNESIUM MUR. : Milk is not tolerated as it cannot be digested and this produces discomfort.

NATRIUM CARB. : Averse to milk because it causes belching, wind and diarrhea.

SEPIA : The patient is worse after taking milk, specially boiled milk. Abdomen bloats up and the patient has nausea even at the smell of milk.

MISCARRIAGE

(SEE ABORTION)

MOLES

(BIRTH MARKS)

These are harmless unless irritating. For irritation the following remedies has been found to be useful :

ACIDUM FLUOR. 200 : Helps in removal of birth marks.

BELLIS P. Q : External use of this remedy is useful in curing the moles.

CALCAREA CARB., SILICEA : Removes disposition to the formation of moles.

LYCOPODIUM 200	: A good remedy for the removal of moles.
RADIUM BROM.	: Irritation of moles is relieved by the use of this remedy.
THUJA OCC. Q	: Should be applied externally, twice a day.

MOODS

ANTIMONIUM CRUD.	: Sentimental and moody.
CROCUS SAT.	: Frequent and extreme changes in moods. One moment he is pleasant, sings and laughs and the other moment, he becomes angry. Sudden changes from happiness to sadness. Anger followed by repentance.
CROTALUS H.	: Clouded perception and memory. Impatient.
IGNATIA AMARA	: Introspective, silent brooding. Sighing and sobbing after shock, grief and disappointment. Extremely changeable moods.
NUX MOSCH.	: Changeable moods from tears to laughter. Confused impaired memory. Bewildered.
PULSATILLA NIG.	: Changeable and contradictory. Mild and gentle. Yielding disposition. Cries easily. Better in fresh air.
SARSAPARILLA	: Despondent, sensitive and easily offended. Ill humoured and uncommunicative. Reserved.

TARENTULA HIS.   : Sudden changes in moods. Ungrateful and discontented.

MOONLIGHT

CALCAREA CARB.   : The patient is worse during new moon.

CLEMATIS ERECTA   : Inflammation of eczema increases with the increasing moon and decreases with the decreasing moon.

KALIUM BROM.   : Epileptic attack comes during full moon.

SILICEA   : All the complaints are worse at new moon.

THUJA OCC.   : Complaints from moonlight. Sleepiness and feeling just bad. ,

MORNING SICKNESS

ARSENICUM ALB.   : Vomiting, worse after eating and drinking. Restlessness. Great thirst for small quantities of water.

IPECACUANHA   : Mouth moist and tongue clean. Constant nausea and vomiting.

LAC VACCINUM DEF.   : Obstinate vomiting and constant nausea with restlessness.

LOBELIA INF.   : Extreme nausea and vomiting.

Faintness and weakness in the epigastrium.

NUX VOM. : Flatulence and vomiting, worse after eating in the morning. Tongue coated.

SYMPHYTUM OFF. : Persistent vomiting with gastric disturbances, bitter taste and constipation.

SYMPHORICARPUS : Persistent vomiting of pregnancy. Nausea during menses. Nausea, worse any motion.

MOSQUITO BITES

AZADIRACHTA IND. : 2% of this remedy is mixed with 98% of coconut oil or baby oil and Margosa Q, and applied to the exposed parts. It removes the possibility of mosquito bites on that part.

LEDUM PAL. 200 : It gives immediate relief from itching, burning and swelling of the skin.

STAPHYSAGRIA 6 : While living in an area infected with mosquitoes, three doses taken daily will avoid mosquito bites.

MOUNTAIN SICKNESS

COCA Q : A mountaineer's remedy. Useful in complaints of mountain climbing such as palpitation, breathlessness, anxiety and insomnia.

MOUTH

ACONITUM NAP., HELLEBORUS NIG., STRAMONIUM
: Chewing motions of the mouth.

AMMONIUM CARB.
: Corners of mouth sore, cracked and burn. Dryness of the mouth and throat.

ANTIMONIUM CRUD., CONDURANGO, PSORINUM, NATRIUM MUR., HEPAR SULPHURIS, HYDRASTIS CAN.
: Blisters in the mouth or cracks near the corner of the mouth and lips as per indication of the remedy. Psorinum is indicated, if the cracks at the corners of the mouth are more chronic. In Nat-m., the sores on the lips and around the mouth are cold.

ARSENICUM ALB.
: Mouth feels dry with burning ulcers inside, which are better by warm mouth washes.

ARUM TRIPH.
: Raw feeling at the roof of the mouth and palate. Corners of the mouth are sore and cracked.

BAPTISIA TINC.
: Ulcers in the mouth with a foul smell. The patient is sleepy and debilitated. Useful for children. Merc. is useful for adults in similar conditions.

BARYTA MUR.
: Children go about with their mouth open, looking stupid.

BORAX 3X	: White fungus like growth in the mouth. Mouth hot and tender. Blisters painful on touch and eating. Painful gum boils.
BRYONIA ALBA	: Mucous membranes of the mouth are dry. Lips are parched and there is thirst for large quantities of water at long intervals.
CAUSTICUM	: Bites the inside of cheeks while chewing.
KALIUM CHLOR.	: Ulcers in the mouth and on the tongue. Saliva ropy.
MERCURIUS SOL.	: Offensive odour from the mouth, fills the whole room. Sweetish metallic taste with excessive saliva. Saliva dribbles from the mouth while speaking. Inflammation of the mouth and throat.
NATRIUM SULPH.	: Small ulcers extremely sensitive, better by holding cold fluids in the mouth.
NITRICUM ACIDUM	: Ulcers in the mouth are accompanied by sharp splinter like pains. Acrid and fetid salivation.
OPIUM	: Mouth remains open during sleep.
RHEUM	: Mouth covered with offensive mucus after sleeping.
RHUS TOX.	: Jaws crack while chewing.
TARENTULA CUB., GRAPHITES	: Mouth cracked at corners.

MUMPS
(INFLAMMATION OF THE PAROTID GLANDS)

More commonly acute inflammation is due to the virus of *mumps*, which produces acute swelling, particularly of the parotid glands, with oedema and mononuclear infiltration of the interstital tissue.

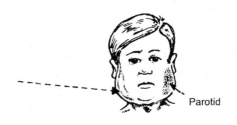

Parotid

ABROTANUM, CARBO VEG.	: Inflammation of the parotid glands and testes is cured by these remedies.
BELLADONNA	: Mania coming on after mumps. It is an excellent remedy for the disease, may be given alternately with Merc-i-r. 3X every 30 minutes.
MERCURIUS SOL.	: Sore pain on touching and from chewing. Whole mouth swollen. Profuse salivation.
MERCURIUS IOD.	: Glands greatly swollen. Swallowing painful. Severe shooting pains in the ears.
PAROTIDINUM 30	: This can be given as a preventive in 200 potency to people not affected by this disease. Usually one dose is sufficient. It may be given in the 30th potency off and on during the disease. It can be given in alternation with any other remedy.
PHYTOLACCA DEC.	: When the affected lesion is hard and painful. Skin pale. Shooting

	pain radeating to the ears on swallowing.
PILOCARPUS M.	: A valuable remedy in limiting the induration of mumps. Saliva pours out in an almost continuous stream from the mouth. May be given alternately with Belladonna or Merc-i-r. 3X.
PULSATILLA NIG.	: Inflammation of the parotid glands and mammae is cured by this remedy.
TRIFOLIUM REP. 200	: Prophylactic against mumps, feeling of congestion in the salivary glands. Pain and hardening, specially of submaxillary glands. Mouth filled with watery saliva, worse lying down. Taste of blood in mouth and throat.

MUSCLES

ACTAEA RACE. (CIMICIFUGA)	: 'Wryneck' i. e. , contracted state of one or more muscles of the neck, making the head appear as if drawn back.
ARNICA MONT., RHUS TOX.	: Removes aching of muscles and tendons. It is a great muscular tonic.
BARTYA CARB.	: Muscles do not develop and are wasted or destroyed at puberty.
BELLIS P.	: A remedy for old labourers, especially gardeners. Removes the sore bruised feelings in the muscles after hard manual labour. Worse

after a cold bath, cold wind, motion and warmth of bed.

BRYONIA ALBA : Aching in every muscle. Pains stitching and tearing, worse by motion and better by rest.

CALCAREA FLUOR. : Inflammation of the muscles and hardness. Slow but effective in action. Takes months to cure.

GELSEMIUM : Complete relaxation of the muscular system. General prostration. Dizziness, drowsiness, dullness and trembling. Tired feeling with muscular weakness. Lack of muscular co-ordination.

HELONIAS : A very good remedy for the hard workers. Tired, sprained muscles, burn and ache.

KALIUM PHOS. : It can be given alternatlely with the above remedies or any other remedy in the atrophy of muscles.

PLUMBUM MET. 200, 1M : Partial or complete destruction and shortening of muscles anywhere in the body. There is no sensation or feeling in that part. Weakness.

RHAMNUS CAL. Q : 10 drops a dose, three times a day is a positive remedy for muscular pains.

MYELITIS
(INFLAMMATION OF THE SPINAL CORD)

ACONITUM NAP. : Fever. Violent pain along the spine. Fear of death. It should be used in the acute or first stage.

ARNICA MONT.	: Inflammation of the spinal cord due to a fall or blow on the spine. Pain, worse on touch.
ARSENICUM ALB.	: Burning pain in the spine. Restlessness with weakness, cramps in the calves. Involuntary urination. Loss of sensibility except to cold. Pain mostly in the hands and feet.
BELLADONNA	: Violent pain along the spine. Tetanic spasms. Fever, when only the upper part of the spine is involved.
CICUTA VIR.	: Violent convulsions. Shrieking cries.
CUPRUM ARS.	: Pain in the lumbar region. Cramps in the calves of legs, relieved by pressure. Numbness of legs. Vertigo.
HYPERICUM PERF. 12X	: Inflammation of the spinal cord, when the nerves have been injured.
PLUMBUM IOD.	: Chronic spinal paralysis. Spinal cord is thickened. Cramps in the calves. Indigestion.
SECALE COR.	: Anus paralysed. Remains open. Stools pass without notice. Pain in sexual organs. Restlessness, sleeplessness and trembling.
STRYCHNINUM PHOS. 3X	: Great rigidity of the lower limbs. Cramps and spasms in the limbs. Anemia of the spinal cord.

NOTE : When the paralysis develops, there is a danger of its becoming complete. At first, there is retention of stools and urine, and later incontinence. Feces and urine may pass involuntarily. Bed sores develop. In rare cases, a slow recovery follows, if the case is treated carefully but partial paralysis may remain, in that case, a remedy for paralysis may be employed.

MYOPIA
(SHORT SIGHTEDNESS)

CARBONEUM SULPH. : Myopia. Color blindness. Absence of the sense of pain in eyes. Painful vision.

PHYSOSTIGMA, PILOCARPUS M. : Increasing myopia is arrested by the use of these remedies. Lenses may be used for myopia, already developed.

NOTE: Best cure is the use of properly and accurately selected lenses. This will arrest further deterioration of eyesight.

MYXEDEMA
(IMPERFECT FUNCTIONING OF THE THYROID GLAND)

(SEE THYROID GLAND)

NAILS BITING

AMMONIUM BROM. : Irritable feeling under the finger nails, relieved by biting them.

ARUM TRIPH. : Biting of finger nails till they bleed.

HYOSCYAMUS NIG.	: Foam in the mouth of the child, who cries at night without waking up. Nail biting.
NATRIUM MUR. 200	: Nail biting in children.
SANICULA AQUA	: Useful for a child suffering from enuresis and weakness.

NAILS MIS-SHAPED

CALCAREA CARB.	: Nails uneven and spotted.
FLUORICUM ACIDUM	: Nails brittle and crumble but grow rapidly.
GRAPHITES	: Both finger and toe nails become thickened like the horn of a cow and grow out of shape. May be black and rough.
THUJA OCC.	: Nails mis-shaped, brittle and crumble easily. May be soft.

NAILS, DISEASES OF

ACIDUM NITRIC. 200	: Inflammation of the nails on account of a tight shoe or under-sized shoe.
AMMONIUM BROM.	: Usually the habit of nail biting is due to nervous irritation. Am-br. is the best remedy for it.
AMMONIUM CARB.	: Nails yellow.
ANTIMONIUM CRUD.	: Deficient growth of nails. Split nails.

BERBERIS VULG..	: Neuralgia under finger nails with swelling of finger joints.
HELLEBORUS NIG.	: Falling of nails without any cause.
HYPERICUM PERF.	: Nails hurt, resulting in pain.
NATRIUM MUR. 200	: Skin around nails, dry and cracked.
OXALICUM ACIDUM	: Nails blue.
SEPIA 200	: Pain under the nails due to fungus growths.
SILICEA	: White spots on nails. Ingrowing toe nails. Yellow hands with blue nails.
SILICEA, THUJA OCC.	: Toe nails grow into the flesh, causing pain.
STANNUM MET.	: Splitting of nails.
THUJA OCC.	: Nails brittle, ingrown toe nails.
WIESBADEN	: Soft nails and nails that grow very rapidly. This tendency is cured.

NAUSEA

AETHUSA CYN.	: Nausea at the sight of food. May be due to indigestion in children. Worse after eating or drinking.
ARSENICUM ALB.	: Cannot bear the sight or smell of food. May be due to respiratory troubles.
BERBERIS VULG.	: Nausea before breakfast.
BRYONIA ALBA	: Nausea aggravated on movement, better by rest.

CARBO VEG.	: Worse during pregnancy and in the morning with weak digestion.
COLCHICUM AUTUM.	: The smell of food causes nausea. even fainting. May be due to excessive flatulence and in pregnancy.
CUPRUM ACET.	: Nausea, retching or vomiting in pregnant women in the morning.
DIGITALIS	: Discomfort even after a small quantity of food or from the mere sight or smell, usually found in patients with heart problems.
IPECACUANHA	: It is a first class remedy for all kinds of nausea, a guiding symptom in the selection of this remedy in any disease. Constant nausea with a clean and moist tongue.
JAMBOSA VULG.	: Nausea better by smoking.
KALIUM CARB.	: Nausea on riding a carriage.
LACTICUM ACIDUM	: Nausea in pale anemic woman, relieved by eating.
NUX VOM.	: Nausea due to indigestion. Wants to vomit but cannot. Worse in the morning.
PODOPHYLLUM	: Nausea with a lot of retching but no vomiting.
PULSATILLA NIG.	: Nausea on looking upwards, worse in a warm room, better in open air.
SEPIA	: Nausea at the smell or sight of food. May be due to uterine problems in women or pregnancy. Nausea in the morning, before eating.

TABACUM 200	:	**Dea**thly nausea worse on opening eyes,least motion and tobacco smoke.
THERIDION	:	Nausea from noise. Patient is very sensitive to noise. Nausea, due to spondylitis.

NAVEL

ABROTANUM	:	Bleeding from the navel of infants with ulceration of the navel.
ALUMINA	:	Navel is abnormally pulled back in the abdomen and there is a depression or a pit at the site of navel.
CALCAREA PHOS.	:	Oozing of blood from the navel of new born.
DIOSCOREA	:	Abdominal pain starts from the navel and then radiates in all directions.
DULCAMARA	:	Cutting pain around the navel.
LYCOPODIUM	:	Navel projects upwards from the abdomen. Great abdominal flatulence.
NUX MOSCH.	:	Pain around the navel extending downwards both ways. Ulceration of the navel in new born babies.
PLUMBUM MET.	:	Sensation as if the navel is being pulled by a string towards the spine. Pain causes a desire to stretch. Strangulated hernia of the navel.

SPIGELIA : Pain around the navel. May be due to presence of worms. Child refers to the navel as the most painful part. Sensitive to touch.

NECK

ACONITUM NAP. : Stiffness of the neck due to exposure to cold winds, worse on movement. Pain extends to the shoulders.

ANTIMONIUM TART. : Stiff neck stretched out, head bent backwards.

BRYONIA ALBA : Painful stiffness of the neck, worse on motion.

CHELIDONIUM : Pain and stiffness of the right side of neck, extending to the right shoulder and scapula.

CIMICIFUGA : Head and neck are pulled back. Rheumatism of the neck muscles.

DULCAMARA : Pain in the neck due to exposure to cold, damp winds or from an uncomfortable position of the head when lying.

LACHNANTHES TINC.Q : Neck is drawn over to one side in sore throat. Rheumatism of the neck. Pain in the nape, as if dislocated.

RHODODENDRON CH. : Pain in the neck due to exposure to dry cold winds, worse before thunderstorm.

RHUS TOX. 200 : Sprain of the neck due to a sudden jerk or an uncomfortable position of the head while asleep.

NEPHRITIS
(BRIGHT'S DISEASE)
(INFLAMMATION OF THE KIDNEYS)

ACONITUM NAP. : Acute nephritis in children with a large abdomen. It is useful, when there is an exposure by sudden cold or getting wet, when perspiring.

APIS MEL. : Swelling on the face, legs and feet. Pale skin. Scanty urine. Pain in the head, back and legs. Kidney region painful. Urine is bloody and contains albumin.

ARSENICUM ALBUM : The urine is dark, loaded with casts and albumin. The patient has a pale skin. He is restless. He sips water in small quantities at shorter intervals and desires warmth. The face is swollen. Convulsions and fear of death. Watery diarrhea. It covers all the stages of this disease.

BENZOICUM ACIDUM : Urine is pungent smelling and dark in color. Sharp pain in kidneys.

CALCAREA SULPH. : Gradual emaciation and debility. Urine contains pus and is burning Anemia.

HELLEBORUS NIG.	: Smell of urine from the body. Convulsions. Unconsciousness, with dilated pupils.
KALIUM CHLOR. 6C	: Nephritis with hemoglobinuria and stomatitis. Urine is dark, scanty and contains albumin, phosphates and bile. Chronic nephritis.
MERCURIUS COR.	: Nephritis in pregnant women. Pedal oedema. Urine is scanty and loaded with casts and albumin. It may contain red sand.
PICRICUM ACIDUM	: Bloody urine with fatty pieces of epithelium. Debility.

NERVES

ACONITUM NAP.	: Sudden inflammation of the nerves due to anxiety or fear worse with noise and light.
APIS MEL.	: Optic neuritis in the first stage.
ARGENTUM NIT.	: Inflammation of nerves. Loss of control and want of balance any-where - mental and physical.
BELLIS P.	: Results of injuries to nerves with intense soreness and intolerance to cold bathing.
CARBONEUM SULPH.	: For atrophy of the optic nerve and optic disc.
CHENOPODIUM AN.	: Affections of the auditory nerve. Hearing better for high pitched sounds. Comparative deafness to the sound of voice. Burning in

ears. Numbness of the auditory nerve.

CIMICIFUGA	: Inflammation of nerves due to reflex disorders.
CINNABARIS 3X	: Pain in the ciliary nerve causing redness of the eyes,canthi and lids. Pain around eyes to temples and orbit of the eyes.
CYPRIPEDIUM	: Nerves shortened by long illness or excessive tea and coffee drinking.
GLONOINUM	: Inflammation of nerves due to heat of sun. Better by motion and uncovering the head. Pulsations all over the body.
HYPERICUM PERF.3X	: Crushing injuries to the nerve sheaths of the spine and other nerves causing tearing, burning and stinging pains. These are cured by this remedy. Slight paralysis caused by entanglement of nerves in the sacrum. Numbness of parts affected and constant drowsiness.
KALIUM PHOS.	: An excellent nerve tonic.
LYCOPERSICUM ESCU.	: Tingling along the right ulnar nerve.
MAGNESIUM PHOS. 12X	: It is a remedy for nerve tension as exhibited in pulse. In severe nerve tension,the wrists also become tense. If it is in both wrists, it shows that the whole nervous system is involved. Three tablets given with hot water 2 hourly will remove the tension. Pain is on the right side, better by heat and pressure.

NAPHTHALINUM	: Paralysis of the optic nerve causing blindness and opacity of the cornea.
PHOSPHORUS	: Atrophy of the optic nerve with cataract and due to paralysis.
RHUS TOX., HYPERICUM PERF., KALMIA LAT.	: Pain along the ulnar nerve, according to the symptoms of the remedy.
SAPONARIA OFF.	: Affections of the 5th nerve. Migraine before menses. Pain in the left temple and eye. Photophobia. Hot stitches deep in the eye.
SPIGELIA	: It cures neuralgia of the 5th nerve. Pain or loss of sensation in the face, forehead, temple and eyes. Deviation of jaw.

NERVOUSNESS
(SEE ANXIETY ALSO)

ACIDUM PHOS. Q	: Weakness on account of nervousness.
ACONITUM NAP.	: A child is scared and nervous to take a bath in a river or lake. A lady becomes nervous on boarding a plane. A solider becomes nervous for taking part in a war because of the fear of death and other horrors of war. A dose of Acon. 30 will give them strength and remove their nervousness.
AETHUSA CYN.	: Nervous dyspepsia from excitement due to good or bad news.

AGNUS CASTUS	: Nervous to perform sexual acts because of lowered sexual vitality.
ANACARDIUM ORI.	: Nervous dyspepsia with pain in the abdomen, relieved by eating. Nervousness and fear of examination in students.
ARGENTUM NIT.	: A child becomes nervous when asked to go to school. A student is nervous before going for an exam. A person becomes nervous before appearing for an interview. A speaker becomes nervous before giving a speech in a gathering. One dose of Arg-n. 30 will produce a soothing effect and will remove the nervousness. Diarrhea due to nervous excitement is also cured by this remedy.
AURUM MET. 200	: Nervous break down. Inclined to commit suicide. Always brooding. Disgust for life. Rapid and constant questioning, without waiting for the reply. The patient becomes almost insane.
BUTYRICUM ACIDUM	: Nervousness for a constant state of fear and worries over trifles.
CAUSTICUM 200	: Nervousness due to worries or grief. Patient is unhappy and inclined to tears. Hopeless. Jumps at the least noise. Forgetful. Very sympathetic and critical of others.
CHINA OFF.	: Becomes nervous on little opposition. He is very sensitive to trifling insults.

COCCULUS IND.	:	The patient is sad and absorbed in himself. Brooding, moody and silent. Sits in a corner burried in his thoughts. Thoughts fixed on a single, disagreeable subject.
GELSEMIUM	:	Nervous diarrhea from excitement, fright and bad news. Depressed. Unable to cope with life. Listless and apprehensive.
HYPERICUM PERF.12X	:	Nervousness of any kind. May be due to an accident. Speech becomes jerky and hesitant. Takes no interest in life.
IGNATIA AMARA	:	Becomes nervous before an interview. A singer becomes nervous about singing before the public for the first time. A speaker becomes nervous before delivering a speech. Give a dose every 2 hours. Nervous breakdown with headache. Trembling. Sleeplessness due to grief or worry is also cured by this remedy.
KALIUM PHOS. 200X	:	One of the greatest nervous remedies. Nervous weakness, tired feeling and nervous depression, mental and physical. Excitement produced is improved by this remedy.
KALIUM SULPH.	:	Very nervous. Sensation of a closely fitted cap on the head. Drops what he holds in his hands, if spoken suddenly.
NATRIUM MUR., ARSENICUM ALB.	:	Nervous prostration. Brain appears tired.

NUX VOM. : Irritable and nervousness due to sedentary habits. Cannot bear light, odor, noise, etc. Does not want to be touched. Fault finding.

PASSIFLORA Q : Sleeplessness produced by nervousness is removed by this remedy. Give 15-20 drops in a dose, repeating often. It will produce a normal sleep.

PHOSPHORUS : Great lowness of spirits. Easily offended. Fearful and restless. Thinks, that he has an incurable heart disease. Looses all ambition to do anything. Cannot concentrate his thoughts.

SILICEA : Nervous and excitable. Sensitive to all impressions. Fixed ideas. Want of grit to appear before the public and say something. This remedy raises spirits and mental stamina, revives hope. Weakness and depression give way to strength and health.

STAPHYSAGRIA : Nervousness, remaining after tooth extraction.

STICTA PULM. Q : Nervous sleeplessness due to pain in sprains and fractures. A few doses puts the patient to sleep.

STRYCHNINUM PHOS. 3X: Nervousness of an inexperienced person, at the time of first sexual act. Want of erection,though healthy creating a feeling of shyness and shame.

TELA ARANEAE : Removes the bad effects of nervousness like fever, headache, cough, excitement, etc. Calms the nerves and makes the patient comfortable.

TRIOSTEUM PERF. 6   : Quitens nervous symptoms.

NERVOUS PROSTRATION
(NEURASTHENIA - BRAIN FAG)

AMBRA GRISEA   : Extreme nervousness, hyper-sensitivness. Coldness and numb-ness, generally of single parts like finger, arm, etc. Dwells upon unpleasant events of the past.

ARGENTUM NIT.   : Inflammation of nerves. Symptoms of incoordination, loss of control and want of balance everywhere, mentally and physically. Trembling of affected parts.

COCCULUS IND.   : Mental weakness. Dwells on the past, disagreeable events.

KALIUM PHOS. 6X-200X   : One of the greatest remedies for nervous prostration and tired feel-ing, specially in young persons. Neurasthenia and brain fag. Marked disturbances in reflex nervous system. Want of nerve power, mental and physical, and depres-sion is wonderfully improved by this remedy.

NATRIUM MUR.   : Dwells upon disagreeable events of the past. She cannot sleep on that account and is always think-ing about it.

PICRICUM ACIDUM : Prostration, weakness and pain in the back. Mental and physical fatigue. Heavy tired feeling. Pin and needle like sensation in the extremities. Lack of will power.

STRYCHNINUM PHOS. 3X: Disinclined to use the brain. Lack of control over muscles and mind. Uncontrollable desire to laugh. It is also an excellent remedy for anemia of the spinal cord.

NETTLE RASH
(SEE URTICARIA)

NEURALGIA

Pain in a severe, throbbing, or stabbing character in the course or distribution of a nerve is known as neuralgia.

ACONITUM NAP. : Neuralgia of the face due to exposure to cold or cold draught. Pain in the joints. Face flushed. Neuralgia of the face especially of the left side.

ARSENICUM ALB. : Periodical attacks of pain, worse by cold and better by warmth. Pain of a burning character.

BELLADONNA : Neuralgia of the face, cheeks, nose, jaws, temples and neck. Rush of blood towards the head.

CHAMOMILLA	: Violent unbearable pains, worse on the left side of face extending to the head and temples. The patient feels pain more than it is in actual. Pain worse on touch. Neuralgia with numbness.
CANNABIS IND.	: Ciliary neuralgia. Pain around the eyes extends to temples,brows and ears. Eye and lids red.
COLOCYNTHIS	: It has symptoms like Mag-p. and is indicated when hard pressure relieves.
GELSEMIUM	: Neuralgia with trembling of the lower extremities. Does not want to be disturbed or spoken to.
KALIUM BICH. 200	: Neuralgia at the same hour everyday.
KALIUM IOD. 3X	: Neuralgia of the left eye with soreness of the head.
KALMIA LAT.	: Neuralgic pains shoot downwards with numbness and sense of coldness in limbs.
MACROTINUM 2X	: Neuralgic pain in the limbs, specially before the start of menses with relief after flow starts.
MAGNESIUM PHOS. 12X	: One of the best remedies in neuralgia, when the neuralgia is on the right side and is relieved by warmth and pressure.
PULSATILLA NIG.	: Facial neuralgia, worse in the evening. Pain with coldness of the affected parts. Thirstless patients.
SANGUINARIA CAN.	: Neuralgia of the right side. Burning pain, worse on motion and touch. Better in darkness and sleep.

SPIGELIA : Neuralgia of the left side, left eye, left chest region, left shoulder, left neck, etc. Pains are shooting and burning. Neuralgia of fifth nerve is prominent.

SYMPHYTUM OFF. 200 : Use it for neuralgia of the knee.

THUJA OCC. 200 : Many neuralgias have psychosis as their base. Therefore, start the case with a single dose of this remedy on the first day, in chronic cases only.

NEURITIS

(SEE NERVES)

NIGHTMARES

ACONITUM NAP. : Nocturnal furious delirium. Restless sleep, with worrying dreams.

AMMONIUM CARB. : Nightmares in heart diseases.

ARTEMISIA VULG. : Walks or does anything else during sleep, semiconsciously.

BELLADONNA : Fears the dark and going to bed. Screams out in sleep.

BORAX : Child cries in sleep frightened and hugs the mother.

CHAMOMILLA : Child starts crying all of a sudden in sleep due to fearful dreams.

CONIUM MAC. : Due to anemia of the brain.

DIGITALIS	: Nightmares in spermatorrhea and heart diseases.
HYOSCYAMUS NIG.	: Twitches and screams while asleep, very weird dreams.
KALIUM BROM.	: Nightmares, when not traceable to any cause. One dose at bed time. Shrieks and trembles.
KALIUM PHOS.	: For walking in sleep, semiconsciously.
NATRIUM MUR.	: Gets up semiconsciously from sleep and sits somewhere in the bed room.
NUX VOM.	: Nightmares due to over loading of stomach or indigestion.
PULSATILLA NIG.	: Restless sleep with troubled dreams.
SILICEA	: Gets up during sleep, walks and sleeps again.
SULPHUR	: For speaking in sleep, semiconsciously.

NIGHT WALKING
(SOMNAMBULISM)

AILANTHUS G.	: Speaking unintelligently, muttering in semiconsciousness, while asleep.
HYOSCYAMUS NIG.	: Child sobs and cries during sleep, without waking.
KALIUM BROM.	: Sleeplessness due to worry, grief and sexual excesses. Grinding teeth. Night walking while asleep.

KALIUM PHOS. 200X	: Walking in sleep. Sleeplessness due to overwork, worry and disease.
NATRIUM MUR.	: Nervous jerking during sleep. Dreams of robbers. Gets up, walks or sits while asleep.
SILICEA	: Night walking. Gets up while asleep. Frequently startles in sleep. Anxious dreams.

NIPPLES

AURUM SULPH.	: Nipples cracked with lancinating pains.
CARBOLICUM ACIDUM	: Tumor of nipples as large as an egg of a hen.
CASTOR EQUI	: Nipples very sensitive. Cannot bear touch. Sore and cracked.
CAUSTICUM	: Eczema of the nipples.
CROTON TIG.	: On nursing, pain in the nipple radiates to the back.
GRAPHITES	: Cracks in nipples, oozing a sticky fluid.
HYDRASTIS CAN.	: Retracted nipples. Ulcerated on account of sucking by the child.
PHYTOLACCA DEC.	: When the child sucks, pain goes from the nipple all over the body. Nipples sensitive and cracked. Sore and fissured, worse by nursing.
RATANHIA PERU.	: Nipples cracked and fissured from nursing.

SARSAPARILLA Q : Nipples short, flat and do not grow properly or are being wasted away. Instead of a projection, a depression exists. Withered and unexcitable.

SULPHUR : Nipples cracked.

NODES

(SEE BONES)

NOSE

ANTIMONIUM CRUD., PETROLEUM : Nostrils ulcerated and cracked.

ARSENICUM ALB. : Acne of the nose.

ARUM TRIPH., AMMONIUM CARB., KALIUM SULPH., PSORINUM, STICTA PULM., TEUCRIUM MAR. : Nose obstructed, must breathe through the mouth. Burning in the nose and constant picking of the nose until it bleeds. Large scabs, high up in the nostrils.

ASAFOETIDA : Numbness of the nose and caries of the nasal bones.

AURUM MET. 200 : Abscess of the nose. Painful ulcers, with fetid discharge.

BARYTA CARB. : Smell of smoke in the nose.

BORAX 3X : Red nose in young women. Red, shining and swollen with throbbing. Tip swollen and ulcerated.

BRYONIA ALBA : Swelling of the tip of the nose.

CALCAREA CARB.	: Dry nostrils, which are sore and ulcerated. Stoppage of nose. Discharge is fetid and yellow.
CAPSICUM	: Tip of the nose shiny red, tickling in the nostrils.
CINA	: Itching in the nose. Patient is often seen rubbing his nose with hands.
HEPAR SULPHURIS 1X	: It often starts secretion and profuse drainage in stuffy colds of the nose. Nose stops up, while going out. Two doses produce the desired results. Painful abscess of the nose.
KALIUM NIT.	: Polypus of the nose, worse right nostril. Nose feels swollen with itching, worse towards morning and afternoon.
LACHESIS	: Red nose of drunkards. Epistaxis. Nostrils sensitive.
LACHNANTHES TINC.	: Bridge of the nose appears as if pinched.
LYCOPODIUM	: Feeling of dryness, ulcerated nostrils. Nose obstructed. Nose congested, when tired.
LYCOPODIUM, PYROGENIUM, FERRUM PHOS., CHELIDONIUM	: Fan like movement of the nose. Flapping of alae nasi. Select the remedy on other symptoms.
MERCURIUS BIN IOD.	: Bones of the nose are swollen.
MERCURIUS SOL.	: Pain and swelling of the nasal bones, caries and ulceration. Yellowish green, fetid pus like discharge from the nose.
NATRIUM CARB.	: Many problems of the external nose, pimples and puffiness. Obstruction of the nose.

POTHOS : Red swelling across the bridge of nose.

SAMBUCUS NIG. : Snuffles in infants. Nose dry and obstructed. Child cannot draw milk from the nipple due to blocking and suffocation. Child wakes up suddenly, nearly suffocated, sits up, turns blue.

SANGUINARIA CAN. : Nasal polypi. Ozena with profuse, offensive and yellowish discharge. Nose feels obstructed. Sneezing.

SILICEA : Itching at the tip of the nose. Bleeding when hard and dry crusts are removed from the nostrils.

TEUCRIUM MAR. : Soft polypus of jelly like consistency.

TRITICUM REP. 1X : The patient is in the habit of blowing his nose always though not suffering from a cold.

TROMBIDIUM : Discharge from the nose while eating or drinking. There are many people whose nose will begin to drip the minute they begin to eat. Fluent discharge from the nose. This is entirely relieved by the use of this remedy.

NUMBNESS

ACONITUM NAP. : Numbness and tingling originating within 48 hours.

AGARICUS MUS.	: Numbness of the legs while cross-ing them. Sensation of cold needles. Sensation as if ants were creeping on the affected parts.
AMBRA GRISEA	: External numbness of the whole body in the morning, with weak-ness. It is indicated in old people and scrawny women. Coldness and numbness usually of single parts like fingers, arms, etc. Numbness worse on pressure.
ARGENTUM NIT.	: Numbness of forearms, specially at night.
ASAFOETIDA	: Numbness of the head. May be accompanied with pain.
AVENA SAT. Q	: Numbness of limbs, as if paraly-sed. 10-20 drops in water will have a tonic effect for this and it also relieves nervous headache and fatigue most assuredly. It also brings about sleep. Strength of hands is diminished.
BARYTA CARB.	: Numbness from knees to scrotum.
BUFO RANA	: Numbness of the brain.
CADMIUM SULPH.	: Sensation of ants crawling on the body and limbs. Paralysed parts feel numb.
CALCAREA PHOS.	: Cold and numb feeling with a crawling sensation in buttocks, back and limbs. Numbness and crawling are characteristic symp-toms of this remedy.
CAUSTICUM	: Numbness and loss of sensation in the hands.

CHAMOMILLA	: Numbness with pain.
CICUTA VIR.	: Numbness of the whole body with coldness of hands.
COCCULUS IND.	: Numbness of arms, first right then left. Numbness of the forearms, specially at night.
CONIUM MAC.	: Numb feeling all over the body.
HYDROCYANICUM ACIDUM	: Sudden numbness and complete loss of sensibility.
KALMIA LAT.	: Numbness with pain, which shoots downwards.
NATRIUM MUR.	: Numbness of fingers. Cannot hold things and drops them.
PHOSPHORUS	: Numbness in arms, legs and tip of the fingers. Burning may be present.
PICRICUM ACIDUM	: Pin and needle like sensation in the extremities. Heavy and tired feeling.
RAPHANUS	: Numbness of the hands, soles and feet.
RHUS TOX.	: Numbness of the extremities often due to overwork and exposure. Crawling sensation in the tip of the fingers. Tingling in the feet.
SECALE COR.	: Sensation of ants crawling and numbness of fingers.
TARENTULA HIS.	: Numbness of the legs.

NYMPHOMANIA
(SEE ALSO SEXUAL DESIRE EXCESSIVE)

Nymphomania is an excessive sexual desire in females.

BARYTA MUR. 3X : Excessive sexual desire often leading to sexual mania. Great feeling of weakness.

CALCAREA PHOS. 6X : Nymphomania with pain and weakness in the uterine region. Leucorrhea like white of an egg.

CHINA OFF. : Desire too strong. Can be satisfied only by masturbation or by sexual intercourse.

FERULA GLAUCA : Violent sexual desire in women.

MUREX PURP. : Pulsations in the neck of the womb excites sexual desires. Least contact of sexual parts causes violent sexual excitement.

ORIGANUM MAJ. : Powerful lascivious impulses, ideas and dreams compelling masturbation. Desire for active exercise. The patient walks to and fro unnecessarily. Dreams even of having sex with brother or son.

PLATINUM MET. : Tingling internally and externally of sexual parts arouses excessive sexual desire.

OBESITY

To control obesity and to reduce fat, individualization of the case is necessary. There is no miracle. Weight gain is the result of several different facts like genetics, hereditary metabolism, inadequate elimination, eating habits and life style. The homeopathic treatment is based upon draining, treating and curing. Drainage means relieving the liver, kidneys and circulatory system of toxins. Fucus is diuretic and detoxifying. It activates burning of fats and sugar. If you forgot to take off your rings before sleeping at night, then next morning you cannot take them off because your fingers are so swollen and after some hours when you pass urine, etc. the fingers become normal. Nat-s. acts as a powerful drainage agent in such cases. The following medicines can be prescribed for the people who are over weight. These will not help people, who just want to lose 5-10 pounds. To get restored to a more normal body and to take off the weight, the patient must know how to eat properly and exercise. Fats should be decreased to minimum in the diet . Fasting and dieting can be more harmful even than being fat.

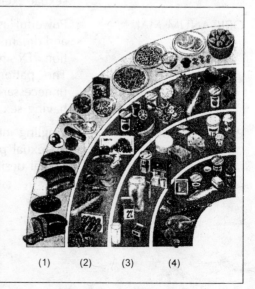

1. Grain Products
Choose whole prain and enriched products more often.

2. Vegetables & Fruit
Choose dark green and orange vegetables and orange fruit more often.

3. Milk Products Choose lower-fat milk prod ucts more often.

4. Meat & Alternatives
Choose leaner meats, poultry and fish, as well as dried peas, beans and lentils more often.

(1)   (2)   (3)   (4)

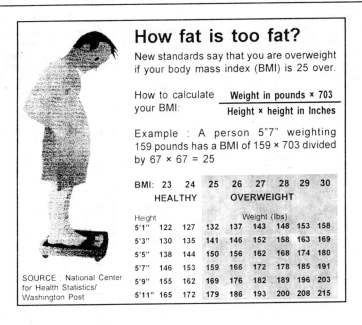

How fat is too fat?

New standards say that you are overweight if your body mass index (BMI) is 25 over.

How to calculate your BMI:

$$\frac{\text{Weight in pounds} \times 703}{\text{Height} \times \text{height in Inches}}$$

Example : A person 5"7" weighting 159 pounds has a BMI of 159 × 703 divided by 67 × 67 = 25

BMI:	23	24	25	26	27	28	29	30
	HEALTHY			OVERWEIGHT				
Height				Weight (lbs)				
5'1"	122	127	132	137	143	148	153	158
5'3"	130	135	141	146	152	158	163	169
5'5"	138	144	150	156	162	168	174	180
5'7"	146	153	159	166	172	178	185	191
5'9"	155	162	169	176	182	189	196	203
5'11"	165	172	179	186	193	200	208	215

SOURCE : National Center for Health Statistics/ Washington Post

AMMONIUM MUR. : Patients having respiratory troubles. Sluggish and have large buttocks and thighs.

ANTIMONIUM CRUD. : Gouty patients with gastric problems and a tendency to grow fat. Tongue thickly coated white.

APOCYNUM CAN. 1X : Abdomen is bloated due to dropsy. Puffiness, elsewhere due to dropsy. By the use of this remedy, the waist can reduce in one month and loss of weight can be upto 20 pounds in one month.

CALCAREA CARB. 200 : Fat people with perspiration on the forehead. Excessive fat on the abdomen. Obesity, specially in children and young people. Excessive appetite. Chilly patients. Thyroid or pituitary dysfunction.

Body Mass Index

The Body mass index indicates whether you are at low, moderate or high risk of developing health problems. It recognizes that there is no one, ideal weight for everyone of the same height. The BMI does not apply to children and teenagers, adults over 65, women who are pregnant or nursing, extremely muscular people or endurance athletes.

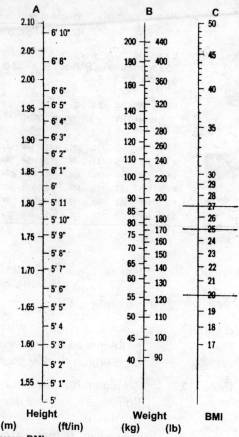

Height		Weight		BMI
(m)	(ft/in)	(kg)	(lb)	

How to find your BMI:

1. Mark an X at your height on graph A.
2. Mak and X at your weight on graph B.
3. Take a ruler and join the two Xs.
4. Extend the line along the ruler to graph C.

- **Under 20** A BMI under 20 may be associated with health problems for some individuals. It may be a good idea to consult a dietitian and physician for advice.
- **20-25** This zone is associated with the lowest risk of illness for most people. This is the range you want to stay in.
- **25-27** A BMI over 27 is associated with increased risk of health problems such as heart disease, high blood pressure and diabetes. It may be a good idea to consult a dietitian and physician for advice.

CALOTROPIS Q	: It decreases flesh and hardens muscles.
FUCUS VES. Q	: Patients with defect in thyroid gland and because of it they are gaining weight and becoming fat. It is a diuretic and detoxifying agent. It burns excessive fats and sugar.
GRAPHITES	: Anemic young ladies with a red face and tendency to obesity due to delayed menses. It suits the males also. Such patients have skin affections and have weeping tendencies.
IODIUM 2X	: Debilitated fat patients having thyroid troubles - feeling hungry always. In such cases, Iodium 2X will reduce obesity. Higher potencies will increase weight.
PHYTOLACCA BERRY Q	: Obesity without any possible defect in the system. A general remedy to reduce weight and fat.
PULSATILLA NIG. Q	: Obesity due to uterine problems. Patient is shy, emotional and thirstless.
THYROIDINUM 200	: Excessive obesity due to imperfect function of thyroid gland. Such patients crave large amounts of sweets.

ODOR (SMELL)

ALLIUM CEPA	: Very sensitive to the odor of flowers.

ANTHRACINUM	:	Bad effects of inhaling foul odors.
ARSENICUM ALB.	:	Odor of sulphur fumes from the throat while coughing.
AURUM MET.	:	Everything smells bad, putrid smell while blowing the nose.
BELLADONNA	:	Sensation of smelling rotten eggs or a gas. Great sensitiveness to odors. Even little and faint odors are unbearable.
BOVISTA	:	Perspiration in the armpits smells like onions.
CALCAREA CARB.	:	Offensive foot sweat.
COLCHICUM AUTUM.	:	Smell of cooking food, especially fish, causes nausea, vomiting and even fainting.
COLOCYNTHIS	:	Perspiration smells like urine.
CROTON TIG.	:	Sensation of smelling stools.
GRAPHITES	:	Smell of burnt hair.
GUAIACUM OFF. Q	:	Unclean odor from the entire body.
KALIUM PHOS.	:	Foul smelling breath.
LACHESIS	:	Bad odor from the mouth, specially during menopause.
MAGNESIUM MUR.	:	Loss of smell and taste, after influenza.
MERCURIUS SOL.	:	Foul breath, bad odor from the armpits and discharges.
NITRICUM ACIDUM	:	Foul smell from the body. Fetid discharge. Urine smells like that of a horse.
NUX VOM.	:	Bad odor from the mouth after eating. Cannot bear strong odors like phenyl, petrol, etc.

PHOSPHORUS CORALLIUM RUB.	: Odor of garlic from the perspiration. Cough from strong odors.
PHOSPHORUS	: Odour of onions, smoke, etc. in the nose. Look for other symptoms of the remedy to select the remedy.
PSORINUM	: A very uncommon, peculiar characteristic of this remedy is that the discharges of the patients are very foul and fetid. The smell can be felt throughout the house. In all diseases, the patient feels unusually well before an attack.
PYROGENIUM 200	: Breath horribly offensive. Taste terribly fetid.
SABADILLA	: Sensitive to all odors.
SANICULA AQUA	: Sensation of smelling rotten fish from the skin.
SILICEA	: Offensive foot sweat.
STANNUM MET.	: Smell of cooking food causes vomiting.
SULPHUR	: Oversensitive to odors. Offensive smell from all discharges.
SULPHUR, PSORINUM	: Bad smell from the body despite cleaning and bathing.
TELLURIUM MET.	: Garlic like smell from the body.
THUJA OCC.	: Loss of smell during an allergic cold.
WIESBADEN	: Offensive body odor like that of rotten eggs.

OEDEMA (SWELLING)

ACETICUM ACIDUM	:	Swelling of feet and legs. Debility.
ANTIMONIUM ARS.	:	Edema of the eyes.
ANTIMONIUM TART.	:	Most cases of pulmonary edema are benefited by the use of this remedy.
APIS MEL.	:	Give in repeated doses for edema glottis. Its acts on cellular tissues and is used for edema of the skin and mucous membranes in dropsical effusions and anasarca due to kidney troubles. The affected parts are of rosy red color and the pains are of a stinging nature. Edema of lower lips.
APOCYNUM CAN.	:	Edema with scanty urine and great thirst. Edema during menses. It is a very good remedy for dropsies.
ARSENICUM ALB.	:	Edema in heart troubles and in drunkards.
AURUM MUR.	:	Edema due to spleen and liver diseases.
BRYONIA ALBA	:	Swelling of the legs during pregnancy.
CACTUS	:	Edema of hands and feet.
EEL SERUM, VESICARIA COM.	:	Edema due to failure of kidneys and suppression of urine.
HYDROCOTYLE A.	:	Edema due to inflammation of the cellular tissues.
KALIUM CARB.	:	Swelling of the upper lip.
PHOSPHORUS	:	Edema due to the inflammation of

the kidney or due to anemia. Edema of the face and eyes.

RHUS TOX.   : Edema of vulva and penis.

SANGUINARIA CAN.   : Oedema glottis with acute pharyn-gitis.

TEREBINTHINIAE   : Dropsical edema in Bright's disease or inflammation of the kidneys.

THYROIDINUM 3X   : Edema of various types without any cause.

VESICARIA COM. Q   : Edema due to suppression of urine in kidney diseases.

OESOPHAGUS

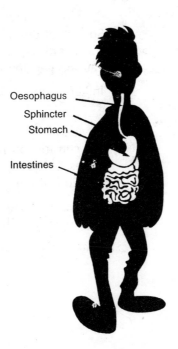

Oesophagus
Sphincter
Stomach
Intestines

ACONITUM NAP., BELLA-: Dryness of the oesophagus.
DONNA, NAJA TRI.

ALUMINA, BAPTISIA TINC.: Constriction of the oesophagus.
PHOSPHORUS   Least solid food gags.

AMMONIUM CARB.,   : Burning in the oesophagus.
CAUSTICUM, CANTHARIS,
PHOSPHORUS,
ASAFOETIDA

ASAFOETIDA 3X   : Flatulence and spasmodic contraction of the oesophagus. Food moves
in the reverse direction, to mouth
from oesophagus.

BAPTISIA TINC.   : Can swallow only liquids. Least
solid food gags.

BAPTISIA TINC.,   : Spasms of the oesophagus.
BELLADONNA
ASAFOETIDA,
IGNATIA AMARA

BARYTA CARB.   : Spasms of oesophagus as soon as
food enters the oesophagus,
causing gagging and choking.

BELLADONNA,   : Inflammation of the oesophagus.
PHOSPHORUS

COCCULUS IND.   : Dryness of the esophagus. Choking constriction in the upper part
of oesophagus. Dyspnea from constriction of the trachea.

CROTALUS H.   : Spasms of oesophagus. Cannot
swallow any solid substance.

PHOSPHORUS,   : Pain in the oesophagus.
AMMONIUM CARB.,
CAUSTICUM

OLD AGE

AGNUS CASTUS 3X : Premature old age due to excessive use of sexual power. Give this remedy thrice daily.

ALUMINA : Old people with lack of vital heat or prematurely old with debility. Sluggish functions, heaviness, numbness, staggering and the characteristic constipation with no desire for stools, for days together.

AMBRA GRISEA : It is a great remedy for the aged with impairment of all functions, weakness, coldness and numbness usually of single parts like fingers, arms, etc. One sided complaints.

ANACARDIUM ORI. : Senile dementia. The patient feels as if he is two persons. Very easily offended. The patient's memory is poor and becomes very absent minded.

BARYTA CARB. : Diseases of old men when degenerative changes begin; cardiac, vascular, cerebral, enlarged prostrate and hardened testes. Senile dementia with confusion and loss of confidence. Loss of memory. Childish behaviour with weakness. Must lie down or lean on something. Very averse to meeting strangers. Weakness due to masturbation or sexual excesses, when young.

BREWER'S YEAST 1X : 2 tablets (2 grains) taken with meals, twice daily brings back youthful looks in people who are growing old before time. This yeast is obtained during the brewing of beer. In the dried form, it is a very good source of vitamin 'B'.

CAUSTICUM

: General health is very poor. The patient feels sad and hopeless but is intensely sympathetic.

CONIUM MAC.

: Difficult gait. Trembling. Sudden loss of strength while walking. Painful stiffness of legs. Urinary problems and weakened memory.

GINKGO BILOBA Q

: It is a nutritional supplement in fight against problems of aging process. Acts as a tonic for the immune system, increases vitality and removes physical fatigue. Improves memory.

LYCOPODIUM 200

: It is also an old age remedy. Weakness of body and mind. Trembling and palpitations. Unable to do mental work. Cannot equal sex with a lady of younger age.

RHODALLINUM 2X

: A remedy for retarding old age. Gastric and rectal problems. Deafness. It helps old age come naturally and normally, without any complication.

SECALE COR.

: In thin and lean women, who are run down and anxious. May be suffering from cataract.

OPERATION

ABROTANUM : A sense of pressure after operation of the chest for pleurisy or other chest diseases.

ACETICUM ACIDUM : It removes weakness after surgery.

CAUSTICUM : Retention of urine after an operation.

CHAMOMILLA : Nausea and vomiting after surgery due to the by use of morphia.

CHINA OFF. : Flatulence with pain after an operation. There is no relief after passing gas.

COLLINSONIA CAN. : It is of special value, when given before operations for rectal diseases. Does not allow complications to arise after the operation.

COLOCYNTHIS : Spasmodic contractions of the urinary bladder after operation of an orifice,entrance or outlets to any aperture. Agonising pain in the abdomen, compelling the patient to bend double.

HYPERICUM PERF. : Relieves pain after operation. Often subsides the use of morphine.

MILLEFOLIUM : For complaints after surgical removal of stones.

PHOSPHORUS 200-1M : A single dose given a day before the abdominal operation will prevent nausea and other distress after the operation.

RAPHANUS : Post operative, gas pains are removed by the use of this remedy.

RHUS TOX., PYROGENIUM : Post operative complications. Look for other symptoms of the remedy.

STAPHYSAGRIA : Abdominal pain, after it's operation.

STRONTIUM BROM. : It relieves shock after an operation and revives the patient, who may have a cold with profuse perspiration and other symptoms of collapse.

STROPHANTHUS HISP. Q : It may be used with advantage after any operation, to remove the weakness occuring from bleeding. It tones up the heart also. Dose, 10 drops three times daily.

OPIUM HABIT

AVENA SAT. Q : Almost specific for removing craving for morphine and opium. Give 20-25 drops in hot water 3 times a day.

BERBERIS VULG. Q : Useful to counteract morphine and opium habit.

CHAMOMILLA : It is useful in antidoting the desire for morphine and opium. It antidotes bad effects like pain and sleeplessness.

COFFEA CRUDA : Antidotes bad effects of narcotics and sleeping pills. Black coffee is better.

PASSIFLORA Q, AVENA SAT. Q	: Mixed in equal parts and given in 20 drop doses three times a day, takes away the craving for morphine and opium.

OPTIC NERVE
(SEE NERVES)

OTORRHEA
(DISCHARGE FROM THE EARS)

CALCAREA CARB.	: Bland discharge of white color.
CALCAREA SULPH.	: Discharge is thick with bloody pus.
GRAPHITES	: Discharge is sticky, fetid and of a light brown color.
HEPAR SULPHURIS	: Discharge is comparatively thick and there is much pain, may be due to an abscess.
KALIUM BICH.	: Ears are swollen; tearing pains. Discharge is thick, yellow, sticky, stringy and fetid.
KALIUM IOD.	: Copious, thick, green discharge.
MERCURIUS SOL.	: For suppuration of the middle ear. Discharge is profuse, green, thick and fetid.
PULSATILLA NIG.	: Thick, profuse, yellow, bland discharge with an offensive odor.

SILICEA : Thin discharge of pus from the ears. May be due to caries of the ear bones if it contains small pieces of bones or may be due to the rupture of a boil in the ear. The pain is negligible.

TELLURIUM MET. 6 : Catarrh of the middle ear. Discharge is acrid, smells like fish pickle. Itching, swelling, throbbing in the meatus. It is the best of all remedies for this disease.

OVARIES

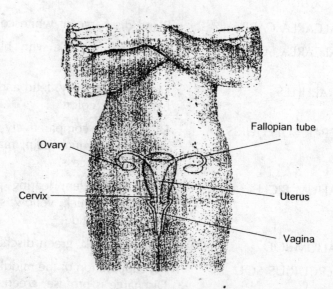

ACONITUM NAP. : Any complaint of ovaries after exposure to dry cold winds.

ALUMEN : Tumors of ovaries with obstinate constipation.

APIS MEL.	: An important remedy for ovarian affections. Congestion in the right ovary causes soreness in the inguinal region with burning and stinging pain; swelling. If there is numbness down the thighs, this remedy is definately indicated. It is also useful in affections of the left ovary. Inflammation of the ovaries in childhood. Suppression of menses due to tumor of ovaries.
AURUM IOD.	: Ovarian cysts.
AURUM MUR. NAT.	: Induration of the ovaries.
BELLADONNA	: Acute ovaritis. Throbbing pains appear and disappear suddenly and appear again. Bearing down sensation. Pain is worse on the right side.
CALCAREA CARB. 200	: Polypi of uterus and ovaries. Cutting pain in the uterus during menstruation. Menses too early, too profuse, too long lasting with vertigo. Feet icy cold. It is a very successful remedy under these conditions.
COLOCYNTHIS	: Ovarian neuralgia relieved by bending double. Cystic tumor.
GRAPHITES	: Swelling and induration of the left ovary with delayed scanty menses. Pain in the right ovary.
HAMAMELIS Q	: Warm mother tincture applied externally over the ovarian region, relieves pain of ovaritis, instantly. It is also useful given orally in case of injuries to the ovaries.

IODIUM : Atrophy of ovaries. Ovaritis. Wedge like pains in the right ovarian region. Dwindling of mammary glands.

KALIUM BROM. : Cystic tumors of the ovaries with increased sexual desire.

LACHESIS : Pain in the left ovary, relieved by discharge from the uterus. Cannot bear tightness about the waist and loins. Tendency of the affection to move from left to right. Chronic enlargement of the ovaries. Tumor or cancer of the left ovary or both ovaries.

LECITHINUM 3X : Ovaries inefficient or not working adequately. Four doses per day for eight weeks.

MEDORRHINUM 1000 : Pain in the ovaries, worse left side or it may move from ovary to ovary.

MERCURIUS COR. : Ovarian neuralgia. Sticking pains in the left ovary.

OOPHORINUM 3X : Complaints, following removal of - ovaries. Ovarian cyst. Atrophy of ovaries.

PALLADIUM MET. : A good ovarian remedy for pain and inflammation. Pain and swelling in the right ovary. Cutting pain in the uterus, relieved after stool. Most indicated in proud ladies, who like flattery.

PHOSPHORUS : Polypi of ovaries with burning, worse lying on painful side and better by taking a cold bath.

SABAL SER. Q, : Ovaries tender and small.
ONOSMODIUM

SILICEA : Cyst in the vagina and ovaries with icy coldness of the whole body.

STAPHYSAGRIA : Ovaritis due to masturbation.

THUJA OCC. : Polypi of the ovaries; ovaritis, worse left side, every menstrual period with profuse perspiration before menses.

XANTOXYLUM A. : Neuralgia of ovaries. Pain in the loins and lower abdomen, worse left side, extending to thighs.

ZINCUM VAL. 2X : Painful affection of the ovaries. Pain shoots down the limbs to the feet. Requires a long time to cure.

OZENA
(DISCHARGE FROM THE NOSE)

ASAFOETIDA : Syphilitic ozena.

AURUM MUR. 12X : Atrophy of nasal mucous membrane accompanied by considerable crusting, discharge and a very offensive odor.

TEUCRIUM MUR. : Ozena with loss of sense of smell. Nasal catarrh of the nose with clinkers and crusts.

PALPITATION

AGARICUS MUS. : Palpitations from sudden noise or on coughing. Nervous palpitation.

BELLADONNA : Palpitations after least exertion with headache and a flushed face.

CARBO VEG. : Palpitations on account of acidity and excessive flatulence in stomach.

CIMICIFUGA : Palpitations with a sinking sensation in the pit of the stomach. Uneasiness and restlessness.

CRATAEGUS OXY. Q, DIGITALIS : Palpitations on account of threatened heart failure.

GLONOINUM : Palpitations with dyspnea. Beats of the heart are very strong and each beat is heard in the ears.

IGNATIA AMARA : Hysterical palpitations.

LACHESIS : Palpitations on least excitement, specially during menopause.

MOSCHUS : Nervous palpitations or nervous excitement. There may not be any organic disease of the heart.

NATRIUM MUR. : Palpitations in anemic patients due to weakness.

NUX VOM. : Palpitations after eating, indigestion and from flatulence.

OXALICUM ACIDUM : Palpitations with dyspnea in organic heart diseases, worse when thinking of it.

TERMINALIA ARJUNA Q : Palpitation in heart diseases, may be due to any heart disorder, dyspnea, nervousness, etc.

VISCUM ALB. : Palpitation during coition.

PANCREAS

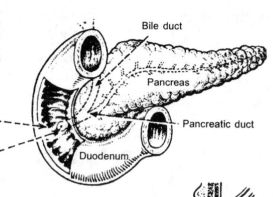

This is the racemose glandular portion of the pancreas producing its digestive secretion which is delivered to the second part of the duodenum.

Anatomical variations occur in this region. Commonly the pancreatic and bile ducts fuse as they enter the ampulla of Vater ....

....but sometimes they enter the duodenum separately.

Microscopically, the exocrine tissue is similar to salivary glands.

ARGENTUM NIT. : Inflammation of the pancreas, flatulence and indigestion. Wind is expelled with noise.

CHIONANTHUS Q : Inflammation of pancreas with liver problems.

FRAGARIA VESCA Q : Stone in the pancreas, for expulsion.

IODIUM Q : Losing flesh while eating well. Cancer of pancreas with vomiting and diarrhea with foamy stools containing fats.

IRIS VERS. : It covers several pancreatic diseases when acidity, indigestion, nausea and vomiting are present. Increases flow of bile.

MERCURIUS SOL., BELLA- DONNA, KALIUM IOD.	: Inflammation of pancreas. Look for other symptoms also.
PEPSINUM 3X	: Imperfect digestion with pain in the gastric and splenic region.
PHOSPHORUS	: Fatty degeneration of the pancreas. Oily looking stools. Excessive bleeding from cancer of pancreas.

PARALYSIS

AGARICUS MUS.	: Exalted notions. Involuntary laughing and crying alternately.
AURUM MET.	: Paralysis due to hypertension.
BARYTA CARB.	: Paralysis of old men, with mental and physical weakness.
BELLADONNA	: Paralysis, insanity, with marked hallucinations and illusions. Depression.
CANNABIS IND.	: When exaltation of ideas is very marked with sleeplessness.
CAUSTICUM 10M	: Paralysis of the left arm and left leg. Paralysis of the ocular muscles, after exposure to cold. Lids seem heavy and there is an inclination to close the eyes. Right side is mostly affected. Paralysis of the right side of face. This remedy is very useful in recent or chronic cases. Repeat after four days, if needed.
CONIUM MAC.	: Slow developing, ascending paralysis.

GELSEMIUM	: Paralysis of various groups of muscles around the eyes, throat, chest, larynx, intestines, extremities, etc. Post diphtheritic paralysis. Polio and Laundry's paralysis. Muttering speech. Numbness.
IGNATIA AMARA	: Hysterical paralysis, specially of the neck.
LATHYRUS SAT.	: Paralytic affections of the lower extremities. Involuntary contraction of the muscles. Paralysis of the eyelids and eye balls. Slow movement of fingers and toes. Infantile paralysis. Paralysis after wasting diseases, with slow recovery of nerve power. Excessive rigidity of legs.
NUX VOM.	: Paralysis as a result of over eating, excessive drinking of liquors, etc.
PLUMBUM MET.	: Paralysis of a single muscle. Cannot raise anything with the hand. Paralysis from over exertion of extensor muscles in piano players. Paralysis of all the four limbs (quadriplegia). Painful paralysis.
SENEGA	: Paralysis of the left side of face with a burning sensation on it. Distinct eye symptoms of a paralytic type.
ZINCUM MET.	: Slow developing, descending paralysis.

PARALYSIS AGITANS
(PARKINSON'S DISEASE)

Parkinson's disease is caused due to the gradual death of dopamine producing brain cells, for some unknown reasons. There is a special kind of protein, called 'Glial-cell Derived Neuotrophic Factor' or G. D. N. F. , and it is believed that this increases the survival and growth of the brain dopamine producing cells.

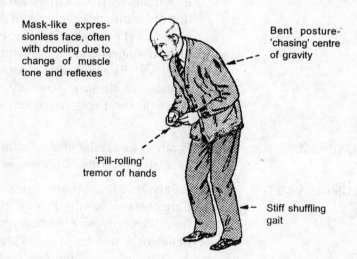

Mask-like expressionless face, often with drooling due to change of muscle tone and reflexes

Bent posture- 'chasing' centre of gravity

'Pill-rolling' tremor of hands

Stiff shuffling gait

AGARICUS MUS.	: Jerking, trembling and stiffness of the muscles. Spine cannot even bear a touch.
AMBRA GRISEA	: Parkinsonism with numbness of the affected parts of the body. Specially indicated in the aged.
ANTIMONIUM CRUD.	: Paralysis with the characteristic, thickly white coated tongue.
ANTIMONIUM TART.	: Chronic tremors of head and hands.

ARGENTUM NIT.	: Use it with Gelsemium on alternate days, when the memory is also impaired with spurting diarrhea and flatulence.
AURUM SULPH.	: Constant nodding of the head.
AVENA SAT. Q	: Best tonic for debility after exhausting diseases, nervous exhaustion and paralysis agitans. Give 20 drops thrice daily, in warm water.
CAUSTICUM	: Unsteadiness of the muscles of forearm and hand. Numbness. Loss of sensation of hands.
COCCULUS IND.	: Staggering gait. Hands tremble while eating or holding things.
CURARE	: Reflexes lessened or abolished in extremities. Weakness of hands and fingers, cannot lift the fingers.
GELSEMIUM	: When this remedy is indicated, there is trembling of the head and other parts of the body. Staggering gait. Start with 30th potency, go on increasing the potency and reducing the number of doses each month. Trembling is the chief indication for the use of this remedy.
HELODERMA	: Parkinson's disease affecting the left side mostly with the feeling of prostration and coldness.
MAGNESUM PHOS. 1000	: Involuntary shaking of the hands. Give it weekly.
MERCURIUS SOL.	: Paralysis on account of overuse of mercury or its preparations.
PHYSOSTIGMA	: Muscular weakness is felt more on movement and in winter. Palpita-

tion of the heart is felt throughout the body.

STRAMONIUM : Parkinsonism. Tremor, muscular weakness and rigidity. Peculiar gait and shaking.

PAROTID GLAND

BELLADONNA : Parotid glands swollen. Sensitive to loud noises. Hearing, very acute.

KALIUM BICH. : Swelling of the parotid gland with sharp pains extending to the ear. Inflammation remaining after measles.

SULPHUR IOD. : Parotid glands enlarged. Parotid hypertrophied.

PELVIS

AESCULUS HIP. 3X : Dragging pain in the pelvis and hips while walking.

BELLIS P. : Sore, bruised feeling in the pelvic region after injuries to the bones under the buttock and pelvic organs. Worse with hot or cold bath, cold wind and motion.

MAGNESIUM SULPH. : Pain in the back, hips and pelvic region.

SEPIA : Bearing down sensation in females. In ladies, hips are like men, narrow pelvis.

PENIS

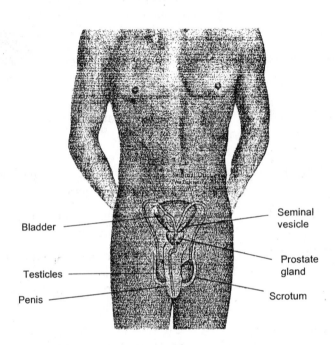

Bladder

Testicles

Penis

Seminal vesicle

Prostate gland

Scrotum

ACIDUM PHOS.	:	Edema of the prepuce and glans penis. Warts on the prepuce. Penis is swollen. Herpes on prepuce.
ANTIMONIUM CRUD., STAPHYSAGRIA, ARGENTUM MET.	:	Thinning and reduction in size of the penis after having attained full girth and length.
CALCAREA CARB. 10M	:	Penis and testicles missing in the child.
CAUSTICUM	:	Itching of penis.
CORALLIUM RUB.	:	Ulcers on glans and inner prepuce with thin, yellow, fetid discharge. Sexual weakness.
DIGITALIS	:	Edema of the prepuce.

GINSENG 3X	: In comparison with age, the penis is weak and does not have hard erections.
GRAPHITES	: Herpes on penis.
HEPAR SULPHURIS	: Ulcers on the external surface of prepuce. Itching of glans, frenum and scrotum.
IGNATIA AMARA, NUPHAR LUT., AGNUS CASTUS	: Penis is small and retracted.
KREOSOTUM	: Burning of penis on sexual intercourse and penetration.
LYCOPODIUM	: Penis becomes small and relaxed due to masturbation and excesses.
MERCURIUS IOD.	: The skin of prepuce becomes tight, obstructing flow of urine and semen. Prepuce cannot be moved up and down.
MERCURIUS SOL.	: Ulcers on glans and inner prepuce. Prepuce irritated. Herpes of the prepuce.
PAREIRA BRAVA	: Violent pain in glans penis and urethritis.
PETROLEUM	: Hole of glans penis is dilated.
QUINIDINUM	: Strengthens the penis and sexual organs.
RHUS TOX.	: Edema of penis.
SABINA	: Cartilaginous swelling of the penis.
SALIX NIGRA	: Pain in penis on erection.
SILICEA	: Eruptions and boils on the prepuce.

SULPHUR   : Stitching pain in penis. Itching of
                             penis when going to bed. Cracks
                             on prepuce.

THYROIDINUM 6   : This remedy is effective in unde-
                             scended testicles in boys.

VIOLA TR.   : Swelling and itching of the pre-
                             puce.

NOTE: **Researchers of the University of California and San
Francisco found that on an average an erected penis
measure 5.1 inches in length and 4. 9 inches in
circumference. Subnormal penis when erected
measures less than 2. 8 inches in length and 3. 5 inches
in girth.**

PEPTIC ULCERS

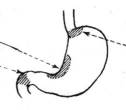

Gastric ulcers are typically sited on the **distal lesser curve**. Chronic ulceration of the first part of the **duodenum is the most common** site of peptic ulceration

A few occur at the cardiac end of the stomach or in the distal **oesophagus**

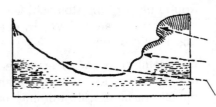

The ulcer is commonly large, 2-3 cm, and oval. It has an overhangng lip at the proximal end.

Frequently it has a terraced structure.

The distal end slopes away from the ulcer bed.

Peptic ulcers are lesions (holes or breaks) in the lining
membrane of the stomach or duodenum. Increased acidic

secretions in the stomach appears to be the major cause but for some people cigarette smoking, stress and some allopathic drugs may also contribute to ulcer development. The allopathic treatment changes rapidly from antibiotics (for treatment of HELICOBACTER PYLORI or H. P. bacteria which is supposed to be one of the causes but they are not sure from where H. P. come) to antiacids to neutralize the acidic symptoms to anti-ulcer drugs to reduce the production of acid. A combination of all the three is also used. In homoeopathy, the following remedies have proved useful and curative.

ALUMINA PHOS.	: It is useful, when the patient vomits food mixed with blood and is suffering from tuberculosis of intestines. Bleeding peptic ulcers. See also acidity.
ANACARDIUM ORI.	: Pain and burning begins after 2-3 hours of taking the meals, when the stomach is empty. Eating gives relief temporarily.
ARGENTUM NIT.	: Use it with the symptoms of Ars. combined with loud eructations.
ARSENICUM ALB.	: Lot of burning in the stomach and epigastric region, worse at night and after eating and drinking.
GRAPHITES	: For long standing peptic ulcers, with pain and pressure.
KALIUM BICH.	: Round ulcer of the stomach. Gastric symptoms are relieved by eating. Peptic ulcers.
LYCOPODIUM 200	: It is useful for peptic ulcers, when the patient passes wind in both directions alongwith burning in the oesophagus. Incomplete burning eructations, rise only to the pharynx and burn there for hours.

PHOSPHORUS	: For duodenal ulcers, when there is vomiting of food mixed with mucus, bile and blood.
ROBINIA	: This remedy is useful, when there is great acidity.
URANIUM NIT.	: Peptic and duodenal ulcers. Eating is followed by flatulence.

Note : Below are some hints for changes in lifestyle for avoiding oesophageal and other gastric ulcers and acidity:

1. **Sleep with your head about 6″ high.**

2. **Do not eat or drink foods with caffeine or alcohol.**

3. **Avoid citrus juices, tomatoes and hot spicy food.**

4. **Eat small meals at shorter intervals, about 6 times each day.**

5. **Do not eat immediately before going to bed.**

PERSPIRATION (SWEAT)

The symptoms of perspiration prove very useful for the selection of a remedy.

ACETICUM ACIDUM	: Sweat drenches the patient in hectic fever but there is no thirst.
ACIDUM FLUOR.	: Itching on account of sweat. Profuse, sour and offensive perspiration.
ALUMINA	: The patient does not sweat at all. Such patients are always constipated; their stools are hard, dry and knotty and the patient has to strain, to expel them.

ARSENICUM ALB.	: Cold perspiration.
BELLADONNA	: Sweating on the covered parts only.
BROMIUM	: Perspiration on palms and on least exertion.
BRYONIA ALBA, SELENIUM MET.	: For continued, profuse sweat. Nothing answers so well in sweating of phthisis.
CALADIUM SEG.	: Sweet perspiration, which attracts flies.
CALCAREA CARB.	: Cold, pale and fleshy patients with excessive general sweat, specially on the head, hands and feet.
CALCAREA PHOS. 6X	: Sweat on the hands, which feels cold. Sweaty head at night.
CALOTROPIS Q	: Increases the skin circulation. Has a powerful effect in producing perspiration.
CARBO VEG.	: Profuse sweat on the forehead. Patient has to wipe it off with his hands.
CHELIDONIUM	: Sweat stains the clothes, yellow.
CHINA OFF.	: Perspiration during sleep or on being covered.
COLCHICUM AUTUM.	: Profuse sweat accompanied with gastric ailments. Bad effects from suppressed sweat.
COLOCYNTHIS	: Perspiration smells like urine.
CONIUM MAC.	: Sweating on head, hands, palms, etc. as soon as one sleeps or just on closing the eyes.
FERRUM PHOS.	: Sweating in acute infectious diseases.

HEPAR SULPHURIS	: Cold and foul foot sweat.
HYROCOTYLE A.	: Perspiration copious.
IODIUM	: Perspiration on little exertion, on account of weakness.
LACHESIS	: Perspiration is absent.
LEDUM PAL.	: Warm sweat on hands and feet, increases with the heat of bed. It is worse on waking.
LYCOPODIUM	: Sweat smells like onions, and it disappears on movements.
MAGNESIUM MUR.	: For foot sweat.
NATRIUM CARB.	: Inclination to perspire easily.
NATRIUM MUR., CHAMOMILLA	: Perspiration while eating. This condition is called gustatory sweating and mostly occurs in diabetes.
NITRICUM ACIDUM	: Sweat all over the body after a meal.
PETROLEUM, SULPHUR, SILICEA, MERCURIUS SOL., STAPHYSAGRIA	: Fetid perspiration.
PILOCARPUS M., HYDROCOTYLE A.	: Very copious perspiration. Pilocarpus has drops of perspiration all over the body.
PSORINUM 200	: There is profuse sweating after the cure of diseases. Sweating feels pleasant.
PULSATILLA NIG.	: Sweating on one side of the face only.
RHUS TOX., SILICEA	: Offensive sweat of axillae and feet as indicated with other symptoms. Perspiration on palms and soles.
SILICEA	: Offensive sweat on icy cold feet.

The foot feels sore. Profuse sweat on head extending to the neck. Offensive sweat in armpits.

STRYCHNINUM PHOS. 3X : Hands and axillae are covered with sticky fetid sweat.

SULPHUR : Sweat smells like garlic in the armpits.

THUJA OCC. 200 : Sweat smells like honey and is only on the uncovered parts, except face.

TUBERCULINUM 200 : Profuse sweating in pulmonary tuberculosis with loss of weight. Sweat stains yellow.

VERATRUM ALB. : Cold perspiration, specially on the forehead in all diseases.

PHARYNGITIS

BELLADONNA : Swelling of uvula and stinging in the throat. Pharyngitis with small bleeding ulcers.

CISTUS CAN. : Dryness of the throat, patient likes to drench it by sipping water. Pain in the throat, worse by inhaling cold air.

ELAPS COR. 6 : For chronic naso pharyngeal catarrh with greenish crusts and bad smell, it is specific.

KALIUM BICH. : Pharyngitis with tough, stringy and ropy mucus. Sensation of a thorn in the throat.

KALIUM MUR. : A routine but a good remedy for the disease. Tonsils are swollen.

LYCOPODIUM	: Difficulty in swallowing. Mucous membrane of the throat appears pale.
MENTHOLUM	: It is curative for pharyngitis. Use 2 doses a day.
NATRIUM MUR.	: Suits the patients of pharyngitis with constipation, dryness of the throat and excessive thirst.
PHYTOLACCA DEC.	: Pharyngitis with small, white ulcers in the throat. Pain in the throat with a bluish look.
SANGUINARIA CAN.	: Pharyngitis, worse on the right side. Throat appears red.
SILICEA	: Pharyngitis with a sore throat and chronic catarrh.
STICTA PULM.	: Coryza with a frequent desire to blow the nose.
WYETHIA	: It is an excellent remedy for pharyngitis in singers and public speakers. Throat is irritable and there is dry hacking cough due to tingling in the larynx.

PHLEGM
(MUCUS)

CAUSTICUM	: Cough with mucus lodged under the sternum which is difficult to dislodge and expel.
CORALLIUM RUB.	: Post nasal catarrh. Profuse secretion of mucus dropping through the posterior nares.

GRAPHITES   : Phlegm with extreme sensibility to strong smells. There are crusts inside the nostrils and cracks on the nose. It is painful to blow the nose.

HYDRASTIS CAN.   : Mucus is yellowish green, thin and acrid. It accompanies coryza, when the nose runs constantly. Post nasal dripping of thick mucus.

KALIUM BICH.   : Mucus is greenish yellow and stringy which can be drawn in long strings or is ball like and sticks on the tongue. It falls at the back of the nose into the throat.

KALIUM MUR.   : Mucus that occurs in the second stage of cold, is thick and white with post nasal dripping.

NATRIUM CARB.   : Catarrh of posterior nares. Hawking much mucus from the throat, worse slightest draught.

NATRIUM MUR.   : Mucus like white of an egg or transparent and is very profuse. There may be loss of sense of smell and taste.

PHYTOLACCA DEC.   : Flow of mucus from one nostril and from the posterior nares.

PULSATILLA NIG.   : Yellow mucus with a stuffed nose and pain above the eyes or in the right cheek bone. The patient has a weeping tendency.

PHOTOPHOBIA
(DREAD OF LIGHT)

(SEE LIGHT)

PHTHISIS

(SEE TUBERCULOSIS)

PILES

(SEE HEMORRHOIDS)

PIMPLES

(SEE ACNE)

PITUITARY GLAND

Anterior pituitary (Adenohypophysis)

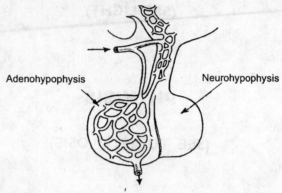

CALCAREA CARB.	:	Dysfunction of the pituitary gland.
HECLA LAVA 3X	:	Tumor of the pituitary gland.
THYROIDINUM 2X	:	Excessive activity of the pituitary gland and fibroid tumors in the pituitary gland.

NOTE: The pituitary gland regulates the release of growth hormone. People who have their pituitary gland removed, do not grow properly.

PLAGUE

IODIUM	:	Acts prominently on connective tissues and constriction of larynx on account of plague.
OPERCULINA TURP.	:	Plague with fever and diarrhea. Lymphatic glands enlarged and indurated. Boils suppurate slowly. Abscesses.

TARENTULA CUB.   : A curative and preventive remedy
                          specially during the period of in-
                          vasion.

PLEURISY

(INFLAMMATION OF THE PLEURA)

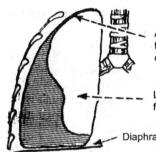

Above the fluid, the fibrin covered layers of pleura are adherent

Lung is collapsed by fluid pressure

Diaphragm depressed by fluid

Pressure of fluid may displace heart to opposite side.

Fluid contains small masses of clot. Its specific gravity is high, >1018, and its protein content>4%. These features distinguish it from a transudate.

ACONITUM NAP.   : It should be the first remedy, to be
                          thought of for chest pains. Bryonia
                          alba should be given, if it fails to
                          relieve in one day.

ANTIMONIUM ARS.   : Pleurisy with sweat and inflamma-
                          tion of the heart.

ARNICA MONT.   : Pleurisy resulting from an injury
                          inflicted by a broken rib. It may
                          yield completely to the use of this
                          medicine. If a supplement is
                          needed, Bryonia and Kali-c.
                          compete for choice.

ARSENICUM ALB.   : Great restlessness. Drinks often but
                          little at a time. Burning pain in the
                          chest, relieved by warmth.

BRYONIA ALBA	: Stitching pain in the chest, worse on any motion and better by rest and cold things. Dry pleurisy.
CANTHARIS	: Great burning in the chest, also in the urethra while urinating.
CHINA OFF.	: Pleurisy with fever and great weakness.
HEPAR SULPHURIS	: Pleurisy complicated with bronchitis. Formation of pus in the chest. Wet pleurisy.
KALIUM CARB.	: Breathlessness. Burning pain in the chest. Cough.
KALIUM SULPH.	: Applicable in the later stages of inflammation. Rattling of mucus in the chest. Yellow expectoration with pus formation.
RANUNCULUS BULB.	: Pain in the muscles of the ribs. Chilliness in the chest while walking in open air. Rheumatic pains in the chest. Pleurodynia.

PNEUMONIA

ACONITUM NAP.	: A remedy for the first stage of pneumonia. High fever preceded by chill. The pulse is hard and the skin is dry. Dry painful cough. The cause may be dry, cold winds. When thick expectoration starts, Acon. ceases to be the remedy.
ANTIMONIUM TART.	: Great rattling of mucus but very little is expectorated and that too,

with some efforts. Threatened paralysis of the lungs.

ARSENICUM ALB.   : Dyspnea. Thirst, drinks often but little. Fever with restlessness.

BRYONIA ALBA   : If the above remedies fail to cure, use of this remedy is indicated. Cough is loose and there are sharp sticking pains in the chest. Breathlessness and the patient does not want to move.

CHELIDONIUM,   : Fan like motion of alae nasi. LYCOPODIUM   Pain under the corner of right shoulder blade is a sure indication for use of Chelidonium.

FERRUM PHOS. 6X   : In the beginning of the disease or in the later stages, when there is bleeding from the lungs. Repeat it every 2 hours. A suitable remedy for fever.

IODIUM 3X   : It can be indicated in any stage of pneumonia. There is cough and difficulty in breathing. The sputum is bloody. Repeat it every hour, when indicated.

IPECACUANHA   : Nausea. Wheezing cough. Chest feels full of phlegm but does not yield to cough. Pneumonia of children.

KALIUM MUR.   : This remedy is alternated with Ferr-p. for good results in this disease. The mucus is thick and white.

PHOSPHORUS 200   : Give one dose if Ant-t. and Bryonia fail. It follows Bryonia very well. This remedy is more often indicated and gives curative results.

TUBERCULINUM 1M   : Broncho pneumonia of children. Hard hacking cough. Profuse sweat and loss of weight. Rales all over the chest.

VERATRUM VIR.   : Extreme congestion of the chest, breathing opprened. Dyspnea. Nausea and vomiting.

POLIO

ACORUS CALAMUS Q   : 10 drops a dose in the morning, daily for a few months.

CALCAREA PHOS. 12X,   : Two grains of each mixed together,
NATRIUM MUR. 12X,   3 doses a day for 3 months. All the
KALIUM PHOS. 12X   medicines should be stopped during this course.

GELSEMIUM 6-CM   : In increasing potencies, it cures polio. Use 6th potency, 2 doses per day for a month, 30 potency 2 doses per day for a month and 200 potency one dose every 5th day for 2 months and CM potency one dose a month for 3 months till cured.

HYPERICUM PERF. 12X   : Two doses a day for 1-3 months in the morning and noon.

LATHYRUS SAT. 30   : Two doses daily for 1-3 months in the evening and at bed time.

THUJA OCC. 200   : Start the treatment with this remedy. No other remedy should be given on that day.

NOTE: Watch the following symptoms for post-polio syndrome for the indicated remedy.

1. Unaccustomed fatigue requiring the patient to rest during mid-day or earlier.

2. New joint and muscular pains.

3. Muscular weakness or loss of muscle use which did not bother while suffering from polio.

4. Respiratory or swallowing problems.

5. Unusual intolerance of cold, which causes muscular weakness, burning pain or discoloration of limbs.

6. Psychological stress.

POLYPUS
(SOFT TUMOR)

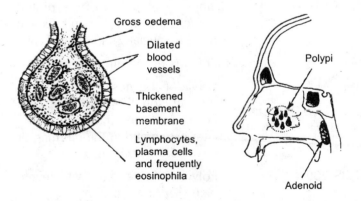

An abnormal growth from the mucous membrane resembling a tumor but not cancerous; commonly found in the nose, uterus, rectum and sometimes in the ear and larynx.

ALUMINA	: Polyp in the left nostril of the nose. The peculiar constipation confirms the use of this remedy.
BERBERIS VULG.	: Polyp of vocal cords.
CALCAREA CARB. 200	: A good remedy for polypus of the nose, ear, bladder, uterus, etc. It should be repeated after 7 days. Mucus polypus, which bleeds easily.
CALCAREA IOD. 3X	: Polypi of the nose and ear.
CALCAREA PHOS.	: A large polypus of the nose extending to the brain.
CHOLESTERINUM	: Polypus of the gall bladder in a pre-cancerous stage. Burning pain in the liver region. General debility.
CONIUM MAC.	: Uterine polyp, which protrudes while passing urine. Bleeding polypus of the nose.
FORMICA RUFA	: Stops development of polypi and reduces the size. It is an effective remedy specially for polypi of ears.
KALIUM BICH.	: Polypus of the air passages.
KALIUM NIT.	: Polyp of the nose or elsewhere, specially on the right side with headache or heaviness of the head after eating and in the morning or towards the evening.
LACHESIS 200	: Polyp of the left ear, with severe pain. Sensitive to air.
LEMNA MINOR	: Nasal polypi. Swollen mucous membranes of the nose. Atrophic rhinitis. Fetid smell. Reduces the obstruction of the nose by reducing the swelling.

MERCURIUS SOL.	: Polypus, blocking the ear which bleeds easily and affects hearing. Right ear is mostly involved.
PHOSPHORUS	: Nasal polyp, bleeding easily. Handkerchief is always bloody. Imaginary odors. Craving for cold drinks. Sneezing.
SANGUINARIA CAN.	: Polypus of the nose or larynx. Smarting and burning in the nose and throat. Nose obstructed. Bleeding from removal of crusts.
SILICEA 6X	: Blockage of nose, nostrils inflamed. Patient chilly. Perforation of the septum.
TEUCRIUM MAR. CM	: It is one of the best remedies for polypus of the nose. Three - four doses repeated after an interval of 15 days usually cures permanently. It cures polypus of the rectum also. Blockage of the nose on the side the patient lies on. It cures polypus of the vagina too. Polyp is soft and of jelly like in consistency.
THUJA OCC. 200	: Polyp of the middle ear and uterus with a chronic tendency.

POLYURIA
(SEE ALSO URINE)

ALFALFA Q	: Polyuria. Frequent urging to urinate.

ALUMINA	: Frequent urination, but one must strain to pass it. Urine burns and is sometimes mixed with yellowish pus.
ARGENTUM NIT.	: Frequent and profuse urination.
CAUSTICUM	: Frequent urination at night. It takes a long time to finish.
CHELIDONIUM	: Frequent desire. Urine is copious. May be milky in color and foaming like beer.
ERYNGIUM AQUA	: Frequent urination, every half an hour. Dribbling and burning in the urethra, before and after passing urine.
IGNATIA AMARA	: Polyuria in hysterical subjects and frequent urination after drinking tea and alcohol.
LEDUM PAL.	: Polyuria. Urine may be copious or little. The stream of urine often stops during urination.
MURIATICUM ACIDUM	: Urine escapes while passing wind. Polyuria day and night with copious urine.
NUX VOM.	: Frequent urination on account of indigestion.
PULSATILLA NIG.	: Specially indicated in ladies. Dribbling of urine. Has to rush to urinate or it escapes.
SABAL SER. Q	: Prostrate gland enlarged. Constant desire to pass urine.
VESICARIA COM. Q	: Polyuria, worse at night. Has to pass urine every 15 minutes or so, due to inflammation of the bladder or a kidney trouble. Blood, pus,

albumin, etc. in the urine is cured by the use of this remedy.

PRE MENSTRUAL SYNDROME
(P. M. S.)

CALCAREA CARB. : PMS with fluid retention, particularly swollen, tender breasts, painful joints, weakness, lack of energy, depression, tearfulness, irritability, anxiety and fear of insanity.

PULSATILLA NIG. : PMS with extreme tearfulness, depression, self pity, anxiety about the future, tendency to gain weight before menses and possibly headache, nausea and dizziness.

SEPIA : PMS with marked indifference to words the loved ones. Irritability, tearfulness, difficulty in concentrating,a desire to get away from everything, extreme anger, fits of screaming, sensation as if the uterus is coming out of the vagina, accompanied by an oily skin and desire for very salty or very sweet food. Such conditions usually occur on approach of menopause.

PREGNANCY

For details of a particular symptom during pregnancy, also see the particular head in this book.

Bearing down	: See PROLAPSUS, UTERUS
Cough	: See DROPSY
Miscarriage	: See ABORTION

AMYGDALUS PER. Q	: This is a very good remedy for 'morning sickness'. Constant nausea and vomiting in pregnant women, also gastric and intestinal irritation.
AGARICUS MUS.	: For weakness of the lower extremities.
ALUMINA	: Craving to eat chalk, lime, soil or charcoal.
ANACARDIUM ORI.	: Dyspepsia and insomnia.
ANTIMONIUM CRUD.	: Loss of appetite. Desire for acids, bitter lemon, pickles, etc.
APOCYNUM CAN.	: It is useful when there is albuminuria or some kidney problems.
ARNICA MONT.	: For mis-step or an accident during pregnancy, when a miscarriage is threatened, repeat every 15 minutes till the desired results are achieved.
BELLIS P.	: Backache and inability to walk.
COCCULUS IND.	: Bleeding during pregnancy due to lack of sleep. Clotted blood with spasmodic colic.
CONIUM MAC.	: Breasts become painful. Constipation.

FICUS IND. Q	: It is a very useful remedy for all sorts of abnormal bleeding before and after pregnancy.
GRATIOLA OFF.	: Vertigo. Dyspepsia, dysphagia, cramps and colic with wind in the abdomen. Constipation or diarrhea, stools are forcibly evacuated without pain.
IPECACUANHA	: Nausea and vomiting in pregnancy.
KALIUM CARB.	: For weakness in general.
LAC DEF.	: Vomiting during the first quarter of pregnancy.
MAGNESIUM CARB.	: Toothache during pregnancy.
MANGANUM ACET.	: Desire for always lying down in the bed.
MUREX PURP.	: Walking difficult in pregnancy because of weakness of all joints. Must lie down from weakness but her symptoms worsen on lying down and after sleep.
NATRIUM MUR.	: Unnatural and excessive craving for salt during pregnancy.
NITRICUM ACIDUM, CALCAREA PHOS.	: Longing for indigestible things like chalk, sand, etc.
PHOSPHORUS	: Albuminuria during pregnancy.
PULSATILLA NIG.	: Give it in 30 potency when the position of the unborn child is not normal i. e. head is not below and is upside or lying sideways. It also avoids displacement of the uterus and keeps it in the right place.
SECALE COR. 6	: Discharge of blood during pregnancy.

SEPIA : It is a good remedy for toothache or constipation during pregnancy. It is also useful when there is always an urgent desire to void urine and if not voided in time, a few drops may escape. It is also useful in vomiting of pregnancy. Unusual bleeding during pregnancy from 5th to 7th month or a habitual abortion from 3rd to 7th month. Constipation during pregnancy

STRAMONIUM : Symptoms of insanity or mania during pregnancy.

SULPHUR : Feeling in the abdomen as if the child is kicking from inside.

SULPHUR 6, CALCAREA PHOS 6X : If a woman repeatedly gives birth to babies who die soon after birth or in early infancy, give these medicines, one dose of each, daily during the last two months of pregnancy. The child should be given Alfalfa Q, 5 drops, three times a day for several months, 10 minutes before each feed.

SYMPHORICARPUS 200 : It is a routine prescription for vomiting during pregnancy. The leading symptom is relief from lying on the back.

SYMPHYTUM OFF. : Persistent vomiting.

THUJA OCC. : Violent movements and kicking of the child inside the abdomen. It compels the mother to urinate on account of pressure on the urinary bladder.

VIBURNUM PRUN. Q   : 5 drops a dose will cure cramps during pregnancy.

NOTE 1: It is said that for obtaining a male child, a woman should take Nat-m. 6X one dose daily and for obtaining a female child, Pulsatilla 6X one dose daily from 3rd to 5th month of pregnancy.

NOTE 2: Aur-m. CM (one dose) given at the time of commencement of pregnancy, usually results in the birth of a male child.

PRICKY HEAT
(SEE SUMMER RASH)

PROLAPSUS

RECTUM

ALOE SOC.   : Prolapse of the rectum with diarrhea, bleeding and tenesmus.

FERRUM PHOS. 6X   : Prolapse of rectum in children.

MURIATICUM ACIDUM   : Prolapse while urinating.

PODOPHYLLUM   : Rectal prolapse after stool, by sneezing, coughing and with diarrhea. Stools of green or yellow color. Worse in the morning. Useful for both women and children.

RUTA G.   : Prolapse at the slightest attempt to pass stool. Prolapse after labor in women.

SEPIA	:	Prolapse of the rectum with weight like a ball in the rectum.

UTERUS

ALOE SOC.	:	Prolapsus of the uterus with diarrhea.
BELLADONNA	:	Bearing down with feeling as if everything will be passed out of the vulva. Fetid discharge.
KALIUM CARB.	:	Prolapse of the uterus after labor. One dose after 7 days, if necessary Not to be repeated often.
LACHESIS	:	Prolapse of uterus during menopause.
LILIUM TIG.	:	Feeling as if all the pelvic contents will pass through the vagina. Dragging from the naval. Constant desire to pass urine.
NATRIUM MUR.	:	Prolapse of uterus with cutting in the urethra. Bearing down pains, worse in the morning.
PODOPHYLLUM	:	Prolapse of uterus after the delivery of a child.
PULSATILLA NIG.	:	Bearing down sensation with pains, worse lying down.
SEPIA	:	It is the most effective remedy in prolapsus uteri, misplacement of the uterus or its inversion, etc. It restores the uterus to the normal position within a few days without manual intervention even in the 30th potency. Higher potencies will work well in chronic cases. Must cross limbs to prevent protrusion of parts.

STANNUM MET.   : It is another strong remedy for prolapse of uterus. It also strengthens the uterine ligaments. Prolapse is worse while passing the stool.

TILIA EUR.   : Bearing down feeling as if everything will protrude out of the vulva. Leucorrhea. Uterine prolapse after labor. Intense sore feeling around the uterus.

PROPHYLACTICS

BACILLINUM 10M   : Preventive against tubercular inheritance. Should be taken for about 2 months, a dose every 4th day.

BAPTISIA TINC.   : Preventive against typhoid.

BELLADONNA   : Prophylactic against simple scarlet fever.

DIPHTHERINUM 200   : Preventive against diphtheria.

GOLONDRINA 1M   : Its use provides immunity against the bites of poisonous snakes.

INFLUENZINUM 200   : Preventive against influenza.

KALIUM MUR.   : Prophylactic against the epidemic of jaundice. 3 doses a day for a week or so.

LATHYRUS SAT.   : Preventive against polio.

MALARIA OFF.   : Preventive against malaria.

MORPHINUM, MALANDRINUM   : Preventive against measles.

PAROTIDINUM   : Preventive against mumps.

PERTUSSINUM	: Preventive against whooping cough.
PSORINUM 1000	: Preventive against itches and scabies mite.
PULSATILLA NIG. 1000	: Triple vaccine for prevention of measles, mumps and chickenpox. One dose every day for three days at bed time. Repeat every 3 or 6 months.
STAPHYSAGRIA 6X	: Preventive against mosquito bites.
VACCININUM, MALANDRINUM	: Preventive against small pox.

NOTE: In case of prophylactics, it may be understood that higher the potency, the longer the immunity. It is said that 10000 potency will give an immunity of about 8 years, 1000 would give about 2-1/2 years protection and 30 would give protection for a few months only.

PROSTRATE GLAND

Approximately 75% of all men over the age of 70 suffer from prostrate problems. Symptoms are usually caused by an enlarged prostrate. In some cases, it is cancer.

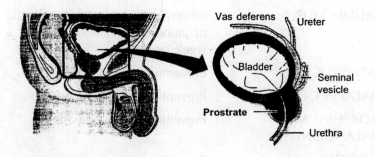

Enlarged prostrate gland

Possibly due to male hormone concentration, the gland grows, putting pressure on the urethra.

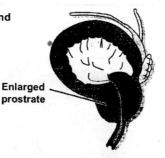

Enlarged prostrate

Symptoms

- Weak urinary stream.
- Frequent urination.
- Urination takes longer than normal.
- If untreated, can cause bladder infections and kidney failure.

What prostrate is

- Cluster of glands about the size of a walnut.
- Surrounds the urethra, the tube carrying urine from the bladder.

- Secretes thick whitish fluid that helps transport sperm.
- Growth of the prostrate gland stops at age 20, starts again after age 50.

Prostrate cancer

Second most common cancer among men.
Symptoms: Similar to those for enlarged gland.

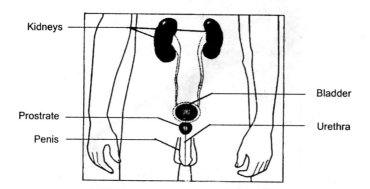

Kidneys

Prostrate

Penis

Bladder

Urethra

Front view of interior of male urinary system and prostrate

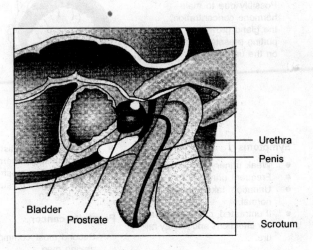

*How the digital rectal examination helps
detect prostrate disease*

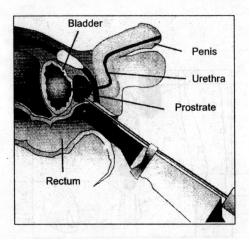

Transrectal ultrasound biopsy of the prostrate

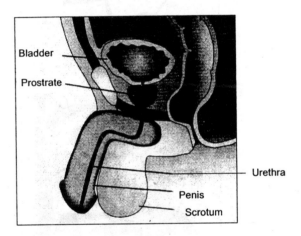

BPH : Enlarged prostrate squeezes urethra and bladder wall is thickened

Stage of prostrate cancer

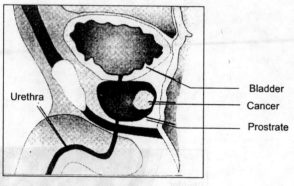

Urethra

Bladder

Cancer

Prostrate

Cancer confined to the prostate

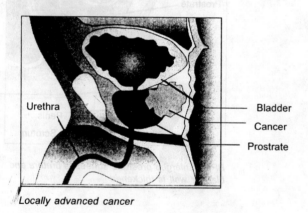

Urethra

Bladder

Cancer

Prostrate

Locally advanced cancer

Lymph nodes

Bones

Cancer spread to other organs (metastatic)

ACIDUM PHOS. Q	: Prostrate fluid passes even when passing a soft stool.
ALFALFA Q	: Enlargement of the prostrate gland and polyuria.
ALOE SOC.	: Involuntary passing of urine in old age due to enlargement of prostrate gland.
ANACARDIUM ORI.	: Prostrate fluid passes while at stool and after having made water.
ARGENTUM NIT.	: Chronic enlargement in old people.
BARYTA CARB.	: Enlargement of the prostrate gland in old people.
CADMIUM PHOS.	: Useful in suspected carcinoma of the prostrate gland.
CHIMAPHILA	: Great urge to urinate. Straining necessary to commence urination. Urine feels hot, when passed.
CISTUS CAN.	: Cancer of the prostrate gland.
CONIUM MAC.	: Discharge of prostratic fluid on every motion with itching of prepuce and enlargement. Urine starts and stops again and again.
CROTALUS H.	: Cancer with bleeding of the prostrate gland.
DIGITALIS	: Constant urging to pass urine which comes in drops with a cutting and throbbing pain in the bladder.
HOANG NAN Q	: Cancer of the prostrate gland. Start with 5 drops thrice daily and gradually increase to 20 drops.
HYDRANGEA Q	: Enlargement of the prostrate gland without any complication, specially in old people. 2 doses of 5-10

drops, morning and evening every day. Very difficult urination. It also works well in 200 and 1000 potency. Urine may be retained, specially in men over 50 years of age.

LYCOPODIUM : Backache before urination, which goes afterwards. Urine is slow to come and the patient strains to pass it. In 1M potency, it is useful curing prostrate cancer.

PARIERA BRAVA : Retention of urine due to prostrate enlargement.

PITUITRINUM : Prostatitis, chronic nephritis and high blood pressure, difficult mental concentration and confusion are removed by the use of this remedy in the 30th potency.

SABAL SER. : Burning in the urethra while passing urine and difficulty in passing urine. Recent or chronic enlargements. Sensation of coldness from the prostrate gland to genitals.

SELENIUM MET. : Discharge of prostratic fluid during stool. Prostratitis in elderly men. Dribbling of prostratic juice during sleep. The use of food articles containing this metal reduces the risk of prostrate cancer. It is found in minute quantities in meat, fish, whole grains, dairy products and vegetables grown in selenium rich soil.

STAPHYSAGRIA : Enlargement with frequent urge to pass urine. Sensation as if a few drops remained.

THUJA OCC.   : Prostratic discharge is thick and
                         green. Inflammation of the gland.

TRIBULUS TER. Q   : 15 drops thrice daily corrects
                         prostratitis and ill effects of mastur-
                         bation.

TURNERA Q   : It cures prostratic discharge, which
                         is chronic and accompained with
                         sexual debility.

NOTE 1: Eating tomatoes reduces the risk of prostrate cancer.
   Tomato contains vitamins A, B complex,C as well as iron
   and potassium. Red tomatoes contain lycopene which
   protects against a variety of ailments.

NOTE 2: Excessive use of aluminium in water or in food is
   believed to be one of the major causes of prostrate
   cancer.

NOTE 3: The prostrate is a small gland about the size of a
   chestnut and is situated just below the bladder. It
   secretes a fluid which transports the sperms during
   ejaculation. Women do not have a prostrate.

NOTE 4: In all urinary problems, the prostrate gland is not
   always concerned. It is best to consult an urologist (i.
   e. a person who specializes in dealing with the urinary
   tract in both sexes and the genital tract in males) before
   getting a treatment.

NOTE 5 : Prostrate cancer patients are being effectively treated
   by using a vaccine prepared from their own cancer.
   Seeatle (New Orleans-USA) researchers make the vac-
   cine by drawing blood from the prostrate cancer
   patients. This vaccine shrinks the prostrate tumor and
   puts an hold on its growth.

PRURITUS

ALOE SOC.	: Intense itching in the anus and the opening of the intestines into it. The patient bores fingers into the anus for relief and gets pleasure in rotating the finger in it.
ALUMINA	: Intense itching all over the body, when getting warm in bed. Must scratch until it bleeds and then becomes painful. Brittle skin on the fingers.
AMBRA GRISEA	: Voluptuous itching of scrotum and pudendum with soreness and swelling. Parts numb but burn internally. Itching in the urethra.
BORAX	: Sensation of distention in the clitoris. Itching during pregnancy.
CALADIUM SEG.	: Pruritus of vulva and vagina during pregnancy.
COLCHICUM AUTUM.	: Pruritus of female genitals. Sensation of swelling in vulva and clitoris.
COLLINSONIA CAN.	: Swelling accompanied with dark redness of genitals and soreness. Pruritus lessens after menses. Swelling of labia and clitoris.
HELONIAS	: Very irritating itching of vulva and vagina.
MEDORRHINUM 1000	: Pruritus with intense itching.
RADIUM BROM.	: For intense itching of the anus, one dose of 30 potency each day.

SEPIA	: Pruritus of vagina and yellow leu-corrhea.
SULPHUR	: Pruritus due to warmth of bed with burning urine. Parts bleed on scratching.
TARENTULA HIS.	: Vulva dry and hot with intense itching.

NOTE: Such patients should take a bath daily but a sudden change in the temperature of water should be avoided. Medicated soaps or ointments should not be used. If necessary, a glycerine soap may be used for bathing and coconut oil may be applied gently on the affected parts and not rubbed. Locally, the parts can be washed with hydrogen peroxide, 1 part of it is mixed with 12 parts of water.

PSORIASIS

Psoriasis can be on any part of the body but is rarely present on the face. The cause is unknown and it responds to homoeopathic treatment very well. Sun rays specially early morning at down are very beneficial as they contain ultraviolet rays. The treatment is lengthy and requires patience. The disease lessens severely in summer and goes into remission from time to time with no apparent reason.

ARSENICUM ALB.	: When other symptoms of the remedy are present and there is irritation of the skin. Its first influence is to make eruptions redder and more inflamed. It is the good sign when using this remedy. There is a burning sensation which is relieved by warmth.

AURUM MUR. NAT. 3X	: Only for psoriasis syphilitica.
CALOTROPIS Q	: Psoriasis of syphilitic patients in the second stage, when mercury has stopped doing further good.
CARCINOCINUM 1M	: A monthly dose as an intercurrent remedy ensures, prompt cure.
CHRYSAROBINUM	: If the nails become dull and develop ridges and pits, the cause being psoriasis. Give T. D. S. Its ointment - 8 grains in an ounce of vaseline can be used externally. Vesicular lesions with fetid discharge and crust formation. Violent itching. Thighs,legs and ears specially affected.
CICUTA VIR.	: Spots with burning pain, when touched. Several irritating eruptions on the ears.
CORALLIUM RUB.	: Psoriasis of palms and soles.
CUPRUM MET.	: Chronic psoriasis. Skin is of a bluish color. Few spots itch, worse in the folds of joints.
GRAPHITES	: If the crusts are sticky and glutaneous, and the patient is constipated and cautious.
HEPAR SULPHURIS 200	: Patient over sensitive to changes in weather, specially dry cold and desires warmth.
HYDROCOTYLE A. 200	: Psoriasis of soles, palms, trunks and extremities with circular patches. Circular spots with scaly edges. The skin is excessively thick and dry.
IGNATIA AMARA 200	: Aggravation of psoriasis after disputes and anger.

KALIUM ARS.	: Discoloration of the skin, after psoriasis has been cured,is removed by this remedy.
KALIUM BROM.	: Worse on the chest and shoulders and in very rare cases, when it spreads to the face also. It is a leading remedy for psoriasis.
MANGANUM ACET.	: Psoriasis with painful cracks and worse at the time of menses.
MERCURIUS BIN IOD. 3X	: Syphilitic and non-syphilitic psoriasis.
MEZEREUM 200	: Psoriasis of palms, itching worse warmth.
PETROLEUM 200	: Once a week, when there is aggravation by cold and in winters. Thick greenish crusts. Burning and itching specially in psoriasis of hands with fissures.
PSORINUM 200	: This is a nosode and it works well. When the skin looks dirty and there is much itching, which is worse by the warmth of bed. Crusts disappear in summer and reappear in winter.
RADIUM BROM. 200	: Circular patches of psoriasis all over the body. Itching, redness, swelling and extreme burning of the skin as if on fire, worse on undressing but better in the open air and by taking a hot bath.
SELENIUM MET. 200	: Syphilitic psoriasis of palms.
SULPHUR 10M	: Start the treatment with this remedy. The patient is dirty and has an aversion to bathing. Burning and itching, dry, scaly,

unhealthy skin. The disease is worse in spring time and in damp weather. No other remedy should be given for 24 hours after Sulphur 10M has been given and repeat it after a month.

THYROIDINUM 3X : It is indicated specially in younger girls. It is also useful in distressing, itching of the disease. It is more indicated in patients with thyroid problem and obesity. Skin is dry.

TUBERCULINUM 200 : Chronic psoriasis with intense itching, worse at night. It is particularly indicated in tuberculous children and in patients having a history of tuberculosis in the family.

DIET : **Long term dietary changes with respect to fat intake may help to produce an improvement. Animal fats should be eliminated while oil of seeds does not produce any adverse effect. Similarly non-vegetarian food should be substituted with vegetarian food. Alcohol should not be consumed during the treatment. It is generally believed that the disease is produced by eating a fish suffering from psoriasis but the exact cause is not known.**

PUBERTY

ALUMINA : Anemia in girls, who have not yet menstruated. Pale and livid complexion. Laziness. Impaired appetite and digestion. Chlorosis.

ASAFOETIDA 3X : Breasts swollen and painful. Milk may appear in them though, patient has never been pregnant.

ASTERIAS RUB. : Pimples on the face during puberty.

AURUM MET. : Palpitations of the heart at puberty. Foul breath from the mouth.

CALCAREA CARB. : Leucorrhea before the appearance of menses.

FERRUM MET. : Polyuria.

KALIUM CARB. : Delayed first menses or menses appear once and since then, have not appeared for months together.

LYCOPODIUM : Non development of breasts even at the age of 18 years.

MANCINELLA : Mentally depressed at puberty. Sadness on account of disappointed love.

MERCURIUS SOL. : Appearance of milk in breasts instead of menses.

ONOSMODIUM 10M : Absent breasts appear and exceedingly small breasts may become normal by its use. Use one dose every 15 days.

PITUITRINUM 30 OR 200, : Delayed symptoms of puberty i. e.
ZINCUM MET. defective development of the breasts, no growth of axillary and pubic hair.

PULSATILLA NIG.   : This is a remedy for many men-
                           strual troubles during puberty. First
                           menstruation is delayed. Uncalled
                           sadness or weeping during pu-
                           berty. It also cures irritability dur-
                           ing puberty.

SULPHUR   : Abdomen having an appearance
                           of pregnancy, but without it.

PURGATIVE

CASCARA SAG. Q   : 15 drops in water, thrice daily
                           restores the normal functions of
                           the intestines.

HYDRASTIS CAN. Q   : In chronic constipation, 3 drops of
                           it in a glass of water in the morning
                           is an effectual purgative. It is best
                           suited to persons, who after an
                           active life have become seden-
                           tary.

LAXATIVE   : A glass of cold water on rising in
                           the morning with a level teaspoon
                           of common salt makes an excel-
                           lent laxative.

PYORRHEA

CALENDULA OFF. Q   : It reduces the inflammation of the
                           gums and also avoids formation of
                           pus. 10 drops in an ounce of water

may be used as a mouth wash and a little of it can be swallowed.

EMETINUM 1X : Thrice daily for three days, go on reducing gradually and stop, when cured.

HECLA LAVA : When there is a thick pus like discharge and foul smell from the mouth.

KALIUM CARB. : All the teeth are loose. Bad smell from the mouth.

MERCURIUS SOL. 200 : It is a remarkable remedy in pyorrhea to avoid extraction of teeth, spongy gums and bad odor from the mouth.

SILICEA : It is an excellent remedy for this disease, in the chronic form. Painful inflammation of the gums with gum boils.

SYMPHYTUM OFF. Q : 2 grams in 8 ounces of water is a good local application for the gums in these cases.

QUARRELSOMENESS

AURUM MET. : Peevish, at least contradiction. Profound depression. Talks of suicide. Over sensitive.

IGNATIA AMARA : Sighing and sobbing with changeable moods. Melancholic and uncommunicative, the symptoms follow shock, grief and disappointment.

NUX VOM.	: Irritable, cannot bear noise or smell. The patient is sunken, fault finding and has a fiery temperament.
PETROLEUM	: Feels that death is near. Irritable, easily offended. Vexed at anything.
SULPHUR	: Lazy, irritable and depressed. Very selfish with no regard for others. Hates standing, dislikes water and washing.
TARENTULA HIS.	: Sudden changes in moods. Ungrateful and discontented.

QUINSY

(ACUTE INFLAMMATION OF TONSILS WITH FEVER)

(SEE THROAT ALSO)

HEPAR SULPHURIS 3X	: Extreme pain in the throat on swallowing, one sided swelling and inflammation about the tonsils, pain often extending to the ear. Three doses a day preferably in water.
HYDRASTIS CAN Q	: Used as a gargle in septic sore throat, in malignant scarlet fever; arrests the destructive process at once.
LACHESIS	: There is no remedy so effective in breaking up an attack of quinsy at its conception or in promoting resolution in the later stages. Very distressing, aggravation after sleeping.

RABIES
(HYDROPHOBIA)

ANAGALLIS 1X, CANTHARIS, XANTHIUM SPIN.	: These remedies are given symptomatically when there isgreat fear of water.
BELLADONNA 30	: After 7 days, one dose in the evening one in the morning, when there is fever and diarrhea.
HYDROPHOBINUM 30	: Rabies on account of bites of mad animals. This remedy should be taken four times a day at an interval of two hours each for 7 days.

RASH

ACONITUM NAP.	: Rash with sharp fever.
AMMONIUM CARB.	: Scarlet rash, miliary rash, scarlatina.
BELLADONNA	: Rose rash.
BRYONIA ALBA	: Rash accompanied with constipation.
IPECACUANHA	: Rash accompanied with nausea and difficult breathing.
NATRIUM SULPH. 6X	: Red wart like eruptions all over the body. Itching, worse while undressing,rainy weather and after bathing.
PHYTOLACCA DEC.	: Measle like rash, rose colored.
PULSATILLA NIG.	: Rash from a disordered stomach.

REGURGITATION

AETHUSA CYN.	: Regurgitation of food after about an hour of eating.
ASAFOETIDA 3X	: Flatulence and regurgitation of liquids with pulsations in the pit of the stomach.
CARBO VEG.	: Regurgitation of fluids with wind, due to indigestion.
CARBOLICUM ACIDUM	: Regurgitation of food with constant belching and nausea.
CHINA OFF.	: Regurgitation of bitter fluid and food, worse after eating fruits. Belching gives no relief.
LYCOPODIUM	: Regurgitation of food with rolling of flatulence.
PULSATILLA NIG.	: Regurgitation of food eaten long before.

REJUVENATION

ANACARDIUM ORI. 200	: Exhausted people, whose spirit is shattered and whose memory has suffered, be it after a serious illness, sexual excesses or the breaking down process of old age. The greedy, suspicious, malicious old man can use this remedy for all his mental and physical health if relief by eating is indicated. It is a leading symptom for the use of this remedy.

CALCAREA PHOS. 6X : Both men and women whose health has been broken down by a town residence, missing sunshine and open air for a greater part of the day and for any reason has become incapable of doing much work and whose spirits are depressed, are benefited much by use of this remedy.

MAGNESIUM PHOS. 10M : It covers the exhaustion and most of the painful ailments, of which old people often complain and a person who looks older than his age.

RESTLESSNESS

ACONITUM NAP. : Physical and mental restlessness. Tossing about, even in sleep. Frequent nightmares. Severe neuralgia with tingling and numbness. Thirst is always present and comes with fever.

AETHUSA CYN. : Violent palpitations. Headache and vertigo. Anxious and weeping.

AGARICUS MUS. : Severe itching. Skin feels as if burning.

ALUMINA : Anxious and confused dreams.

AMBRA GRISEA : Excited and very talkative.

ANAGALLIS : Cross and irritable, wanders aimlessly. Bewildered and confused.

APOCYNUM CAN. : Unable to sleep with restlessness.

ARANEA DIAD.	: Wakes with feeling as it arms and legs were swollen and heavy. Extreme coldness, day and night. Poor sleep.
ARNICA MONT.	: Sleepless and restless when overtired.
ARSENICUM ALB.	: Weakness and exhaustion, worse each night. Periodical burning pains with a cold skin and extreme anxiety.
BELLADONNA	: Hot red skin with a flushed face, dry mouth and throat. Excited mentally. Restless sleep. Acuteness of all senses.
CALCAREA CARB.	: Restless sleep at the time of periods.
CANTHARIS	: Anxiety and restlessness ending in rage.
CAUSTICUM	: At night, tearing pain in bones and joints. Loss of energy. Restless legs at night.
CHAMOMILLA	: Peevish and restless with colic, especially in children.
COCA	: Nervousness and nocturnal restlessness while teething.
COFFEA CRUDA	: Great nervous agitation with sleeplessness.
IODIUM	: Fever with flushed cheeks. Apathetic.
KALIUM BROM.	: Restless sleep with nightmares. Grinds teeth in sleep.
MAGNESIUM MUR.	: Sleeps during the day but restless at night because of heat. Bad nightmares.

NATRIUM CARB.	: Anxious and restless during thunderstorm.
PASSIFLORA	: Restless and wakeful resulting from exhaustion.
PHOSPHORUS	: Restless and fidgety. Wakes up frequently at night. Depressed and over sensitive.
PULSATILLA NIG.	: The first sleep is restless. Tired in the afternoon, wide awake in the evening. Thirstless, peevish and chilly.
RHUS TOX.	: Extreme restlessness. Constantly changing position. Joints are tender and ache. Great apprehension at night.
SECALE COR.	: Insomnia with restlessness. Fever and anxious dreams.
ZINCUM MET.	: Depression with restlessness. Coldness and spinal weakness. Restlessness during periods and menopause.

RHEUMATISM
(SEE UNDER GOUT)

RICKETS
(SEE UNDER BONES)

This disease is due to vitamin D deficiency which is found in milk. Sunshine is a good source of vitamin D. Children suffering from this disease have abnormalities in shape and structure of their bones. The usual symptoms are restlessness and slight fever at night, free perspiration about the head, enlarged liver and spleen, delayed dentition and badly formed teeth.

RINGWORM
(HERPES CIRCINATUS)

APIS MEL. 1000 : Ringworm with itching and burning, better by cold applications. Give one dose only.

BACILLINUM 200 : One dose should always be given at the commencement of the treatment. No other medicine for 24 hours.

CHRYSAROBINUM 3X : Vesicular ringworm. Foul smelling. Discharge and crust formation. Violent itching. Thighs, legs and ears are mostly affected. Scaly eruptions around the eyes and ears with pus beneath.

COD LIVER OIL : Application of the plain oil at bedtime on the affected skin has proved to be very useful in removing the madening itch.

DULCAMARA : Ringworm of the scalp. Thick brown crusts which bleed on scratching. Ringworm on the face, genitals and hands. Eruptions appear red.

GRAPHITES 200 : Eruptions oozing a sticky liquid, honey colored. Worse in the bends of limbs, groins, neck and behind the ears.

HEPAR SULPHURIS	: When the disease extends to the forehead, face and neck. Worse in dry, cold winds.
HYDROCOTYLE A. Q	: Dry eruptions. Great thickening of the skin. Scales. Psoriasis in circular patches on trunk, extremities, palms, soles.
KALIUM SULPH. 6X	: Ringworm of scalp or beard with abundant scales.
RADIUM BROM.	: It is better in open air and worse in bed and undressing.
RHUS TOX.	: Ringworm lesion oozes an offensive moisture with violent itching. Ringworm of scalp in children extending to face, neck and eyes.
SEPIA	: Ringworm is worse in open air and cold weather. Ringworm on moustaches. Itching not relieved by scratching. Eruptions every spring.
SULPHUR	: It may be used off and on during the treatment of the disease, if disease is not yielding properly. Also when there is acidity alongwith ringworm.
TELLURIUM MET.	: It is a remedy of great importance in the cure of this disease. It should be given 24 hours after the use of Bacillinum, four times a day. It is more indicated when ringworm is on the face. Body odor and sweat smell like garlic.

SACRUM

AESCULUS HIP.   : Aching, aggravated by walking or standing with blind piles.

ALOE SOC.   : Drawing and heaviness aggravated in the evening with bleeding piles and diarrhea.

BAPTISIA TINC.   : Pain in the sacrum, around the hips and legs. Sore and bruised, worse humid heat, indoors and in fog.

BERBERIS VULG.   : Violent pain, aching, bruised, dragging or pressing, aggravated by lying or sitting or stooping with rectal problems.

HELONIAS   : Sensation of weakness, dragging and weight in the sacrum and pelvis with great weakness and debility. Tiredness and pain in the back. Patient feels better, when he is kept busy or when his attention is engaged in some work.

LACHESIS   : Pain in coccyx, worse on rising from a seat, better by sitting perfectly still.

SABINA   : Pain from sacrum to pubes.

SEPIA   : Dragging pain with uterine disorders or loaded urine.

TELLURIUM MET.   : Pressing or bruised pain, stabbing like on motion, worse by coughing, laughing, stooping with rectal problems.

SALIVATION

AMMONIUM CARB., KALIUM CARB.	: Constant spitting due to excessive saliva.
ARSENICUM ALB., PULSATILLA NIG.	: Saliva bitter.
ARSENICUM ALB., NUX VOM.	: Saliva bloody. Saliva like cotton.
ARUM TRIPH.	: Saliva produces burning and rawness of lips.
KALIUM CARB., BARYTA CARB.	: Saliva runs out from the mouth during sleep.
COFFEE BERRIES	: Chewing of coffee berries cures excessive salivation when all other remedies fail.
HYDROPHOBINUM 200	: Constant spitting. Saliva tough and ropy. Throat is sore.
IRIS VERS.	: Saliva in the corners of the lips when talking. May accompany nervous headache. Profuse flow of ropy saliva.
KREOSOTUM	: Excessive saliva during pregnancy.
MERCURIUS SOL.	: Saliva fetid.
NITRICUM ACIDUM	: Saliva profuse and bloody.
PILOCARPUS M.	: Saliva pours out in an almost continuous stream. Many children suffer from this, during teething.
SYPHILINUM, STRAMONIUM	: Dribbling of viscid saliva. In Syphilinum saliva runs out of the mouth while sleeping.

SCABIES

(SEE ECZEMA AND ITCHING)

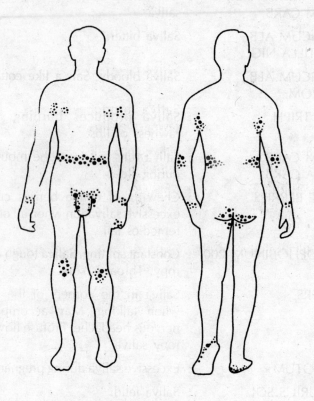

Distribution pattern of scabies

Parts most commonly affected are hands, between the fingers, wrists, axillae, genitalia, beneath the mammae and inner aspect of thighs.

SCALDS
(SEE BURNS)

SCALP

AETHUSA CYN.	: Feeling of hair being pulled from the scalp.
ARSENICUM ALB.	: Scalp itches intolerably and is covered by dry scales. It is very sensitive and even brushing of the hair is not tolerated.
BERBERIS VULG.	: Sensation of a tight cap pressing upon the whole scalp.
CALCAREA CARB.	: Eczema capitis or milk crusts on the scalp of children.
COLOCYNTHIS	: Pain and soreness of the scalp, better by heat and pressure.
NATRIUM SULPH.	: Scalp is sensitive to combing of hair. The patient does not want to comb her hair.
PHYTOLACCA DEC.	: Rheumatism of the scalp. Pain comes, everytime it rains. Scaly eruptions on the scalp.
SULPHUR	: Scalp dry. Itching. Scratching causes burning.
VINCA MINOR	: Eczema of scalp with great itching and a desire for scratching. Spots ooze moisture which mattes the hair together.

SCAPULA

AMMONIUM MUR.	: Icy coldness between scapulae not relieved by warmth or covering. Better in open air.
BARYTA CARB., RHUS TOX.	: Pain between the scapulae or shoulder blades.
CHELIDONIUM	: Constant pain under the lower inner angle of the right scapula.
CHENOPODIUM	: Intense pain between angle of right shoulder blade near the spine and through the chest. It has pain in the left shoulder blade also.
COLOCYNTHIS	: Sharp pain in the right deltoid and chest, better by pressure and warmth.
KALIUM CARB.	: Sharp, cutting pains in the right scapula, early in the morning and better on motion.
KALMIA LAT.	: Deltoid rheumatism, specially right.
LACHNANTHES TINC.	: Chilliness between scapulae.
LYCOPERSICUM ESCU.	: Sharp pain in the right deltoid and chest.
PHYTOLACCA DEC.	: Shooting pain in the right shoulder and scapula.
RANUNCULUS BULB.	: Muscular pain along the lower angle of scapulae, increased by cold air.
STICTA PULM. 30	: Pain in the right deltoid and chest, worse by sudden changes in weather.
SULPHUR	: Pain in the left shoulder and left shoulder blade.

SCARLET FEVER

AILANTHUS G. : The skin appears hot, purple or livid. Semi-consciousness, delirious, weak pulse and general prostration. Diarrhea and dysentery.

AMMONIUM CARB. : Lack of proper eruptions. Taking a chronic form. Throat swollen. Body red.

BELLADONNA : Covers many symptoms of the disease like sudden onset, rarely with a chill but sometimes with convulsions in very young children. Sore throat. Temperature from 101° F to 105° F. Frequent vomiting followed by a rash first on the neck and chest. Face flushed. Rash is seldom seen on the face.

RHUS TOX. : Symptoms of Belladonna but with blister like eruptions on the body.

STREPTOCOCCINUM : Antifebrile action. Septic conditions of the disease. Rapidly brings down the temperature and other symptoms.

SCARS

ACIDUM FLUOR. : Old scars become red around edges and itch.

ACIDUM SULPH. : For removal of scars left after healing of a wound.

CALCAREA FLUOR. 6X	: Use it for birth marks, scar marks and hard skin.
CROCUS SAT., LACHESIS	: Old healed scars of wounds, open again and again with a tendency to suppurate.
GRAPHITES	: For formation of a smooth scar after an operation. Old hard scars.
HYPERICUM PERF. 12X	: Slight paralysis due to entanglement of nerves in the scar. It removes effects of pain and bruises or injury to an old scar.
KALIUM IOD., PHYTOLACCA DEC.	: Scars left after the healing of an abscess or pimples.
MALANDRINUM	: For removal of scars of vaccination.
SILICEA	: Scars left after drying up of pimples, blotches or ulcers are removed by the use of this remedy. Scars of vaccination.
STAPHYSAGRIA	: Burning pain in the scar of an abdomen, after its operation.
VARIOLINUM 1000, THUJA OCC. 1M	: For the removal of ugly scars left after cure of small pox and chicken pox.

SCHIZOPHRENIA (MIND)
(SEE ALSO INSANITY)

A common type of mental disorder characterized by a disorder in perception, content of thought, thought processes (hallucinations and delusions), and extensive withdrawal of the individual's interest from other people and the outside world.

AETHUSA CYN.   : Sees cats and dogs and tries to jump out of the window, to escape their bite.

AILANTHUS G.   : Feels as if rats or insects are crawling over his body.

ALUMINA   : Confused. He sees something new and thinks he has already seen it. He says something and thinks he has already said it. Never smiles or laughs.

ANACARDIUM ORI.   : The patient has two wills, good and evil. Cannot take decisions. Fears he is being prusued by someone , enemies or thieves. Fears everything and everybody. Hears voices calling his name. Does not like to work and lacks self confidence.

ARGENTUM NIT.   : Fearful and nervous. Impulses to jump out of the window. Brain fag with general debility and trembling. Vertigo. Fear of death. Feeling of strangulation in the throat.

ARSENICUM ALB.   : Fears that thieves have entered his house. Searches them or hides himself due to their fear. Feels happy at others misfortune.

AURUM MET. 200   : Feeling of self condemnation and utter worthlessness. Disgusted of life. Hypertension. Talks of suicide but is afraid of death. Constant questioning, without waiting for a reply.

BELLADONNA	:	Eyes are blood shot. Attack others in self-defence or if somebody acts against his will.
BRYONIA ALBA	:	Thinks, talks and dreams always about business.
CALCAREA CARB.	:	Unable to acquire knowledge due to non-development of brain. Obstinate. Forgetful and confused. Talks to himself or appears to be talking to a person, who is not there. Sad and full of worries.
CAMPHORA	:	Fears darkness and strangers. Thinks of ghosts and fears them.
CANNABIS IND.	:	Imagines, he is hearing a love song, closes his eyes and is lost in the ideas of love. Thinks he has not taken any food for several days, though he has taken it a few minutes ago. Imagines he is enjoying the luxuries of paradise.
CANNABIS SAT.	:	Hears, somebody superior commanding him to commit suicide. Tries to obey the super human orders.
CAUSTICUM	:	He is terribly afraid, as if he has committed a crime and will be arrested, and jailed soon.
CHAMOMILLA	:	Very sensitive and irritable, therefore suffers from this disease, as a consequence.
CHLORALOSUM	:	Night terrors at night and in darkness. Sleeplessness.
CICUTA VIR.	:	Thinks, he was living in a strange place though living in his own house. Hate friends and relatives.

CICUTA VIR., STICTA PULM., LAC CAN.	: Sensation as if flying in air or walking several feet above the ground.
CIMICIFUGA 200	: Mania, due to suppressed neuralgia.
COCCULUS IND., COCA	: Delusion of something rolling on the wall or floor.
CROCUS SAT. 200	: Pleasant mania, sings and laughs, now happy and affectionate then currently becomes angry. Sudden changes from hilarity to melancholy.
CUPRUM ACET.	: Wrong concept of others. Fear of an attack on him. Sleeps late at night, at about 2 A.M. He is afraid that the police has come to arrest him. Hallucination of all kinds of figures and premises, when shutting eyes and during sleep.
CYCLAMEN, OLEANDER	: Thinks he is as pure and all others are impure. Walks away from everybody or grabs his clothes so that they do not touch another person . Takes a bath, if somebody touches him. One object appears double.
FERRUM IOD.	: Wrong impression about his height. Thinks he is so tall that he can touch the roof.
GRATIOLA OFF.	: It is a useful remedy,specially for women,when mental troubles arise on account of suppression of hurt pride.
HELLEBORUS NIG.	: Stupefied drowsiness during which he sees spirits and souls, and talks

	to them. Cannot be aroused from the stupor despite shaking him vigorously.
HELONIAS	: Very irritable and sad. Cannot withstand the least contradiction. Patient must do something to engage the mind and is better when kept busy and mind engaged.
HYOSCYAMUS NIG.	: Suspicious, quarrelsome and obscene. Strips himself before others. Jealous. Suspects he is being poisoned, refuses to take the medicine or food. Talks to imaginay persons. Desire to remain in bed always.
IGNATIA AMARA 1M	: Complaints after disappointment in love or due to grief. Changeable mood. Silent brooding. Melancholic, sad and tearful. Sighing and sobbing.
KALIUM PHOS. 6X	: Extreme depression. Very nervous. Anxiety. Lethargic. Does not want to meet people. Extreme lassitude. Night terrors. Loss of memory. Shy, weak and tired. This remedy causes mental and physical improvement in a wonderful way. For insomnia use 200X potency.
LACHESIS	: Suspicious. If he sees two persons talking, he thinks that they are talking about him, tries to listen to their conversation secretly. Dreams that God or angels are commanding him and he must obey. Suspects that enemies are pursu-

ing him. Very inclined towards religion.

LYCOPODIUM 200 : Sad. Afraid to be alone. Apprehensive. Weak memory and confused thoughts. Sadness in the morning on rising. Spells or writes wrong words. Lack of confidence.

MEDORRHINUM : Suspects someone talking or whispering behind her back or someone following her. Feels as if committed a sin but is not afraid of going to jail. Very selfish and hasty in manners. Hopeless of recovery. Cannot speak without weeping.

MELILOTUS ALBA : Suspects that everybody is looking at her. Runs away from the scene.

MERCURIUS SOL. : Feels something unusual in his openings of the body, cold water in the eyes, ice ball in the ear, a vegetable plug in the throat, etc.

MERCURIUS COR. : Mistrustful. Loss of will power. Wary of life. Desire to kill his own child. Filthy and bad smell from the body and breath.

NATRIUM MUR. 200 : Psychic, on account of a disease or due to grief, fright, anger, etc. Depressed. Consolation aggravates. Wants to be alone and cry. Tears with laughter.

NATRIUM SULPH. 1M : Complaints due to head injury. Lively music makes him sad.

NUX MOSCH. : Feels as if he has two heads. Feels that people are playing and stops to watch them.

NUX VOM.	: Irritable and vindictive. Cannot bear light, noise, odors, etc. Does not want to be touched. Fond of non-vegetarian food and alcohol.
PALLADIUM MET.	: Thinks that he is not getting the respect he deserves while he is a fool.
PETROLEUM	: Feels another person is sleeping with her in the bed. Shrieks on this account.
PLATINUM MET.	: Very proud of herself and feels that all others are inferior to her in wisdom, wealth and height.
PSORINUM	: Sensation as if the head is floating and the body on the ground, both separated.
PULSATILLA NIG. 200	: Weeping, yielding, gentle and mild. Easily consoled and discouraged. Religious minded. Sad and weepy, before menses.
SABADILLA	: Thinks she is pregnant where as she is not. Will sleep with her legs elevated for fear of abortion.
SEPIA 200	: Aversion to the family members even to husband and children. Lacks natural affection.
STAPHYSAGRIA	: Insanity on account of insults and anger. Depressed without a cause. Insanity from sexual sin of a forced intercourse.
STRAMONIUM	: Talks with spirits. Visions of animals, black dogs, etc. Must have light and company. Imagines a crowd of bedbugs is pursuing him.

Attempts to stab and bite. Thinks all others are smaller than him in height. Feels as if a part of his body is missing . Delivers prophecies. Claps hands. Religious mania. Wants to pray all the time. Childhood mania. Suppressed violence or fear of violence to him.

SULPHUR : Thinks, he has a large sum of money in the bank or feels that a large sum of money is due to him from somebody. Untidy herself but feels very beautiful. Very selfish with no regard for others.

TARENTULA HIS. : Restlessness. Moves around constantly, without an aim. Foxy. Destructive impulses. Becomes violent on contradiction. Very lustful. Schizophrenic patients who have a dirty body and clothes. Sensitive to music. Wants hair brushed or head rubbed.

THUJA OCC. 200 : Feels as if his soul and body were separate. Music causes weeping and trembling.

TUBERCULINUM : Mania. Symptoms always changing. Wants to roam and travel. Depressed. Fear of dogs and animals. Desire to use foul language, curse and swear. Cruel and destructive. Insomnia, Irritable, especially when awakening. Nocturnal hallucinations. Awakens frightened.

VERATRUM ALB. Religious mania. Wants to pray all the time. Destroys things and tears up his clothes. Mania from childhood. Walks briskly in the room without any aim, looking upon the ground.

ZINCUM MET. : Weak memory. Very sensitive to noise. Melancholic, lethargic and stupid.

SCIATICA

AESCULUS HIP. : Sciatica with backache. Walking, stooping or rising from a seat is very painful.

AMMONIUM MUR. : Feels shortness of the left hip. Limps while walking. Pain worse while sitting but better on lying down.

ARSENICUM ALB. : Sciatica on account of certain fever and after. Pain is of a burning character and is better by hot applications.

CARBONEUM SULPH. : Sciatica, flying pains, returning regularly for a long time. Chronic sciatica.

CAUSTICUM : Left sided sciatica with numbness. Constant desire to move the foot.

CHAMOMILLA : Sciatica in very sensitive patients, who feel the pain much more than what it actually is. Numb feeling. Pain worse by motion and at night.

COLOCYNTHIS 200 : Remedy of the first choice for sciatic pain. Dull pain shoots down the hip to the feet through the thighs. Pain is relieved by heat and

	hard pressure but worse on movement.
EUPATORIUM PERF. 200	: Shooting pain along the course of left sciatic nerve. Pain in the hip bones with a tired feeling.
GINSENG 6	: It is considered as specific for sciatica, when there is a frequent desire for micturition. Feeling of contraction and stiffness in the affected parts.
GNAPHALIUM	: Sciatica pain, worse by rest. Numbness alternates with pain. It is specially useful when the pain is associated with numbness. It's peculiar symptom is that, the pain is worse lying and walking but better by sitting.
GUAIACUM OFF. Q	: Gouty, tearing, lancinating pains and feeling of contraction in the affected limb. Pain is worse by pressure, motion, heat, cold wet weather and from 6 P.M. to 4 A.M.
INDIUM MET. 200	: Sciatica with modalities like Rhus-t. It is a very good remedy for this disease.
KALIUM BROM.	: Left sided sciatica, better by motion.
LYCOPODIUM 1M	: Sciatica, worse right side.
MACROTINUM 2X	: A good remedy for sciatic pains. It should be tried first, when no definite remedy can be chosen.
MAGNESIUM PHOS.	: Right sided sciatica, better by warmth. Pain comes and goes rapidly.

MEDORRHINUM 200 : When other remedies fail, patient feels better in knee chest position.

PHYTOLACCA DEC. 200 : Pain runs down the outer side of limb, specially on the right side, like electric shocks.

RANUNCULUS BULB. Q : Chronic sciatica. Apply tincture to the heel of the affected leg also.

RHUS TOX. : Pain worse right side, cold weather and at night. Sciatica brought about by an exposure to moist weather.

SYPHILINUM 1000 : Sciatica, worse at night. Gradually better from sunrise to sunset and the pain gradually increases at night.

SEA SICKNESS
(SEE TRAVELLING SICKNESS)

SEMEN

ACIDUM FLUOR. : Semen reddish brown.

ACIDUM MUR. : Semen bloody.

ANACARDIUM ORI. : Semen passes during a hard stool.

CONIUM MAC. : Absence of sperms in semen.

DAMIANA Q : Sperms are absent in the semen.

LACHESIS : Semen milky with a strong odor.

MERCURIUS SOL. : Semen bloody.

NATRIUM PHOS.	: Odor of stale urine in semen.
PHOSPHORUS	: Sudden ejaculation.
SARSAPARILLA	: Bloody seminal emissions.
SELENIUM MET.	: Dribbling of semen after stool and micturition. Suffering after seminal emissions like headache, etc. Semen is thin and odorless.
TRIBULUS TER. Q	: For correcting semen and sperms. Sperms are absent or are in low count. Weak and thin semen. Poor mobility of sperms and other abnormalities like coiled tails, pairing, etc. are corrected by the use of this remedy.

NOTE: Semen is a mixed product of various glands. Prostate gland secretes a thin and slightly alkaline fluid which forms a part of the semen. Spermatozoa are produced in the testicles and are stored in the seminal vesicles. Sperm count in semen is 60-150 million/cc^3 out of which 80% should be mobile or moving.

SENSATIONS

ACONITUM NAP.	: Sensation of ants crawling on the abdomen.
AGARICUS MUS.	: Sensation of cold needles pricking the body and hair being pulled from scalp.
AILANTHUS G., ALUMINA	: Sensation as if something was crawling on the legs, under the pants.

ALUMINA SIL.	: Sensation of ants crawling under the head.
BORAX, GRAPHITES	: Sensation of a cobweb on the face.
CANNABIS IND.	: Sensation of being transparent and dual existence.
CHINA OFF.	: Sensation of sand in the eyes.
CISTUS CAN.	: Sensation of ants running through the whole body.
COCCULUS IND.	: Sensation as if worms were crawling in the stomach.
COCCUS C.	: Sensation of hair in the throat.
CROCUS SAT.	: Sensation of an imaginary pregnancy. Sensation of a child moving in the abdomen.
DAPHNE IND.	: Sensation as if limbs were separate from the body.
DULCAMARA	: Sinking sensation.
HYPERICUM PERF.	: Sensation of crawling in hands and feet.
LAC CAN. 200, STICTA PULM.	: Sensation as if walking on air.
LACHESIS	: Sensation as if someone was following him.
NITRICUM ACIDUM	: Sensation of splinters everywhere in the body. Sensation of biting by dogs.
PETROLEUM	: Sensation of somebody else sleeping in bed with her.
PYROGENIUM	: Sensation of a cap on the head.
STRAMONIUM	: Sensation as if limbs were separated from the body.

SULPHUR : Sensation of hot needles pricking the body.

THERIDION : Sensation of something moving around in the abdomen.

THUJA OCC. : Sensation of something alive in the body.

WILDBAD AQUA : It has a peculiar sensation as if all the joints were loose.

SEPTIC INFECTION
(SEPTICEMIA)

CALENDULA OFF. : It is a remarkable healing agent when applied locally on an open wound, which may be septic.

ECHINACEA Q : Symptoms of blood poisoning and septic conditions generally. Septic pustules. Foul discharges with emaciation. Useful in bites of co-bra snake, where it is given in 200 potency every 15 minutes and is also applied externally in tincture form. Puerperal septicemia.

LACHESIS : Low forms of diseases when the system is thoroughly poisoned, the prostration is profound. Modalities usually guide to the selection of this remedy. Worse after sleep and bluish purplish ap-pearance of the skin in boils, car-buncles, blisters, dissected wounds, etc.

PYROGENIUM 200   : It is the great remedy for septic states with intense restlessness, in septic fevers specially puerperal, dissecting wounds, sewer gas poisoning and after effects of miscarriages. All the discharges are horribly offensive. Chronic complaints that date back to the septic conditions and septic fevers.

STAPHYLOCOCCINUM 200: Septic infection in case of acne, abscesses, boils, etc.

SEXUAL DESIRE, EXCESSIVE

AGARICUS MUS.   : Itching and irritation of genitals makes her restless and she has a strong desire to embrace everybody.

ASTERIAS RUB.   : Excitement of sexual instinct with nervous agitations.

BARYTA CARB. 200   : Excessive sexual desire in children or in old persons.

BARYTA MUR.   : Excessive sexual desire for intercourse in ladies.

BUFO RANA   : Produces sexual over stimulation in healthy males.

CALADIUM SEG.   : Excessive sexual excitement due to pruritis of vulva and vagina during pregnancy or due to worms in the vagina.

CALCAREA PHOS.   : Suckling of a child causes sexual excitement. Sexual excitement before menses.

CANTHARIS	:	Irritation of vulva causes excessive sexual desire leading to sexual mania.
GRATIOLA OFF.	:	It is a very good remedy for females with excessive sexual desire, compelling her to masturbate.
HYOSCYAMUS NIG.200	:	She talks about obscene, nonsensical and vulgar things. Exposes her genitals.
LACHESIS	:	Desire increased during menopause.
MUREX PURP.	:	Violent excitement of the sexual organs. Desire easily excited even by the touch of parts.
ORIGANUM MAJ. 3X	:	Increased sexual desire in young girls, who are forced to masturbate. Desire for intercourse daily.
PHOSPHORUS 200	:	The patient exposes her genitals. Unbearable sexual desire forces her to vices. Desire again after coition. Constant wish for coition. Desire is worse during menses and pregnancy.
PICRICUM ACIDUM 6	:	There is a strong sexual desire with terrible erections.
PLATINUM MET. 200	:	Tingling inside the vagina and pruiritis causes excessive sexual desire, specially in virgins. Wishes to embrace everybody.
PULSATILLA NIG.	:	Sexual excitement during menses.
SEPIA 200	:	Leucorrhea causes increased sexual desire.
SILICEA	:	Excessive sexual stimulation.
STAPHYSAGRIA	:	Desire diminished after excessive masturbation or after excessive

indulgence.

STRAMONIUM 200 : Excessive sexual desire during the lying in period in women after labor and during menstrual periods.

STRYCHNINUM : Excessive desire for coitus in females turns "on" due to any touch on the body.

TARENTULA HIS. : Sexual desire increased during menses and mania. Wants coition again and again.

VERATRUM ALB. : Uncontrollable, excessive sexual desire during menses.

ZINCUM MET. : Excessive sexual stimulation with a desire to masturbate.

SEXUAL WEAKNESS

ACIDUM PHOS. Q : Sexual power deficient. Spermatorrhea. Parts relax during an embrace. Glans penis swollen. Semen is discharged, shortly after or even before an erection occurs.

AGNUS CASTUS Q : Lowered sexual vitality resulting in mental depression. Lacks courage for sexual act. Parts cold and relaxed. Loss of semen on straining. Testicles painful. No erection. Patient has no desire for intercourse, remains sad and sterile.

BUFO RANA : Partial impotence. Premature ejaculation and involuntary ejaculation.

CALCAREA.CARB.

: Increased desire for intercourse. Irritability and weakness after the intercourse. Ejaculation, too early.

CONIUM MAC.

: Male has a weak organ with intense desire and enormous thoughts, but is unable to perform. He ejaculates at the very thought of the presence of a woman. Erection is weak, lasts for a short time or the penis relaxes in the act of embrace. This condition can occur in both sexes as a result of frequent indulgence or excessive abstaining. It is a good remedy for old bachelors and old maids. A man's eyes wonder as virility declines, cannot perform without considerable help from the partner.

DAMIANA Q

: Sexual coldness and absence of sperms in semen. Impotence and sexual weakness in old people.

GRAPHITES

: Increased desire, decreased ability. Too early or no ejaculation. Decided aversion to coitus.

LECITHINUM 3X

: Male power lost or enfeebled. Absence of desire for sex.

LYCOPODIUM 200

: A man has lived a life of luxury and excesses. Has been unfaithful to several ladies in his younger days but now in advanced age has weak, thin semen and ejaculates earlier than his sex partner causing embarrasement; a dose of 200 or higher potencies will give satisfying results.

NUX VOM. 200	:	Parts relax during an embrace. Bad effects of excessive wine, women and high living. Testicles painful. Backache.
ONOSMODIUM	:	Sexual weakness in both sexes. Depressed sexual life in a woman, sexual desire completely destroyed in women and diminished in men.
SABAL SER. Q	:	Sexual desire is lost or diminished in both sexes on account of nervousness and some sort of fear.
SARSAPARILLA	:	Seminal emissions are bloody. A very bad smell emits from the genitals.
SELENIUM MET.	:	Increased desire with decreased performance. Sexual weakness due to thin and weak semen, which is without smell. Dribbling of semen involuntarily. Irritability after sexual intercourse. Penis relaxes during intercourse. Desire for sex absent.
SULPHUR	:	Erections are infrequent. Loss of semen at first contact. Organs cold, relaxed and powerless.
TITANIUM MET.	:	Sexual weakness with early ejaculation of semen in coitus.
TRIBULUS TER. Q	:	Sexual weakness and partial impotency due to over indulgence and advancing age. Corrects the bad effects of masturbation and spermatorrhea. A near specific for early ejaculation, 10 drops a dose.
YOHIMBINUM Q	:	Stimulates sexual desire in both the sexes.

SHOULDER

CAUSTICUM : Pains specially in the left shoulder with numbness. Contracted tendons with tearing in the shoulder joints and weakness. Better by warmth, specially of bed.

CHELIDONIUM : Pain in the arms and shoulders. Constant pain under and lower angle of right scapula. Pain at the lower angle of left scapula. Pain is worse by motion and touch, better by rubbing.

CHENOPODIUM AN. : Intense pain between the angle of right shoulder blade near the spine and through the chest.

FERRUM MET. : Rheumatism of the shoulder, worse while sitting still and after cold washing while overheated. Midnight aggravation of pain is the characteristic of this remedy.

PHYTOLACCA DEC. : Pain and soreness in the shoulders accompanied with restlessness. Specially shooting pain in the right shoulder with stiffness and an inability to raise the arm. Pain flics like electric shocks and is worse in the morning, in wet weather, and better in dry weather and warmth.

RHUS TOX. : Pain in the tendons and joints of the shoulders. Pain due to over work and excessive use of hands, arms and shoulders. Pain is tearing in charater and there is tingling in the arms. Pains may extend to the neck. Worse while sitting, better by movement and pressure.

SHYNESS

BARYTA CARB.   : Shy. Aversion to strangers. Loss of confidence in himself. Suited both to children and old persons.

COCA   : Bashful and shy while sitting in society. Feels ill on such occasions.

KALIUM PHOS.   : Shyness, disinclined to converse.

SIGHING

CALCAREA PHOS.   : Involuntary sighing.

CIMICIFUGA   : Sighing with sadness.

IGNATIA AMARA   : Hysterical sighing. Frequent with sadness and sobbing. Even crying and weeping does not stop it. Sighing continuous after crying.

NATRIUM PHOS.   : Sighing and a desire for deep breathing during menses.

OPIUM   : Long sighing respiration.

SINKING SENSATION

AMBRA GRISEA : Sinking sensation is felt after passing stool and thinking of unpleasant happenings of the past.

CIMICIFUGA : Sinking sensation with a waving sensation in the head and darkness before the eyes. It is generally connected with uterine affections.

DULCAMARA : Sinking sensation with mental confusion. It is generally found in patients living or working in damp places and in basement dwellers.

HYDRASTIS CAN. : Constant sinking sensation and depression. The patient is sure of death and desires it; patient is constipated.

IGNATIA AMARA : Sinking sensation with a sensation of emptiness in the pit of the stomach which is not relieved by eating. Involuntary sighing.

LAC CAN. 200 : Sinking sensation in the epigastrium.

PODOPHYLLUM : Sensation of sinking is felt in the abdomen with weakness and during pregnancy.

SULPHUR : Sinking greater at 11 A.M. Depressed. The patient is very selfish, thin and weak.

SINUSES

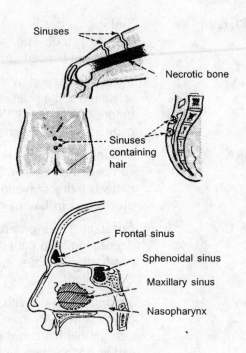

KALIUM BICH.	: Aching and fullness between the eyebrows in the forehead. Semi-lateral headache in small spots. Mucus stretchy and is greenish yellow in color. Nostrils blocked.
MENTHOLUM	: Pain over frontal sinus, descends to eyeballs. Supra orbital pain over the left eye.
PULSATILLA NIG.	: Sinus with facial tenderness, which is sensitive to touch. Excessive yellow mucus with sneezing. Yellow, green phlegm.

SANGUINARIA CAN.	: Sinusitis. Pain in the right eyebrow.
SEPIA	: Sinusitis. Stinging pain from within outwards and upwards, specially on the left side of head or forehead.
SILICEA 200	: A dose every 7th day for sinus left after an abscess.
SPIGELIA	: Sinusitis. Pain beneath frontal eminence and temples extending to the eyes. Headache starts from the nape of the neck and extends to the left eye.
STICTA PULM.	: In sinusitis which is dry. Pain over both the eyebrows after an exposure.

NOTE: Sinuses are the cavities in certain facial bones and sinusitis is the inflammation of those cavities. Sinusitis most often occurs after a cold and is accompanied by pain in the forehead and under the eyes.

SKIN

ACIDUM SULPH.	: Red and blue skin due to any cause.
AETHUSA CYN.	: Black and blue spots all over the body or the whole body may be of blue or black in color.
ANACARDIUM ORI.	: Skin of the soles cracks.
ANACARDIUM ORI., ARSENICUM IOD., SULPHUR IOD.	: Lichen planus. Fungal disease of the skin. Discoloration of skin with itching.
ANTIMONIUM CRUD.	: Urticaria and measle like eruptions.

ANTIMONIUM TART.	: Bluish red or violet marks left after pustular eruptions.
ARNICA MONT., LACHESIS	: Skin black or blue.
ARSENICUM ALB., ACIDUM SULPH.	: Black or blue spots on the skin.
BELLADONNA	: Eruptions like scarlatina with a very red skin.
CALCAREA CARB.	: Red spot on the skin.
CHINA OFF.	: Skin is very sensitive to touch but tolerates hard pressure.
CONIUM MAC.	: Skin is green.
DIGITALIS	: Abnormal redness of skin, measle like eruptions.
GELSEMIUM	: Measle like eruptions on the skin.
GRAPHITES	: Persistent dryness of the portions of skin, not effected by a disease.
HYPERICUM PERF.	: Red lines or streaks on the body.
KALIUM ARS.	: Discoloration of the skin after psoriasis and lepra.
KALIUM SULPH.	: Ailments accompanied by profuse scaling of the skin.
LACHESIS	: The patient is able to withstand hard pressure on the skin but he cannot bear light pressure, not even pressure caused by the tightness of clothes.
LEDUM PAL.	: Prolonged discoloration of the skin after injuries.
LUPULUS H.	: Sensation of insects crawling under the skin.

LYCOPODIUM	: Specific for discoloration of the skin by sun rays, uterine troubles and dyspepsia.
LYCOPODIUM, SEPIA, THUJA OCC.	: Yellowish spots on the skin.
MERCURIUS SOL.	: Skin constantly moist.
MYRISTICA SEB.	: Bluish red streaks on the arms, legs, etc.
NATRIUM MUR.	: Skin is greasy and oily, especially on the hairy parts. Face appears greasy and shiny.
NITRICUM ACIDUM	: Sensation of splinters in the skin.
OPIUM	: Sweaty skin.
PHOSPHORUS	: Yellow or brown patches on the abdomen.
PHYTOLACCA DEC.	: Scarlatina like rash.
PLATANUS OCCI.	: Skin like that of a fish, dry and horny.
PLUMBUM MET.	: Skin of the face is shiny and greasy.
PSORINUM	: Skin is oily because subcutaneous glands secrete excessively. Scratching causes pain. Patient likes cold climate.
RADIUM BROM.	: Cancer of the skin. Great burning, itching and restlessness, better by a hot bath.
RANUNCULUS BULB. Q	: Vesicular and pustular eruptions. Blister like eruptions on the palms and anywhere on a little pressure.
SECALE COR.	: Skin is shrivelled, numb and dusky blue due to blotches. It is a remedy for old people with shrivelled skin.

SULPHUR IOD. 3X   : It is specific for Barber's itch and obstinate skin diseases.

SULPHUR   : Any disease, as a result of suppression of skin disease. Such a disease will come out and be cured by the use of this remedy. Skin is dry and rough. Skin looks dirty as patient is averse to washing.

SYPHILINUM 1000   : One dose a month for ulceration of the skin. Reddish brown eruptions with a bad odor. Extreme emaciation of the skin.

THUJA OCC.   : Brown spots on the skin.

THYROIDINUM   : Ichthyosis, fish like skin.

VINCA MINOR   : Redness and soreness of the skin from slight rubbing.

SKIN—OILY

BRYONIA ALBA   : Skin is greasy, specially on the face. The skin is hot and the face has a yellow appearance.

MERCURIUS SOL.   : Skin remains constantly wet, moist and greasy. There is excessive perspiration, worse at night.

NATRIUM MUR.   : Skin is oily, specially on the hairy parts. A healthy skin is clean and glowing, neither too dry nor too oily. The following homoeopathic lotions are natural prescriptions for a beautiful and healthy skin.

1. Wash the face with luke warm water.

2. Towel dry.

NORMAL TO DRY SKIN

Gently massage into the skin the following lotion with the finger tips in a circular motion.

BERBERIS AQ. Q	- 5 ml.
HYDROCOTYLE A. Q	- 5 ml.
ECHINACEA Q	- 5 ml.
MUSTARD OIL	-30 ml.

Mix thoroughly and keep in a tight stoppered bottle.

OILY SKIN

BERBERIS AQ. Q	- 5 ml.
ECHINACEA Q	- 5 ml.
CITRUS VULG. Q	- 2 ml.
WATER	- 30 ml.

Mix thoroughly and apply gently.

SLEEP

ARSENICUM ALB.	: Sleeps with hands over the head.
BAPTISIA TINC.	: Sleeps while being spoken to.
BELLADONNA	: Sleeps with hands under the head.
CINA	: Child sleeps on hands and knees or on the abdomen.
KALIUM CARB.	: Can sleep only on the right side.

LACHESIS	: The patient sleeps into aggravation of his disease. The symptoms become worse after sleep, whether during the day or night.
LYCOPODIUM	: Sleeps in the knee chest position.
LYCOPODIUM, NAJA TRI.	: Cannot lie on the left side.
MEDORRHINUM	: Sleeps on abdomen or knee elbow position.
MERCURIUS SOL.	: Cannot sleep on the right side.
NUX VOM.	: Sleep is unrefreshing. Wakes up feeling tired. He feels sleepy after eating in the evening.
PLATINUM MET., CHAMOMILLA	: Sleeps with legs apart.
PODOPHYLLUM, ACETICUM ACIDUM	: Can sleep only on the abdomen and finds relief on doing so.
RHODODENDRON CH.	: Cannot sleep unless the legs are crossed.
STANNUM MET.	: Sleeps with one leg drawn up and the other stretched out.
STAPHYSAGRIA, PHOSPHORUS, KALIUM CARB., RHUS TOX.	: Sleepy after eating. Look for other symptoms of the remedy.
SULPHUR	: Talks, jerks and twitches during sleep. Wakes up singing. Wakes up frequently and becomes wide awake suddenly. Cannot sleep between 2-5 A.M.

SLEEPLESSNESS
(SEE INSOMNIA)

SLEEPY
(SOMNOLENCE)

BAPTISIA TINC.	: Falls asleep while being spoken to.
CHLORALOSUM	: A useful remedy for prolonged drowsiness, which may continue for a number of days. It is also useful for drowsiness and sleep of drunkards, whose faculties are only partially depressed.
CIMEX LECT.	: Irresistible sleepiness.
GELSEMIUM	: Patient is sluggish and always feels sleepy. He does not like to discuss matters but likes to be alone and undisturbed.
HYPERICUM PERF. 3X	: The patient constantly feels drowsy.
INDOLUM	: Wants to sleep all the time. Aversion to work.
LYCOPODIUM	: Feels sleepy soon after taking dinner.
NATRIUM SULPH.	: Sleepy while reading.
PULSATILLA NIG.	: Sleepy while eating.
STAPHYSAGRIA, KALIUM CARB., PITUITRINUM	: Feels sleepy after eating.

SLIPPED DISC
(ALSO SEE SPONDYLITIS AND BACKACHE)

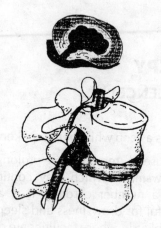

A herniated disc

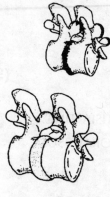

Drop in pressure

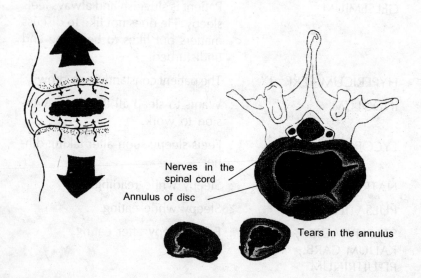

Nerves in the spinal cord

Annulus of disc

Tears in the annulus

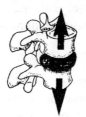

Decompression : two verte-bra beginning to be pulled apart, showing direction of distraction

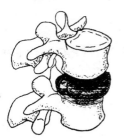

Distraction reaches maximum point

Discs are gelatinous cushions in between each vertebra and are surrounded by tough fibrous mass called "annulus fibrosis".

ACONITUM NAP. : In the early stages, on exposure to cold dry winds with sudden onset. Worse on movement and at night.

AMMONIUM CARB. : Prolapse of the disc. Pain in the lumbar region of the back, worse on sneezing and coughing.

APIS MEL. : Burning bruised pain, worse by heat, covering and movements. Cool air gives relief.

ARNICA MONT. 1M : Spine is very sensitive. Spasms in the muscles of neck and back. Bruised pain, worse on movement.

BELLADONNA : Violent cutting or tearing pains in the neck, spine or hips. Restless-ness, worse by resting. Burning with pain.

BRYONIA ALBA : Pain in the neck, back and limbs, better from heat and pressure, worse on movement.

CAUSTICUM : Tearing pain in the limbs and in the hollow of knee. Better in damp weather and by warmth.

CHAMOMILLA	: Sensitive patients, feel pain more than it actually is. Feeling of numbness.
HYPERICUM PERF. 3X	: Spinal concussion. Loss of power or function in the spinal cord due to a fall, severe blow or severe jerking. Pain in the nape of neck, pressure over sacrum. Pain in coccyx. Pain radiates up and down the back and extremities.
KALIUM BICH.	: Pain in the lumbar region of the spine while sitting. Pain in the fingers and wrists. Patient is irritable. Pain worse by cold.
KALIUM CARB.	: Stabbing, sticking or cutting pains. Worse on movement and better by hard pressure. Pain from back to thighs.
LEDUM PAL.	: Shifting pain accompanied by stiffness. Worse by heat and movement and better by cold applications.
NUX VOM.	: Pain on account of over exertion. Movement or turning in bed hurts. Cramps in the calves and soles at night.
RHUS TOX.	: Backache due to over exertion, hard exercise or due to an exposure to cold or wet, when sweating or warm. Pain and stiffness is worse at rest but better on movement for a short time.

SMALL POX

HYDRASTIS CAN. Q   : This remedy reduces the symptoms of small pox, abolishes the distress and shortens its course. Its use lessens the danger and greatly mitigate its consequences. Use 10 drops every hour till its curative effects appear.

SOLANUM XANTH. Q,   : When small pox is prevalent in the
MALANDRINUM   locality, 10 drops of either remedy given every hour is stated to be a sure preventive against small pox. Such a locality should be left immediately and even after shifting to a far off place,10 drops of it should be taken twice daily for 7 days.

SMELL
(SEE ODOR)

SNEEZING

ACONITUM NAP.   : Common cold with much sneezing in the early stages of cold. Due to suddden exposure to cold, dry winds.

ALLIUM CEPA   : Frequent and violent sneezing during coryza. Worse coming into a warm room.

AMMONIUM PHOS. 3X	:	Sneezing only in the morning with excessive running from the nose and eyes.
ARSENICUM ALB.	:	Ineffectual desire for sneezing or actual sneezing, better by hot applications. Burning discharge from the nose.
ARSENICUM IOD.	:	Burning, copious, watery discharge with sneezing. The discharge burns the nostrils and the lips. The patient is better in the open air and with cold applications.
CYCLAMEN	:	Excessive sneezing with itching in the ear.
GELSEMIUM	:	It indicates tendency to morning sneezing without any cause.
GLYCERINUM	:	Sneezing worse in the evening.
HEPAR SULPHURIS	:	Sneezing due to cold, dry winds.
NAPHTHALINUM	:	Sneezing and inflamed eyes. It is both curative and preventive of sneezing.
NATRIUM MUR. 200	:	Violent sneezing with coryza. Loss of sense of smell and taste. Sneezing, worse at about 10 A.M. or after rising from sleep in the morning. Discharge from the nose is either watery or like the white of an egg. Nose stopped up.
OPIUM	:	Violent sneezing, when well selected remedies fail.
SAPONARIA OFF.	:	Violent sneezing, with sharp, burning taste and severe sore throat, worse right side. Symptoms are worse in a warm room.

SILICEA	: Sneezings aggravated in the morning with a chronic tendency.
SULPHUR	: Sneezing while lying on a pillow filled with feather or synthetic materials.
TUBERCULINUM 200	: In several cases, it cures sneezing or atleast cuts short the treatment.

SNORING

CHINA OFF.	: Snoring specially in children.
HIPPOZAENINUM	: Noisy breathing and snoring, specially in the aged. May be due to chronic nasal catarrh and ulceration of nasal sinuses.
LEMNA MINOR	: Snoring due to nasal polyp and nasal obstruction.
OENANTHE CROC. 6	: Snoring; in epileptic patients and during menstruation.
OPIUM 200	: Stertorous breathing and deep snoring, specially in old people.

SNOW

ACONITUM NAP.	: Profuse watering of the eyes due reflection of snow in bright sunlight, is cured by the use of Acon. 30. A dose or two will suffice.
CALCAREA PHOS.	: Symptoms are aggravated during the season, when the snow is melting.

CICUTA VIR.	: Any bad effect on the eyes due to exposure to snow.
MERCURIUS SOL.	: Symptoms aggravated during snow storm.
SINAPIS NIG.	: Coryza and sneezing with itching and burning in the eyes.

SOLES

ANACARDIUM ORI.	: Cracking of the skin on the soles.
ANTIMONIUM CRUD.	: Soles are covered with corns and callosities, which are very tender. The patient cannot walk on this account.
BARYTA CARB.	: Soles get tender due to foot sweat.
BORAX	: Stitches in the soles.
CALCAREA CARB.	: Burning in soles, although knees and feet feel cold. Cold extremities in winter but burn in summer.
CALCAREA SULPH.	: Burning and itching in soles.
CHAMOMILLA	: Burning in soles at night.
CROCUS SAT.	: Pains in the soles.
LEDUM PAL.	: Soles tender while walking.
LYCOPODIUM	: Soles are swollen and painful.
MEDORRHINUM	: Cannot walk on soles. Walks on heels. Soles are very tender. Pain in the heels.

NATRIUM SULPH.,   : Burning in the soles.
SANGUINARIA CAN.,
SULPHUR, LILIUM TIG.

TARTARICUM ACIDUM   : Soles are painful.

SPEECH

HYOSCYAMUS NIG.   : Becomes speechless on account of
                         fear.

HYPERICUM PERF. 12X   : Speech becomes jerky and
                         hesitant due to nervousness of any
                         kind that may be due to shock or
                         an accident.

KALIUM CYAN.   : Power of speech lost but intelli-
                         gence intact. The patient can
                         express himself in gestures.

LACHESIS   : Speech difficult or lost due to
                         stiffness of the tongue and diffi-
                         culty in protuding it.

LAUROCERASUS Q   : Loss of speech due to violent pains
                         in the stomach.

LYCOPODIUM   : The patient uses wrong words in
                         his speech.

STANNUM MET.   : Talking causes a very weak feeling
                         in the throat and chest.

STRAMONIUM   : Speech difficult on account of
                         spasms of the tongue.

SPERMATORRHEA
(SEE EMISSIONS)

SPINAL STIMULANT

HERACLEUM S. 3C

: Use of this remedy increases the functional activity of the spine. It is a stimulant for the spine.

SPINE

AESCULUS HIP.

: Constant dull backache across the sacrum and hips, worse on walking and stooping.

AGARICUS MUS.

: Tingling and burning in the spine as if cold needles were thrust into the spine. Twitching in various parts of the body, specially eyelids. Stiffness of the entire spine. Numb feeling in the spine.

ALUMINA

: Pain on account of degeneration of the spinal cord. Feels as if walking on cotton. Patient is constipated.

ARGENTUM NIT.

: Useful in hardening and wasting of the spine.

ARNICA MONT.

: Spine is very sensitive. Spasms in the muscles of the neck and back. Find bed too hard.

BELLADONNA	: Constant backache with burning of the spine.
CALCAREA CARB. 200	: Caries of the spinal cord.
CIMICIFUGA	: Sensitiveness to pressure on the upper and lower cervical verte-brae. Pain shifts about from one part to the other and is sometimes accompanied by nausea. Pain in the lumbar region, the patient cannot lean back on a chair. Weakness in the legs.
COCCULUS IND	: Paralytic weakness of the spine and that of motor nerves, when the lumbar region is affected. Weakness in the small of back, which gives out while walking. Weakness of the entire lower extremities. Knees give out while walking. Soles feel asleep. Thighs ache. Weakness of the cervical muscles. Can hardly hold the head. Heaviness of the head.
CONIUM MET.	: Ill effects of bruises and shocks to the spine. Pain, worse on walking on an uneven surface. Paralysis from below upwards. Vertigo from turning the head sideways. Gradval loss of power in the legs.
FORMICUM ACIDUM	: Pain in the spinal cord.
GELSEMIUM	: Deep seated muscular pain, stiffness of the neck and nape. Numb feeling in the feet.
HECLA LAVA 3X	: It is of great use in rachitis - inflammation of the spine.

HYPERICUM PERF. : Pain on account of injuries to the spine, pain shoots up with local soreness when injuries are in the upper portion. Burning pain. Impotency due to injuries to the spine.

NATRIUM MUR. : Great sensitiveness between the vertebrae, relieved by pressure and lying on a hard surface. Restlessness with debility and morning aggravation.

NUX VOM. : Backache in the lumbar region. Burning in the spine worse 3 to 4 A.M. Has to first sit up in order to turn in bed. Spinal weakness due to sexual excesses. Sudden loss of power in legs in the morning.

PICRICUM ACIDUM : Weakness and pain in the back, in the lumbar region due to degeneration of the spinal cord. Pin and needle feeling in the extremities. Heavy tired feeling.

PULSATILLA NIG. : Body feels stiff. Back feels as if bandaged tightly.

SILICEA : Inflammation of the lower parts of spine.

STRYCHNINUM PHOS. 3X : An excellent remedy in anemia of the spinal cord. The patient is disinclined to use the brain. Lack of control, uncontrollable desire to laugh. Aching and burning in the spine. Mid dorsal region tender on pressure.

SULPHUR : Pain in the spine on a little movement due to suppression of menses.

TARENTULA CUB.	: Caries of spine (Pott's disease).
THERIDION	: Degeneration of spinal cord with vertigo.
THIOSINAMINUM	: Wasting away of spinal marrow, which causes lightning pains, is improved by the use of this remedy.
ZINCUM MET.	: Pain in the spine, worse sitting. Burning in the spine. Dorsal vertebrae mostly affected.

CONCUSSION OF THE SPINE : See Bruises.

CURVATURE OF THE SPINE:

CALCAREA CARB.	: For patients who are fat, chilly and pale.
CICUTA VIR.	: Bending of head, neck and spine, backwards.
PHOSPHORUS	: In dark eyed patients with a pigeon like chest (i. e. narrow chest).
SILICEA	: When the patient is thin and weak.

NOTE: A prolonged back rest, on a hard bed, without a pillow, helps remove the curvature in a shorter time.

ABSCESS OF THE SPINE :

BACILLINUM 200	: Start the treatment with this remedy and it need not be repeated for atleast a week.
CALCAREA SULPH.	: Abscess, discharging pus, specially of yellow color.
PYROGENIUM 200	: Abscess turning septic. Give only one dose a week.

| INFLAMMATION OF | : See Myelitis. |
| THE SPINE | |

| INFLAMMATION OF | : See Meningitis. |
| MEMBRANES OF THE SPINE | |

TUMOR OF THE SPINE (SPINE BIFIDA) :

| BACILLINUM 200 | : Do not repeat it before a week. |
| CALCAREA PHOS. 6X | : Then give this remedy three times a day. |

NOTE: If the tumor is too large due to the fluid in it, put a bandage or any other support to avoid it from hanging down and putting weight on the spine. If inspite of the treatment, the size of the tumor increases, refer the case to a competent surgeon.

SPITTING
(SEE SALIVA)

SPLEEN

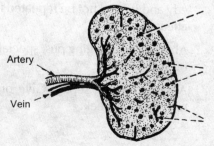

Slow circulation through red pulp which forms the bulk of the spleen tissue.

The white pulp consists of aggregates of lymphoid tissue just visible to the naked eye.

Artery

Vein

Capsule

ACETICUM ACIDUM	: Enlargement of the spleen with emaciation.
AGARICUS MUS.	: Pricking and stitching pains in the splenic region.
ARANEA DIAD.	: Enlargement of spleen due to fevers, specially malaria. Patient feels cold with pain in the long bones. Coldness is not relieved by anything.
CALCAREA ARS. 200	: Enlargement of the spleen in infants.
CEANOTHUS A. Q	: Enlargement of spleen with fever. Pain deep in the spleen. Patient is chilly. Jaundice. Increase in white blood cells in spleen (leukocythemia).
CHINA OFF.	: Enlargement of spleen with fever.
FERRUM ARS.	: Enlargement of the spleen with fever.
FERRUM IOD.	: Enlargement of the spleen without fever.
FRAGARIA VESCA	: For expulsion of stone from the spleen. It also prevents formation of calculi.
LACHESIS	: Violent pain in the splenic region with hemorrhage.
POLYMNIA UVE.	: Acute splenitis. Enlargement. Fever and pain.
QUERCUS Q	: Giddiness with chronic spleen affections. Dropsy of the spleen. Stitches under the left free ribs.
SQUILLA MAR. 3X	: Cough with pain in the spleen under the left free ribs.
TARAXACUM	: Pain and soreness in the splenic

		and hepatic regions. Sensation of bubbles bursting in bowels.
TINOSPORA CORD.	:	An east Indian remedy for splenic affections. Chronic cases of fever with an enlarged spleen.
URTICA URENS Q	:	Pain in the splenic region, in the gouty subjects and after intermittent fevers. Eliminates gravel from spleen. Enlargement of the spleen with localised pain in the splenic region.
WIESBADEN	:	Violent pain in the region of spleen. Much emission of flatus after great rumbling and fermentation in the abdomen.

SPONDYLITIS - CERVICAL

ACIDUM PHOS.	:	A important remedy. Pains tearing.
COCCULUS IND.	:	Cervical spondylitis. Rheumatic stiffness of the neck. Cracking of the cervical vertebrae.
DULCAMARA	:	Pain in the small of back, stiffness and lameness across the neck and shoulders.
KALIUM IOD.	:	With numbness, worse at night.
LACHNANTHES TINC.30	:	One dose in the morning and one in the evening.
MAGNESIUM PHOS. 12X, CALCAREA FLUOR. 12X, KALIUM MUR. 12X	:	Take 2 tablets (2 grains) of each. One such dose 4 times daily.

THERIDION : Degeneration of the spinal cord causes vertigo. Worse closing of eyes.

SPOTS

ARSENICUM ALB. : Blackish spots. Rough, dry, scaly, burning skin.

BELLADONNA, BERBERIS AQ., TARENTULA CUB., TELLURIUM MET. : Red spots.

BERBERIS VULG. : Circumscribed pigmentation, following an eczema.

CALCAREA CARB. : Red spots on the skin.

GRAPHITES, SULPHUR : White spots.

HELLEBORUS NIG. : Blue and bruised spots.

LACHESIS : Bluish purple spots. Face pale.

LYCOPODIUM : Moles. Freckles, worse left side of the face or body.

NATRIUM CARB. : Yellow spots on the face.

SECALE COR., PHOSPHORUS : Black and blue livid spots, ecchymosis.

SEPIA : Freckles. Brown spots on the face. Yellow spots on the chest.

SILICEA : Rose colored spots or blotches.

THUJA OCC. : Brown spots or blotches on the face.

SPRAINS

ACONITUM NAP.	: If the sprain in the neck has been caused by exposure to a cold wind, a few doses will remove the trouble if used within 24 hours of the neck pain.
AGNUS CASTUS 6C	: Another general but a good remedy for sprains and stretching of the muscles.
ARNICA MONT. 30	: It is the first remedy to be used for a sprain.
BELLADONNA 200	: Three doses of it in a day will remove the pain and sprain after failure of Acon.
BELLIS P.	: It is an excellent remedy for sprains in the conditions, when the sprain has been removed but the pain remains. It combines the properties of Arnica and Hypericum.
BOVISTA	: It is a good remedy for swelling of the foot after sprains.
CALCAREA CARB., NATRIUM CARB., PETROLEUM	: These are useful in old sprains according to the totality of symptoms.
DULCAMARA 200	: A dose a day for sprain in the neck, when days are hot but nights are cold.
LACHNANTHES TINC.	: It removes stiffness on account of the sprain in the neck.
RHUS TOX. 200	: Sprain in the neck. Give four doses in a day. It will relieve the patient from the neck pain.

RUTA G.

: As soon as the sprain occurs, bathe the place with warm water in which a few drops of Ruta have been added. This treatment if applied right away generally cures, and does away the need to use any other medicine. It may also be used for formation of nodules after sprains.

SQUINT OF THE EYES

ALUMEN : Internal squint of the right eye.

ALUMINA : Squint of either eye due to loss of power of internal rectus.

BELLADONNA : Squint due to convulsions.

CINA, SPIGELIA : Squint with worm symptoms.

CYCLAMEN : Convergent squint.

GELSEMIUM : Internal squint of either eye.

HYOSCYAMUS NIG. : Chronic squint.

STRAMONiUM : Internal squint of either eye with protruding eyeballs.

NOTE: Eye squints can be cured with practice under the supervision of an eye specialist, before the child is 3 years old. Glasses may be needed.

STAMINA
(VITALITY)

COCA 3X

: It increases stamina in athletes, sportsmen and players. It gives them greater power of endurance and relieves breathlessness. Give 2 doses at an interval of one hour before the start of a game, etc. Given after the occasion, it calms down muscles and gives relief and reduces palpitations and dyspnea. Useful in various complaints of mountain climbing.

STERCULIA A. Q

: It gives power to endure prolonged physical exertion without taking food and without feeling fatigued. 10-100 drop doses, three times a day. This is better than 'dope' used by the athletes and sportsmen for increasing the stamina. Dope (testosterone) is a steroid prepared from the male sex hormones. Zinc-p. 3x antidotes its ill effects, where as dope is illegal for its use and its presence can be tested in blood, use of Sterculia is not illegal and its presence in blood is hard to determine.

STAMMERING

This disease usually starts between the age of 2 and 7 years and is four times more common in boys than girls.

This must be overcome by practice and determination of the patient.

BOVISTA : Specially adapted to stammering in children and old maids.

BUFO RANA : Stammering on account of extreme anger.

CUPRUM MET. : Constant protrusion and retraction of the tongue like a snake with stammering.

HYOSCYAMUS NIG. : It is very useful if the patient doubts, that he will not be able to speak correctly.

MERCURIUS SOL. : Stammering on account of trembling or other defects of the tongue.

STRAMONIUM : Benefits after a prolonged used. It is also used if stammering is a result of parkinsonism.

NOTE: The remedies listed above should be tried one at a time for one month. If there is no response try further for two months. Take one dose twice daily. Take into account the totality of symptoms of the patients.

STERILITY - FEMALE
(INFERTILITY)

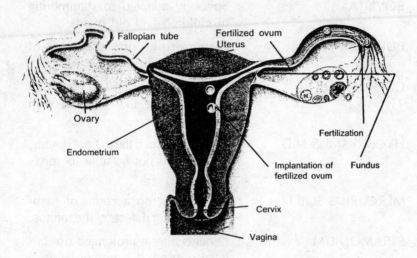

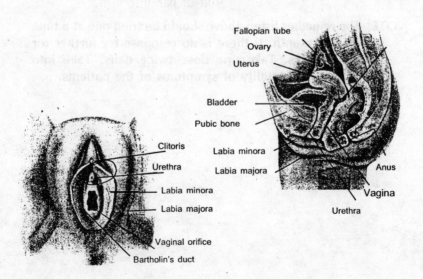

ABROMA RADIX Q : It should be given in 5 drop doses, three times a day, from the first day of menstrual flow for seven days. It will cure dysmenorrhea if present and will bring on conception if intercourse is performed after cessation of menses.

AGNUS CASTUS : Give only one dose a day - 5 drops in water in case sterility is due to scanty menses or leucorrhea. Such ladies have a strong dislike for intercourse.

ALTERIS FAR Q. : This remedy tones up the uterus if sterility is due to anemia, prolapse, leucorrhea, rectal distress, premature and profuse menses with labor like pains.

AURUM MUR. NAT. 3X : Sterility on account of organic defects in the uterus and prolapse. Cervix is hardened. Ulceration of the womb and vagina. Inflammation of the uterine membrane.

BORAX : It favours early conception on correction of diseases connected with menses. Leucorrhea like white of an egg, its warm liquid destroys the mobility of sperms.

CALCAREA CARB. : Sterility with copious menses and increase of fat in the abdomen.

EUPIONUM 3 : One or both the fallopian tubes are blocked.

KALIUM PHOS. 6X, CALCAREA FLUOR. 6X : Alongwith the indicated remedy, a dose of these remedies combined together (3 grains each) helps. In cases of weak uterus give Vib-p.

Q, a dose a day. It is a uterine tonic.

LACHESIS	: Fallopian tubes are blocked, specially the right side. Burning in the right ovary. Uterus is bent.
NATRIUM CARB.	: In obstinate cases of sterility, when cervix is hardened. Vaginal walls are defective in growth.
PHOSPHORUS	: Excessive sexual desire. Menses too early but scanty and long lasting. Polypus of the uterus. Discharge corrosive.
PLATINUM MET.	: Increased sexual desire. Pain in the ovaries and uterus. Leucorrhea.
SABAL SER. Q	: Sterility due to enlarged ovaries which are tender. Breasts shrivelled, shrunken or withered. Married late and had suppressed sexual desire, may have been lead astray and avoided conception.
SEPIA	: Irregularity of menses. Yellow leucorrhea. Constipation. Expulsion of wind from the vagina during intercourse. Bearing down sensation and a dislike for intercourse.
THYROIDINUM 3X	: This remedy is sometimes very useful in conception especially in cases of glandular disorders, inflammation of the uterus or where even surgery failed to induce conception.
TURNERA Q	: Sterility on account of coldness to sex. Ladies are indifferent to sex.

XEROPHYLLUM	: Vulva inflammed with terrible itching.

NOTE 1: Sterility in females is usually due to the diseases of the uterus, like menses, leucorrhea, abnormality of the ovaries, fallopian tubes, etc. Correction of these defects generally leads to conception.

NOTE 2: 'Vitamin A' helps homoeopathic treatment when no such defect is the cause.

NOTE 3: It has been observed that the reproductive organs do not mature fully before the age of 19 years. If such people start their sex life earlier than this, 60 percent of such adolescent girls develop a scar on the immature cervix which blocks the movements of eggs from ovaries to the uterus through the fallopian tubes. Such women either do not conceive or the pregnancies are ectopic, meaning the position of the baby in the uterus will not be normal.

STERILITY - MALES

PHOSPHORUS	: Irresistible sexual desire but no ability to perform.
SELENIUM MET.	: Impotence. Semen is thin, cold and odorless. On attempting coition, penis relaxes. Increased desire with decreased ability.
THUJA OCC. 200	: Has suffered from syphilis or gonorrhea and is impotent.
TRIBULUS TER. Q	: Discharge too quick. Partial impotence on account of advanced age. Weak semen. Sperms absent or too count low. Poor mobility of

sperms. It cures almost all the abnormalities of the spermatoza like coiled tail pieces,pairing,etc. which render the patient incapable of fertilizing the egg. Give 10-15 drops thrice daily. Results are usually achieved in 4-6 months.

TURNERA Q : Impotency. Absence of sperms. 10 drops in water thrice daily.

STERNUM

AURUM MET. : Nocturnal paroxysm of pain behind the sternum.

CAUSTICUM : Mucus under the sternum, which the patient cannot raise. Pain in the chest with palpitations.

MERCURIUS SOL. : Rheumatoid pain behind the sternum and around the joint.

TARAXACUM : Pain behind the sternum, under the breast.

STEROIDS

To antidote the bad effects of excessive use of steroids, the following medicines may prove useful:

BARYTA PHOS. 200 : When steroids have stopped young people from normal growth to his or her full height.

CALCAREA PHOS. 6X : People who require long term use of steriods, should also take this remedy to reduce the risk of 'osteoporosis' and if it has already started.

CHELIDONIUM 6 : When heavy use of steroids has caused liver damage and hardening of arteries.

CORTISONUM 200 : To antidote the bad effects of cortisone.

HYOSCYAMUS NIG. 30 : When steroid use has made a person, highly suspicious of all.

OOPHORINUM 1M : To antidote the bad effect of steroids prepared from female sex hormones.

ORCHITINUM 1M : To antidote steroids prepared from male sex hormones like "testosterone" and other anabolic steriods.

SAPONINUM 200 : To antidote bad effect of steroids prepared from plants.

NOTE: If the steriod hormone therapy is to continue for more than a few days,the patient should have a low salt diet, restricted fluid intake and a high protein diet.

STINGS

AMMONIUM CAUST. Q : Give this remedy by inhalation in case of unconsciousness due to a snake bite. It is a powerful cardiac stimulant.

APIS MEL. Q-30	: If there is very rapid swelling and a lot of burning, apply the Q externally and give 30 potency internally. Use it in scorpion bites.
ARNICA MONT. Q	: Wasp sting, apply externally.
CEDRON Q	: Painful effects of poisonous stings are antidoted by this remedy.
DRONA Q	: An east Indian drug is also very useful for scorpion bites. Give 5 drops orally and apply on the affected part.
GUACO 6	: Antidotes scorpion bites and snake bites.
LEDUM PAL. Q-200	: Stings of scorpions. Apply externally and give 200 internally. Bee stings and other stings are antidoted by this remedy.
URTICA URENS Q	: Apply externally, it gives instant relief.

STOMACH

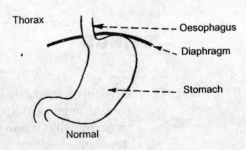

Thorax — Oesophagus — Diaphragm — Stomach — Normal

AMMONIUM CARB.	: Pain at the pit of the stomach with heartburn.

ASAFOETIDA 3X	: Pulsations in the pit of the stomach.
CADMIUM SULPH.	: Stomach cancer, with constant vomiting of black fluid.
CAMPHORA	: Pressive pain in the pit of the stomach, coldness followed by burning.
COLCHICUM AUTUM.	: Burning or icy coldness in the stomach and abdomen. Pain in the stomach and flatulence.
DIOSCOREA	: Sinking at the pit of the stomach. Pain along the sternum and extending to the arms. Eructations of sour and bitter wind.
GAULTHERIA Q	: Severe pain in the stomach and epigastrium with prolōnged vomiting.
KALIUM CARB.	: Flatulence in the stomach. Sensation of a lump in the pit of the stomach. Sour eructations. Constant feeling as if the stomach is full of water. Throbbing and cutting in the stomach. Any bang, shock, bad news or fear is felt in the stomach.
NUX VOM.	: Nausea in the morning after eating. Weight and pain in the stomach. Worse sometimes after eating. Stomach region is very sensitive to pressure.
ORNITHOGALUM Q	: Cancer of the stomach, specially of its lower part causing painful contractions. Distention of the stomach. A single dose of 10-15 drops, repeat only after seeing the results.

PTELEA   : Debility of the stomach or lack of normal function. Stomach does not contract normally causing slow movement of food from the stomach. Stomach remains loaded with food for an abnormally long time. Stomach symptoms accompanied with pain in the limbs.

PULSATILLA NIG.   : Perceptible pulsations in the pit of the stomach.

TUBERCULINUM 1M   : Carcinoma of the stomach.

STOOL

ALOE SOC.   : Sense of insecurity in the rectum when passing flatus, not sure whether gas or stool will come.

ARGENTUM NIT.   : Stools greenish, expelled with noisy flatus. Desire for passing stool immediately after eating.

ASAFOETIDA   : Watery stools with a very bad smell. Pain in the abdomen before passing it.

CALCAREA PHOS.   : Stool green, slimmy ,hot, sputtering and undigested. Flatus is fetid.

CHAMOMILLA   : Stools green ,watery and offensive.

COLCHICUM AUTUM.   : Painful, scanty, transparent and jelly like stools. Feels faeces in the rectum but cannot pass them.

COLOCYNTHIS   : Desire for stool while eating or drinking. Jelly like stools.

CROTALUS H.	: Thin, offensive and black stools, like coffee grounds.
GRAPHITES	: Liquid, brownish, undigested stools which are very fetid and passed with wind, preceded by colic.
KALIUM PHOS.	: Desire for stools while eating or drinking.
MERCURIUS SOL.	: Never "get done" feeling after passing the stool.
NATRIUM SULPH.	: Large quantity of stool, which is yellow in color and watery. Loose morning stool. Involuntary stool while passing flatus.
NUX VOM.	: Frequent, ineffectual desire for stools.
PODOPHYLLUM	: Great straining for passing the stool with prolapse of the intestines.
PSORINUM	: Stools dark brown, watery with an intolerable, offensive smell.
PULSATILLA NIG.	: Two or three normal stools a day.
RHEUM	: Offensive and sour smelling stools. The patient smells sour. This condition sometimes, occurs with children.
SULPHUR	: The patient has to rush to the toilet early in the morning on rising. The urge is very strong. Alternately, there is great straining before and after passing the stool and a constant bearing down feeling in the rectum.
TANACETUM VULG.	: Desire for stool, immediately after eating or drinking.

VERATRUM ALB. : Patient wants to swallow his own stool or urine. It happens in mentally deranged persons.

STUDY

AETHUSA CYN. : Student does not want to go school for studies . He is unable to think and concentrate.

ARGENTUM NIT. : Student does not want to go school for studies. Fear of failure in an examination.

COLCHICUM AUTUM. : Bad effects of keeping awake overtime, for studies.

CONIUM MAC. 1M : Student is not inclined to study and takes no interest in studies.

STYES

HEPAR SULPHURIS 200 : To be used when there is pus formation.

PULSATILLA NIG. : It is also a useful remedy, specially when the styes are on the upper lid.

STAPHYSAGRIA : It is useful in all cases of styes whether on the upper lid or on the lower lid of the eye. Very effective in obstinate cases when styes recur, every now and then.

SUMMER RASH
(PRICKLY HEAT)

APIS MEL.	: Swellings here and there like blisters with itching.
SULPHUR	: Rash of red color due to the heat of the sun. Simple rash.

SUN ALLERGY

ANTIMONIUM CRUD.	: Cannot bear the heat of sun.
BRYONIA ALBA, GLONOINUM, NATRIUM CARB.	: Heat of sun aggravates all symptoms.
COCCULUS IND.	: Sun allergy, rash and vertigo.
GELSEMIUM	: Heat of the sun causes depression.

SUN HEADACHE

GLONOINUM	: Throbbing headache increases and decreases with the sun.
LACHESIS	: Headache while going out in strong sunlight.

SUN STROKE

GELSEMIUM 200 : Among the remedies for prevention of sun strokes, this one is most important. It covers all symptoms of a man who feels played out and is specially indicated in hot and damp weather. Give one dose to a person going out when the sun is hot and who cannot bear the heat of the sun:

GLONOINUM 10M : Due to sun stroke, face turns pale, fixed eyes, strenuous respiration, high fever and sometimes unconsciousness. One dose of 10M removes these symptoms.

NATRIUM CARB. : Chronic effects of sunstrokes.

NATRIUM MUR. 200 : It is a very good remedy for sun stroke and acts splendidly. A dose every 15 minutes.

NOTE: Move the patient to a shaded, cool place immediately in case of sun stroke.

SUPPRESSION OF DISEASES
(AILMENTS DUE TO SUPPRESSION)

ABROTANUM : Rheumatism after suppression of diarrhea.

AMMONIUM MUR. : Hemorrhoids due to suppression of leucorrhea.

CAUSTICUM : Diseases like asthma, etc. arising on account of suppression of skin diseases like itching of skin or eczema.

MEDORRHINUM 1M : Bad effects following suppression of gonorrhea.

OLEUM AN. 200 : Asthma due to wetting of feet or chilling them, when perspiring.

PLATINUM MET. : Mental problems due to suppression of menses. Physical symptoms disappear as mental problems develop.

SARACA IND. Q : Headache due to suppression of menses, better as the flow starts.

SILICEA 200 : Convulsions due to suppression of the foot sweat.

SULPHUR 200 : Skin problems when suppressed with ointment, etc. cause some other problem, specially respiratory. In such cases, a dose of Sulphur 200 everyday in the morning for four days will bring out the original diseases, which can then be cured by the indicated remedies. Insanity due to suppression is also cured by this remedy.

THLASPI BURSA Q : After effects of suppressed uterine diseases.

ZINCUM MET. : Mania due to suppression of eruptions.

SWALLOWING

ANACARDIUM ORI.	: Swallows food and drinks hastily. Food descends the wrong way.
ANACARDIUM ORI., MERCURIUS SOL., PHYTOLACCA DEC.	: Choking when eating or drinking.
BAPTISIA TINC.	: Can swallow liquids only.
BELLADONNA	: Food regurgitates through the nose.
CARBOLICUM ACIDUM, CROTALUS H.	: Solids are only swallowed.
CUPRUM ACET.	: Liquids descend with a gurgling sound.
DIPHTHERINUM 200	: Swallows without pain but fluids are either vomited or are returned through the nose.
HYOSCYAMUS NIG., PLUMBUM MET.	: Cannot swallow liquids.

SYPHILIS

Hard chancre—
a raised
button like
nodule

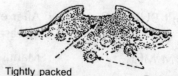

Tightly packed
lymphocytes and
plasma cells

Peri-and
endarteritis

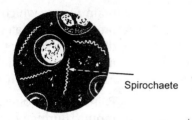

Spirochaete

ACIDUM NITRIC. : It is useful in the early stages of the disease, when the urine smells like that of a horse. It is also useful in babies and children, who have inherited the disease from their parents. Blisters in the mouth and under the lips.

ASAFOETIDA 3X : It has been found to affect favourably deep ulceration and caries of bones in deep syphilitic organisms. There is extreme sensitiveness and terrible throbbing. Nightly pains guide to the use of this remedy.

AURUM MUR. NAT. : It is used when syphilitic eruptions have developed on the body, appearing like psoriasis.

AURUM MET. : It is useful when mercury has been over used but without any further improvement in the case. It is one of the best remedies for pain in bones, specially at night.

CALOTROPIS Q : Psoriasis in syphilitic patients in the second stage, where mercury cannot do any further good.

CARBO ANIMALIS : It is useful when blotches develop on some parts of the body.

FERRUM MET. : In treating a case of syphilis with

brain tumor, which is likely to be present in the later stages of this disease, never use this remedy and if already used, do not repeat. It can cause brain hemorrhage.

KALIUM IOD. : Pain in small joints. Blisters in the mouth. Burning in parts. Larynx is painful.

MERCURIUS DUL. 2X : It is useful in cases of syphilitic women. There are eruptions at the mouth of vagina and vulva and also on the pubis.

MERCURIUS SOL. 2X : This remedy is used in all the stages of syphilis. There are ulcers on the tongue and mouth. All discharges are foul. It is also useful for pains of syphilis. It is useful in males.

SYPHILINIUM 1000 : In primary syphilis, this has little or no effect at all, at this time mercury should be given in high potency. Syphilinum will be useful as a remedy to bring about a reaction in the system. This remedy is of great use in old syphilitics, where convalescence is particularly long after an acute disease. A single dose will bring back his appetite, strength, sleep and cause a rapid gain in weight.

DIET : **In all syphilitic cases, alcohol in every form should be prohibited. A pure vegetarian diet should be suggested.**

TALKATIVENESS

CANNABIS IND.   : Excessive loquacity. Talks nonsense but cannot help it. Talks extempore on any subject but without making any sense and understanding.

LACHESIS   : He does most of the talking in a meeting or a society. Makes speeches in a selective language. He monopolizes all the talks during discussions. He can discuss all the subjects in the world, without any knowledge on all those subjects.

PODOPHYLLUM   : Irrelevant and incessant talking during high fever.

STANNUM MET.   : Talking causes a weak feeling in the chest and throat.

STRAMONIUM   : Ceaseless talking without any aim.

TASTE

ACONITUM NAP.   : Everything tastes bitter, except water.

ARSENICUM ALB.   : Only water tastes bitter, other things taste normal.

BOVISTA, SULPHUR   : Tastes, like blood.

CALCAREA CARB.   : Everything tastes sour. Sour eructations.

CHELIDONIUM   : Taste, bitter.

CHINA OFF.	: Everything including water tastes bitter. Sour eructations.
COLOCYNTHIS	: Taste, very bitter. Acrid eructations. Canine hunger.
CYCLAMEN, CARBO VEG.	: Taste, sweet.
HYDRASTIS CAN.	: Peppery taste.
IODIUM	: Taste of soap.
LYCOPODIUM	: Everything tastes sour.
MURIATICUM ACIDUM	: Everything tastes sweet, even the bitter things.
MYRISTICA SEB.	: Coppery taste.
NATRIUM MUR.	: Taste of food remains long after eating. Loss of taste.
NUX VOM.	: Taste in the mouth is bitter but everything tastes normal.
PULSATILLA NIG.	: Nothing tastes well including water. Mouth is dry but without thirst.
PULSATILLA NIG., CARBO VEG.	: Taste, greasy.
RHEUM	: Taste sour after sleep.
SANGUINARIA CAN., RUMEX	: Even sweets taste bitter.
TRIFOLIUM REP.	: Taste of blood in the mouth and throat.
VERATRUM VIR.	: Water tastes sweet.

TEA

KALIUM HYDRIOD.	: Cough in tea tasters due to inhaling of fungus, is cured by the use of this remedy.
KALIUM HYPOPHOS.	: Bad effects of excessive tea drinking are removed by the use of this remedy.
THEA SIN.	: Removes bad effects of excessive tea drinking like sleeplessness, headache and dyspepsia.

TEETH

ARNICA MONT. '	: For pain and ulcers due to dentures and false teeth.
CALCAREA PHOS. 6X	: Teeth develop slowly in children. First teeth decay rapidly. Diarrhea sour during dentition.
CALCAREA REN.	: Lessens tendency to accumulation of tartar on teeth.
CHAMOMILLA	: Original first teething difficult in children. Foul odour from the mouth. Diarrhea during dentition. Irritability in children.
FRAGARIA VES.	: Removes tartar from the teeth.
KREOSOTUM	: Teeth become black and decay. Gums become spongy. Restlessness in children. Caries of the teeth.

PHYTOLACCA DEC.	: Desire to bite and press the teeth together.
PLANTAGO Q	: For local use in toothache, in hollow of teeth. Decay of teeth. Pain and soreness.
SILICEA 10M	: Fistula of teeth at their roots.
STAPHYSAGRIA	: Teeth turn black and crumble, specially in children.
SULPHUR	: Milk teeth of the child do not break till they are quite old, for long age, sometimes upto 14 years of age. Teething takes place irregularly.
THUJA OCC.	: Decay of teeth from roots. Gums receede, upper part of the teeth remains intact.

TOOTHACHE

ACONITUM NAP. Q	: Insert a cotton swab drenched with it, in the tooth cavity. It reduces pain within minutes. Facial neuralgia, pain due to decayed teeth.
ANTIMONIUM CRUD.	: Toothache in the hollow of a tooth.
ARNICA MONT.	: Toothache from wearing false teeth.
BELLADONNA	: Throbbing, shooting pain extending to the head due to an infection.
CHAMOMILLA	: Toothache is caused by taking warm water in the mouth but is not relieved by cold things. Pain is

maddening. Decay of a tooth is generally the cause.

CHEIRANTHUS C. : Ill effects of cutting wisdom teeth. Deafness, otorrhea, nose stopped up at night due to irritation of cutting the wisdom teeth.

COFFEA CRUDA : Maddening toothache, better by holding cold water in the mouth. Facial neuralgia from decayed teeth.

GUNPOWDER : Toothache after extraction of abscessed teeth.

HECLA LAVA 3X : Toothache in carious teeth or due to abscess of gums with swelling.

MAGNESIUM CARB., SEPIA : Toothache of pregnancy.

MAGNESIUM PHOS. 6X : Toothache, better by hot applications.

MERCURIUS SOL. : Pulsating pain due to inflammed gums and sockets of the teeth. Pain in the hollow of teeth.

PHOSPHORUS : Toothache in "washer women".

PLANTAGO 2X : Dilution cures toothache within 15 minutes. Use internally and externally.

SILICEA 6X : Toothache, worse by hot or cold things.

SPIGELIA : Tearing pain in the carious teeth extending to the molar bone of the affected side.

STAPHYSAGRIA : Toothache due to unhealthy and decaying gums. Teeth turn black. Pain worse with hot or cold things.

TOOTH EXTRACTION

TRILLIUM PEND. Q   : A cotton plug drenched with it, is inserted in the hollow from where the tooth has been extracted,stops bleeding at once. Can be used internally.

TEETH GRINDING

ASAFOETIDA   : Grinding of teeth in hysteria.

BELLADONNA   : Grinding of teeth while sleeping.

CINA   : Grinding of teeth in children having worm symptoms.

TEMPERATURE

CACTUS 3X   : Persistent subnormal temperature due to any cause is cured by its use.

CAMPHORA Q   : Subnormal temperature with an icy cold body and sinking of strength. Give in drop doses on sugar and repeat often.

CHININUM SULPH.   : Subnormal temperature after cure of malaria, with weakness.

MILLEFOLIUM   : Continuous, high temperature without any reason.

SULPHUR 200	: Continuous temperature, not high, which did not become normal after cure of a disease. A single dose does wonders in such cases.
TUBERCULINUM 100	: Continuous temperature, neither very low nor very high, generally found in patients of tuberculosis.

TEMPLES
(CAROTIDS)

In pulsating carotids, one of the following remedies will be found useful as per the symptoms of the remedy.

ACONITUM NAP., BELLADONNA, CACTUS, GLONOINUM, VERATRUM VIR.

TESTICLES
(MALE REPRODUCTIVE GLANDS)

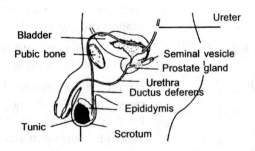

ACIDUM PHOS. 1C	: Testicles tender and smaller; sexual weakness.
ACONITUM NAP.	: Inflammation of the testicles with fever and restlessness. Bruised pain. Painful erections.

ANTIMONIUM CRUD.	:	Atrophy of testicles.
ARGENTUM MET.	:	Pain in the testicles, as if crushed.
AURUM MET. 200	:	Chronic enlargement with pain in the cord and testicles. Swelling. Hydrocele. Atrophy and undeveloped testicles.
BARYTA CARB.	:	Testicles harden in an advanced age. Sexual weakness. Testicles hard,enlarged and burn.
BELLADONNA	:	Inflammation with redness. Great sensitiveness of the nervous system. Intolerable pain. Testicles hard. Nocturnal sweat on testicles.
BRYONIA ALBA	:	When born with hydrocele.
CALCAREA CARB. 10M-50M	:	Penis and testicles missing in a child. One dose every fortnight.
CLEMATIS ERECTA	:	Chronic inflammation of the testicles because of incomplete cure of gonorrhea. Testicles indurated a with bruised feeling; testicles hang heavy or are retracted with pain in the spermatic cord, worse right side.
CONIUM MAC.	:	Testicles enlarged and hard due to injuries of the testicles.
HAMAMELIS	:	Inflammation with local sensitiveness and pain of the spermatic cord runs into the testicles. Testicles, large and painful.
IODIUM	:	Testicles become small due to impotency.
LYCOPUS Q	:	Pain in the testicles of patients suffering from valvular heart disease.

MERCURIUS BIN IOD.	: Chronic enlargement due to syphilis.
MERCURIUS COR.	: Orchitis of right testes with pain extending to the scrotum and abdomen.
MEZEREUM	: Testicles enlarged and hanging with very strong sexual desire.
NUX VOM.	: Constrictive pain in testicles with inflammation.
PULSATILLA NIG.	: Acute inflammation. Pain from abdomen to testicles. Orchitis due to gonorrhea.
PULSATILLA NIG., RHODODENDRON CH.	: Pain and swelling of the right lobe of testicles.
PULSATILLA NIG. 200, CONIUM MAC. 30	: Sacrocele or flesh tumor of the testicles.
SILICEA 6X, NATRIUM MUR. 6X	: 2 grams of each mixed together and given thrice daily, is very useful for orchitis.
SPONGIA	: Swelling of the spermatic cord and testicles with pain and tenderness.
THYROIDINUM 1X	: Testicles undeveloped. 2 doses a day over a long period are stated to be effective.
ZINCUM MET.	: Pain and swelling of the left testes.

TETANUS
(LOCK JAW)

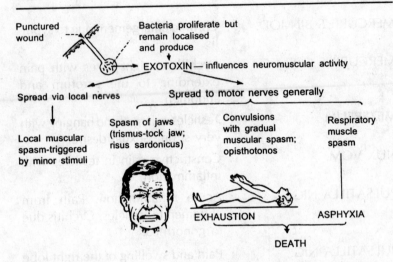

CAMPHORA Q	: Tetanus with deathly coldness.
CICUTA VIR.	: A useful remedy in tetanic convulsions, rigidity and jerking followed by prostration. Breathing is oppressed with lock jaw and oesophageal spasms.
HYDROCYANICUM ACIDUM	: There is lock jaw, impeded respiration and frothing at the mouth. The body becomes rigid and bent backwards.
HYPERICUM PERF.	: It is the best remedy for prevention of tetanus by punctured wounds or when nerves are injured, especially nerves of toes and fingers, more so when tips of toes and fingers are involved. It is also used when the symptoms of tetanus have developed. Persistent painful spasms of some voluntary muscles, stiffness of the jaw and muscles of the oesophagus and neck. In the later stage, muscles of the back, extremities and penis become rigid.

LEDUM PAL. 200 : Tetanus due to bad effects of anti-tetanus shots. Give one dose daily. After each injury, give it in a similar way for three days to avoid tetanus. It is also a remedy for prevention and cure of tetanus when punctured wounds are produced by sharp pointed instruments or bites. It is more indicated, when the wounded parts are cold. Tetanus with twitching of the muscles. It suits ill effects of infections.

MAGNESIUM PHOS 1M : It is considered as specific against tetanus. It also removes ill effects of the disease.

NUX VOM. : It is a leading remedy for tetanic convulsions with distortion of the eyes and face with dyspnea.

PASSIFLORA Q : 20 drops of it, given in alteration with Hypericum with a gap of 20 minutes is a very effective treatment for tetanus.

STRYCHNINUM : Tetanus with explosive nervousness. The pain and sensations come suddenly and return at intervals. Muscles relax during and between paroxysms of tetanic convulsions. Corners of the mouth are drawn up.

VERATRUM VIR. : Tetanic convulsions.

THALASSEMIA

Thalassemia is of two kinds :

1. Thalassemia major which is transmitted to the genes of the child from either parent. It is an inherited abnormality of

hemoglobin and erythrocyte or the oxygen carrying red blood cells. The bone marrow is defective and red blood cells are not produced. It is very difficult to cure. Blood transfusions at intervals have to be done and this can lead to a fatal build up of iron in the patients body and no remedy, so far, is available to help remove the excessive iron build up.

2. Thalassemia minor : The patient's genes are different from that of the parent. This may be cured by use of the following remedies but for some period blood transfusion be allowed to continue till the indicated remedy starts to act.

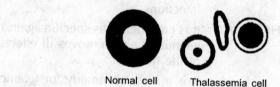

Normal cell   Thalassemia cell

BUTYRICUM ACIDUM 1X : A salt of Butyricum acid can cure cell anemia -thalassemia.

CALCAREA ARS. : Its use increases hemoglobin and red blood cells.

LACHESIS 200 : After transfusion of blood, this remedy will stop its further decomposition. The interval between the blood transfusion is increased and the progress of the disease is retarded.

NATRIUM CACODYL. 1X : It increases the number of red blood cells almost to double.

PHOSPHORUS 30-200 : It stops further disorganization of blood. Skin is very pale and jaundice may be present.

PLUMBUM MET. : Rapid reduction in number of red blood cells causing great paleness of the skin. Cramps in the calves. Twitching of muscles.

THIOSINAMINUM : This may prove useful in the treatment of the disease as it cures wasting of the spinal marrow-tabes dorsalis.

THINKING

AETHUSA CYN. : The patient does not apply his mind to thinking. He decides things without thinking. Student has no mind to study.

CAMPHORA : Pain better while thinking of it.

CANNABIS IND. : Always absorbed deep in thinking without any subject, with eyes closed.

CAUSTICUM : Thinking of complaints aggravates, specially hemorrhoids.

COCCULUS IND. : Dwells on the past, disagreeable events.

COFFEA CRUDA : Always absorbed in thinking, now on one subject and after a while on another subject. Full of ideas and quick to put them in action.

GELSEMIUM : Ailments increase while thinking of them.

MEDORRHINUM : Worse while thinking of ailment.

NITRICUM ACIDUM : Thinks and speaks always of the bad events in the past, without any use.

ONOSMODIUM : Cannot think, lack of concentration on the topic.

THIRST

ACONITUM NAP.	: Thirst for large quantities of cold water, during fever.
APIS MEL.	: Thirst absent with a swollen throat.
ARSENICUM ALB.	: Unquenchable thirst. Drinks often, but little at a time.
BELLADONNA, AETHUSA CYN.	: Absence of thirst during fever or otherwise.
BRYONIA ALBA	: Thirst for large quantities of cold water at long intervals.
GELSEMIUM	: Light thirst in fever or absence of thirst.
LILIUM TIG.	: Drinks often and much.
MERCURIUS SOL.	: It has a peculiar symptom of intense thirst with profuse saliva in the mouth.
NATRIUM MÜR.	: Unquenchable thirst, during chill.
ONOSMODIUM	: Craving for ice cold water and cold drinks, wants to drink often.
PHOSPHORUS	: Desire for icy cold water, vomits out as soon as it becomes warm in stomach.
PHYTOLACCA DEC.	: Thirst alternates with thirstlessness.
PULSATILLA NIG., LYCOPODIUM	: Inspite of the dryness in the mouth, there is no thirst.
RHUS TOX.	: Thirst for large quantities of water. Dry mouth and throat. Craves milk.
TUBERCULINUM	: For children constantly drinking water, this remedy should be considered first.

THROAT

ACONITUM NAP.

: Acute, painful, sore throat, whose onset is sudden and causes anxiety. Skin is hot, dry and there is great thirst; the throat is dry, rough, constricted, burning and tingy. Hoarseness, accompanys. Movement and warmth relieves and damp,cold weather aggravates. The patient suffers more at night and with rest. Patient feels thirsty for cold drinks.

APIS MEL.

: Back of the throat is bright red, severely swollen with burning and stinging pains. The patient is irritable or depressed and is better from fresh air, exercise, stimulants and warmth around the neck. Throat, uvula and tongue are swollen. The throat is fiery red.

ARGENTUM NIT.

: Sensation of a splinter in the throat.

ARSENICUM ALB.

: Dryness and burning in the throat. Dry mouth and thirst for small quantities of water at short intervals.

ASAFOETIDA 3X

: Sensation of a lump rising in the throat, in hysterical patients.

BARYTA CARB. 200

: Tonsils swollen. Smarting pain, worse on swallowing saliva. Solid diet painful to swallow, can swallow liquids only.

BELLADONNA

: Sore throat in the early stages of fever. Throat red, hot and swollen.

Swallowing difficult. Dryness of the throat.

CAPSICUM : Sore throat of smokers and drinkers. Burning in the throat.

DOLICHOS : Pain in the throat as if a splinter is embedded in the throat, worse on swallowing.

DULCAMARA : Raw, burning acute sore throat with thick saliva and a hoarse voice. Thirst for cold drinks. Sore throat can be due to exposure to cold damp weather or cooling down rapidly after sweating, better by movement and warmth, worse by rest and at night.

EUPHRASIA 6 : In coryza and cold with sneezing and watering of eyes; there is soreness of the throat also.

GELSEMIUM : Sore throat with a bad taste in the mouth. Pain extends to the neck and ears. Swallowing hurts and drinking is difficult. Feels cold and hot alternately, due to fever. The head feels heavy as if tied with a band.

HEPAR SULPHURIS : In chilly patients, it helps preventing the tendency to sore throat and throbbing pain in the throat. Sensation of a plug or a splinter in the throat while swallowing. Patient perspires though feeling chilly.

KALIUM CARB. : Sticking pain in the throat as from a fish bone.

LACHESIS : Purple color of the throat with soreness. Any pressure around the throat even that of a neck tie is unbearable. Swallowing of saliva

or liquids is painful. Left side affected most.

MAGNESIUM CARB.   : Soreness of the throat, before
menses.

MANGIFERA IND.   : Acute problems of the throat.
Sensation of suffocation, as if the
throat would close.

MENTHOLUM   : It is curative in many troubles of
the throat like catarrh, pharyngitis,
laryngitis and pain.

MERCURIUS SOL.   : Sore throat. There is a lot of saliva
in the mouth and the patient has
to spit often.

NATRIUM PHOS.   : Inflammation of any part of the
throat.

PHYTOLACCA DEC. Q : 8-10 drops in about 100 ml of luke
warm water, 2-3 times a day used
for gargling gives good results in
cases of sore throat. The throat feels
narrow,rough with the sensation
of a lump. Throat is dark red in
color.

RHUS TOX.   : Pain in the throat with restlessness.
Sensation of swelling in the throat.
The patient usually craves cold
milk.

SABADILLA   : Soreness of the throat begins from
the left side. Much tough phlegm,
must be swallowed as it is hard to
be spitted out. Throat and fauces
are dry

SPONGIA   : The patient has to clear the throat
constantly.

SULPHUR   : The patient is lethargic with offensive breath. Wants to uncover feet

because they burn. Feeling of a lump and burning in the throat.

TEREBINTHINIAE 1X : Dryness in the throat of speakers and singers. Inflammation of the whole respiratory tract.

WYETHIA : A very good remedy for pharyngitis. Irritable throats of singers and public speakers. Constant desire to swallow saliva and clear throat.

THUMB

BORAX : Pain in thumb. Throbbing pain in the tip of the thumb.

NATRIUM MUR. 1000 : The child has a chronic habit of sucking the thumb. Repeat every 15 days.

THYROID GLAND

Thyroid disease either under production (hypothyroidism) or over production (hyperthyroidism) of hormones is often hereditary and is on account of defective immune system, stress or changing hormone levels.

Hypothyroidism results in easy weight gain, tiredness, forgetfulness, dry coarse hair and skin, heavy menstruation and constipation.

Hyperthyroidism includes nervousness, irritability, bulging eyes, scanty menses, diarrhea and warm moist palms.

Goitre or swollen thyroid gland can occur in both the forms of the disease.

Homoeopathy treats such diseases successfully, and though it is a lengthy treatment, it surely is not for the whole life.

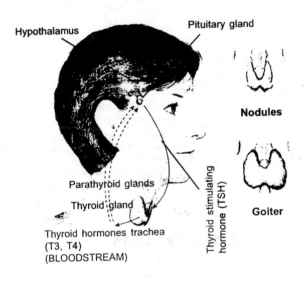

Three steps control the way your thyroid gland functions:

1. First, hormone released from your hypothalamus travels to your pituitary gland (see diagram). This hormoen signals the pituitary gland to release another hormone, Thyroid Stimulating Hormone (TSH).

2. Second, TSH travels from your pituitary gland to your thyroid gland. TSH triggers your thyroid gland to make the hormones thyroxine (T4) and triiodothyronne (T3).

3. Third, thyroid hormones T4 and T3 are release from your thyroid gland into your bloodstream. T4 and T3 travel throughout your body and regulate the rate at which many defferent organ systems work.

Hypothyroidism results when your thyroid gland is underactive–it does not produce enough thyroid hormones for your body to function at the right level. Some of the symptoms of hypothyroidism include fatigue, weight gain and intolerance to cold. Treating hypothyroidism is simple. Medication can replace the thyroid hormones your body is missing.

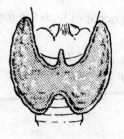

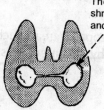

The thyroid is
shrunken, white
and firm

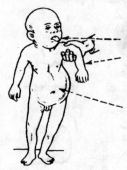

Clinical signs
Protruding tongue

Dwart with short limbs
Coarse dry skin.
Lack of hair and teeth
Mental deficiency.

Pot belly — often umbilical hernia
Changes are irreversible unless treat ment
is given early.
Two forms are recognised:
(1) endemic and (2) sporadi c cretinism.

HYPOTHYROIDISM (MYXEDEMA)

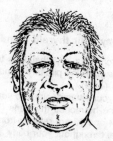

Imperfect or complete loss of function of the thyroid gland
or under production of thyroid hormones.

TUBERCULINUM 1M, CM : Start the treatment with this medicine. No other medicine should be
given for the next 24 hours.

BARYTA IOD. 3X : When the inflammation is accompanied with inflammation of the tonsils.

BELLADONNA 1X : Thyroid secretions become poisonous and spread throughout the body via the blood stream. Extreme thyroid toxemia.

CALCAREA CARB. : Increase of fat in the abdomen. The patient is fat, flabby, fair colored and perspires easily. Thyroid dysfunction.

CALCAREA FLUOR. : Stony hardness of the inflammed glands.

CALCAREA IOD. 3X : Thyroid enlargement about the time of puberty.

CISTUS CAN. : Inflammation, swelling and suppuration of the gland.

FERRUM PHOS. 6X : Inflammation, face flushed and bright red. Menses too profuse and too frequent.

IODIUM : Inflammation and enlargement of the gland.

KALIUM CARB. : Imperfect or complete loss of function. Do not repeat too often in old, gouty and tubercular patients.

KALIUM IOD. 3X : Inflammed hard gland with swelling. It also protects the thyroid gland in case of radiation.

PETROLEUM 200 : Tendency to thyroid diseases.

SEPIA : Low thyroid hormones with low blood pressure and a tired feeling.

THYROIDINUM : Its effects are striking in this disease. The patient craves sugar and is inclined to excessive obesity and weight gain. Arrested mental and physical development.

HYPERTHYROIDISM (EXOPHTHALMIC GOITRE)

Over production of thyroid hormones.

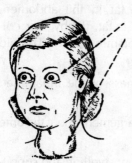

Clinical signs

- Exophthalmos-not always present.
- Prominent thyroid.
- BMR increased.
- Skin warm and sweaty : heat intolerance.
- Weakness, hyperkinesia and emotional instability.
- Loss of weight.
- Glucose tolerance diminished, glycosuria.
- Rapid pulse.
- Cardiac arrhythmia and failure in older patients.
- TSH low.

BROMIUM : Enlarged parotid gland and goitre. Dilated blood vessels on the throat.

FUCUS VES. : Obesity and non-toxic goitre. Protrusion of eye balls. Thyroid enlargement.

IODIUM 2X : Rapid emaciation not withstanding a good appetite. Obesity. Great debility. Slightest exertion produces perspiration. Loss of breath on going upstairs. Goitre is cured with Iodium CM, one dose given for four nights after full moon.

LYCOPUS : Useful in cases of exophthalmic goitre with heart diseases.

NATRIUM MUR. 200 : Exophthalmic goitre. Increased nervousness. Excessive sweating with weight loss. Increased bowel activ-

PETROLEUM 200   : Tendency to thyroid diseases and goitre. Gastric acidity and skin eruptions. Excessive hunger.

NOTE: Thyroid problems can somewhat be determined by self examination in the following way:

1. **Exact problem can only be found out by a clinical laboratory test under the supervision of a endocrinologist.**

2. **Under a hand mirror, focus on the area of the neck just below the Adam's apple and immediately above the collar bone, tipping the head back. Take a drink of water and swallow. Check any protrusions on the neck while swallowing. If there are any bulges, there may be an enlarged thyroid gland or a thyroid nodule.**

TIME OF MODALITIES

ACONITUM NAP.   : Worse at midnight and a little before midnight.

APIS MEL.   : Worse from 4 P.M. to 6 P.M.

ARSENICUM ALB.   : Worse at midnight from 1-2 A.M.

BELLADONNA   : Worse about 3 P.M.

CALCAREA CARB.   : Worse about 2 P.M.

CARBO VEG.   : Worse from 4 P.M. to 5 P.M.

COLCHICUM AUTUM.   : Worse at sunset and sunrise.

DROSERA   : Worse during midnight, at about 3 A.M.

HEPAR SULPHURIS   : Worse from 5 P.M to 6 P.M.

HYPERICUM PERF.   : Worse from 3 A.M to 4 A.M.

KALIUM BICH.   : Worse between 2 A.M. to 3 A.M.

KALIUM CARB.   : Worse at about 3 A.M. This time

is characteristic of this remedy and many cases have been cured on this indication only.

LYCOPODIUM	: Worse from 4 P.M. to 8 P.M.
MEDORRHINUM	: Worse from day light to sunset.
MERCURIUS SOL.	: Worse whole night and extremely worse before midnight.
NATRIUM MUR., GELSEMIUM	: Worse 10 A.M. to 11 A.M.
NUX VOM., THUJA OCC.	: Worse before 3 A.M.
PULSATILLA NIG.	: Fever is worse at about 4 P.M.
RHUS TOX.	: Worse around midnight when resting and at about 7 P.M.
SULPHUR	: Worse at 11 A.M.
SYPHILINUM	: Worse at sunset and sunrise.
THUJA OCC.	: Worse before 3 A.M.

TINNITUS
(SEE EAR - NOISES)

TIRED FEELING
(FATIGUE   SYNDROME)

ARGENTUM MET.	: It is good for business men, students, etc., who feel tired both mentally and physically after work and reading.

ARNICA MONT.	: Fatigue of the body and mind on account of overwork. Body tired and feels, as if beaten.
CALCAREA CARB.	: Tired state, mental and physical due to overtaxing the brain and body.
CHELIDONIUM	: Least exertion tires and he is averse to movement.
CONIUM MAC.	: General feeling of tiredness. The body feels as if bruised by blows. Specially suited during menopause. Debility and weakness of the body and mind is more in the morning, in bed.
ECHINACEA Q	: Tired feeling during acute or sub-acute disorders with tendency to malignancy.
LACTICUM ACIDUM	: Even the brain is fagged and the slightest exertion or mental effort brings on headache.
MAGNESIUM CARB.	: More tired on rising than on retiring. Especially suited to old persons and during menopause. Whole body feels tired, especially legs and feet.
NATRIUM MUR.	: Great debility, weakness and tiredness is felt in the morning in bed.
ONOSMODIUM	: Muscular prostration with numbness. Acts as if born tired, worse motion, better lying on the back.
PICRICUM ACIDUM 6	: Heavy tired feeling. Pins and needle like sensation in extremities. Muscular debility. Heaviness of the legs, can hardly lift them.

Desire to lie down. Tired feeling in the back.

SEPIA : Fatigue from a little exertion.

STERCULIA A. Q : 5 drops in a little water thrice daily, removes the tired feeling due to any cause.

TANACETUM VULG. : Nervous and tired feeling, like half dead, half alive all over. Abnormal lassitude.

TUBERCULINUM : Patient is always tired. Motion causes intense fatigue. Aversion to work.

TOBACCO HABIT

ARSENICUM ALB. : Antidotes the bad effects of chewing tobacco.

CALADIUM SEG. : Removes headache and mental states of smokers. Tobacco heart and asthmatic complaints. Modifies and changes craving for tobacco.

IGNATIA AMARA : Antidotes the bad effects of smoking. Ignatia patient cannot bear tobacco.

LYCOPODIUM 200 : It is useful in impotency of smokers.

LYCOPUS : Helpful in palpitations and rapid heart of smokers. Reduces the heart rate and lowers the blood pressure.

PHOSPHORUS	: Removes sexual weakness caused by tobacco.
PLANTAGO MAJ. 200	: Causes an aversion to tobacco, one dose every 15 days. Removes depression and insomnia of chronic nicotinism.
SEPIA	: Cures neuralgia and dyspepsia of smokers.
TABACUM 1000	: A dose a week removes craving for tobacco.

NOTE 1: A study of 200 male smokers was revealed in London Observer on 26-7-98 that smoking reduces the size of penis erection in the same way as it effects the heart by damaging the blood vessels. Smoking impairs the ability to stretch,said Dr. Clive Bates.

NOTE 2: It has been observed that babies born of women who smoke during pregnancy are more sick and have a high risk of sudden death. It is now, an established fact that many new borns of such women contain carcinogens in their body.

TONGUE

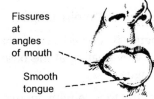

Fissures
at
angles
of mouth

Smooth
tongue

Associated changes
Atrophic glossitis

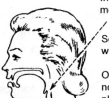

Incoordinate
movements in pharynx

Sometimes actual
web forms

Occasionally carci-
noma is a late com-
plication

Dysphagia-
the Brown-Kelly-Pater-
son or Plummer-Vinson
syndrome

ANTIMONIUM CRUD.	:	Thickly coated, white tongue as if white washed.
APIS MEL.	:	Swelling of the tongue with inflammation. Cancer.
ARGENTUM NIT.	:	Tip of the tongue painful. Bleeding from papillae of the tongue.
ARSENICUM ALB.	:	Tongue blackish or bluish and cracked.
AURUM MET.	:	Cancer of the tongue.
AURUM MUR.	:	Tongue hard like leather.
BORAX	:	Aphthae. White fungus like growths in the mouth and tongue. Leukoplakia.
BRYONIA ALBA	:	Tongue dry.
BUFO RANA	:	Bluish black with cracks.
COLCHICUM AUTUM.	:	Sensibility of the tongue is lost.
CUPRUM MET., LACHESIS	:	Constant protrusion and retraction of the tongue like a snake.
GALIUM APARINE	:	Nodulated tumors of the tongue.
GRAPHITES, APIS MEL., CANTHARIS	:	Burning blisters on the tongue.
GUACO	:	Paralysis of the tongue.
HYDRASTIS CAN.	:	Dirty yellow and moist tongue.
KALIUM MUR.	:	The tongue is coated white or there is a grey coating at the base of the tongue.
KALIUM CYAN. 200	:	Cancer of the tongue with agonizing neuralgia. Ulcer of the tongue with indurated edges.
LATHYRUS SAT.	:	Burning pain at the tip of the tongue with tingling and numbness.

LEMON JUICE	: Relieves pains of tongue cancer when used as a mouth wash - 5 ml to 200 ml of water.
LITHIUM MUR.	: Numbness of the tongue.
LYCOPODIUM	: Ulcers on the tongue.
MERCURIUS SOL.	: Furrow in the middle of the tongue. A tumor under the tongue. It is the main remedy for inflammation of the tongue.
NATRIUM PHOS.	: Blisters on the tip of the tongue. Thus, moist coating on the tongue.
NATRIUM MUR., NATRIUM PHOS.	: Blisters on the tip of the tongue.
OLEANDER	: Parched tongue.
PIPER NIGRUM	: Cramps in the tongue and heaviness of the tongue.
PODOPHYLLUM	: Coated white.
PULSATILLA NIG.	: Dry without thirst.
PTELEA TRI.	: Red and prominent papillae of the tongue.
RHUS TOX.	: Triangular red tip.
RUTA G.	: Cramps of the tongue.
SANICULA AQUA	: Ringworm on the tongue.
SEMPERVIVUM TECT. 2X-30	: It is useful in removal of malignant ulcers of the mouth and cancer of the mouth and tongue.
TARAXCUM OFF.	: Tongue mapped, covered with a white film, feels raw, comes off in patches. Red sensitive spots on the tongue.
THUJA OCC.	: A cyst under the tongue (ranula). White painful blisters close to the

root of the tongue. Biting of the tongue.

VERATRUM VIR.   : Tongue white or yellow, with a red streak in the middle.

VIBURNUM PRUN.   : Cancer of the tongue.

TONIC

A person in good health should not take any tonic. Good health means that the person has no disease. If a healthy person takes tonics, these will have no effect or may even produce an adverse effect. The habit of taking a tonic is simply ridiculous, when a person is healthy.

ALFALFA Q   : Acts as a tonic in digestive functions toning up the appetite resulting in greatly improved mental and physical vigor,with weight gain. Corrects tissue waste.

ARSENICUM IOD.   : In chronic coronary artery diseases and myocardial infections.

ASPIDOSPERMA Q   : A great lung tonic.

AVENA SAT. Q   : 10-20 drops a dose in a little water is a tonic for the nervous system. It brings about sleep. Relieves nervous headache, fatigue and numbness of limbs.

CACTUS Q,   : 10-15 drops of these medicines
CRATAEGUS OXY. Q   mixed together and given every four hours works as a heart tonic and strenghtens the heart.

CALCAREA ARS.	: Excellent heart tonic. Relieves pain, palpitation and dyspnea in dilatation of heart and weak valves.
CALCAREA PHOS. 6X	: A general tonic for weak children, specially during teething. A tonic during pregnancy. In anemia of children and after acute and chronic wasting diseases.
CASCARA SAG. Q	: It is an intestinal tonic,palliative in constipation and helps in removing indigestion. Give 15 drops every three hours.
CHAMOMILLA	: For whining, restless and irritable children.
CHINA OFF., CHININUM ARS., CARBO VEG.	: For debility, remaining after influenza and cold.
CHININUM ARS.	: A general tonic with very marked beneficial and prompt effects. The symptoms of general weakness, weariness and prostration are cured by it.
CRATAEGUS OXY. Q	: Acts upon heart muscles. There is giddiness, lowered pulse, air hunger and low blood pressure.
DIGITALIS	: It is a great cardiac tonic in feeble muscular walls of the heart. Palpitation, breathlessness and vertigo.
ECHINACEA	: Blood poisoning.
GENTIANA LUTEA Q	: Acts as a tonic in increasing appetite.
LECITHINUM	: It has a favourable influence upon the nutritive conditions and specially upon the blood. It acts as a tonic in anemia and during

convalescence. It increases the quantity and quality of milk in nursing women.

NATRIUM SULPH. 6X : Tonic in rheumatism, specially when the patient feels changes of temperature from dry to wet, with weak ankles and knees, pain from hip to toe. A person wearing a ring overnight cannot take it off in the morning due to swelling of the finger.

NUX VOM. : For irritability. Overworked dyspeptic males.

PICRICUM ACIDUM : Mental and physical prostration.

PULSATILLA NIG. : For contradictory, changeable, lachrymose females.

SECALE COR. : In thickening of the coats of arteries producing hypertension, angina pectoris, right heart disease, with cold and blue extremities. Patient is better in cold and with cold applications.

STAPHYSAGRIA : For residual pain, nervousness after tooth extraction.

STERCULIA A. : Fatigue. Regulates the blood circulation. Regulates cardiac rhythm and gives strength to a weak heart. 3-10 drops three times a day.

TURNERA Q : 10 to 40 drops a dose, thrice daily acts as a tonic in sexual weakness and removes frigidity in females.

VANADIUM : A true digestive tonic after sub-acute and acute gastroenteric inflammation.

VERATRUM ALB.   : A useful heart tonic when there is cold sweating on the forehead.

VIBURNUM PRUN. Q   : It is a great uterine tonic. Strengthens the muscles of the uterus and removes tendency to habitual abortions.

YOHIMBINUM Q   : Excites sexual organs and stimulates the function of lactation.

ZINCUM MET.   : For old people and also for paralysis. Often for cerebral thrombosis.

TONSILS

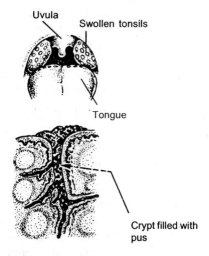

Uvula

Swollen tonsils

Tongue

Crypt filled with pus

AMMONIUM MUR.   : Internal and external swelling of the throat and tonsils, can hardly swallow anything. Phlegm is sticky.

BARYTA CARB.   : Scrofulous children, who are physically dwarfish and do not grow and develop normally. Tonsils always swollen. Catarrh of posterior nares. Takes cold easily. Suppurating tonsils from every cold. Smarting pain, when swallowing. Can swallow only liquids. Stinging pain in the tonsils. A great remedy for such conditions, both in children and old people.

BELLADONNA : Enlarged tonsils with redness. Burning, dryness and a sense of constriction in the throat. In such cases, it should be considered as the first remedy.

BRAIN 3X (LERVEAU) : It is an excellent remedy for sequel or surgical removal of tonsils.

CALCAREA CARB. 1M : It is another remedy for ailments after surgery of tonsils. Give it once a month, till cured.

CALCAREA SULPH. : Abscess on the tonsils.

GUAIACUM OFF. Q : Acute tonsillitis with a sore throat, worse heat and touch.

HEPAR SULPHURIS : Tonsils inflammed with danger of pus formation. Sensation of a thorn in the throat and ulcers on the tonsils are cured by this remedy.

LACHESIS 200 : Tonsils sore and swollen, worse left side. Septic conditions. Painful with hawking. Purplish or livid color. Swallowing saliva or liquids is painful. Cannot bear anything tight around the neck. Slightest pressure internally or externally on the neck or even touch annoys.

MERCURIUS IOD. 2X : It is an excellent general remedy for tonsillitis, when there is inflammation and pain in the tonsils, worse right tonsil.

MERCURIUS SOL.	: Tonsillitis with bad breath and painful swallowing.
NITRICUM ACIDUM	: Tonsillitis,where the throat is so painful that the patient really cannot swallow anything,is cured by this remedy.
PHYTOLACCA DEC.	: Inflammation of the tonsils, with pain in the throat. Tonsils become dark red and blue. The patient cannot swallow hot drinks. Hoarseness is usually present.
PYROGENIUM 200	: For septicemia of tonsils.
STREPTOCOCCINUM 1000:	For all problems and ailments after tonsillectomy (removal of tonsils). The patient is pale; blue or dark rings around the eyes. No appetite and listlessness. Give one dose every month for six months.
TUBERCULINUM	: Always keep this remedy in view when treating frequent tonsillitis and enlarged tonsils with hard, dry cough and loss of weight.

TRANQUILIZER

Tranquilizers are drugs are that promotes tranquility by calming, soothing, quieting or pacifying without sedating or depressing effects.

COFFEA CRUDA	: Sleepless, on account of mental activity; flow of ideas, with nervous excitability.

KALIUM PHOS. : One of the greatest remedies of the nervous system. Want of nerve power. Mental and physical depression on account of excitement, overwork and worries. For insomnia use 200X and otherwise 6X.

PASSIFLORA Q : It has a quietening effect on the nervous system. In cases of insomnia, it produces normal sleep without any disturbances in cerebral functions. Large doses of 60-100 drops are required, repeat several times.

PISCIDIA Q : It is a nerve sedative. Brings normal sleep in cases of insomnia due to worry, nervous excitement, spasmodic cough. Pain of irregular menstruation. Regulates the flow. Neuralgias and spasmodic affections. Use 50 drops a dose as required.

XANTOXYLUM A. 3X : Its specific action is on the nervous system, specially in nervous patients of spare habits. Insomnia. Frightened. Mental depression.

TRAVELLERS

BELLIS P. : A good remedy for travellers, who have muscular soreness. Ill effects of cold food and drinks, when the body is heated. Railway spine.

TRAVELLING SICKNESS

ARNICA MONT.	: Fatigue after travelling by air or a long distance.
BAPTISIA TINC.	: Shipboard fevers.
BELLADONNA	: Air sickness in aviators. Give as a preventive, before boarding an aeroplane.
BELLIS P.	: A good remedy for railway travellers and other travellers who get backache and muscular soreness on travelling. Railway spine.
BORAX	: Great fear of travelling in a plane, when it descends to land.
CHINA OFF.	: Fatigue after loss of blood or other vital fluids.
COCA	: Many complaints of mountaineering are covered by this remedy. Palpitation, dyspnea, anxiety and insomnia.
COCCULUS IND.	: Nausea and vertigo from riding in a car, boat (on looking at a boat in motion), also sea sickness.
LAC DEF.	: Car sickness.
NITRICUM ACIDUM	: Marked improvement in all symptoms while riding in a carriage.
NUX VOM.	: Problems of digestion in air travellers.
PETROLEUM	: Ailments from riding in cars, carriages and ships.
PLATINUM MET.	: Constipation of travellers who are constantly changing food and water.

| SANICULA AQUA | : Nausea and vomiting from riding a car. |
| TABACUM | : Sea sickness. Faint, sinking feeling in the pit of the stomach. Nausea. |

TREMBLING
(PARALYSIS AGITANS-TREMORS)

ABSINTHIUM	: Feeling of trembling in the heart and tongue.
AMBRA GRISEA	: Trembling of single parts of the body, like hands, arms, etc. in old age. It is a great old age remedy and cures many diseases related to old age.
ARGENTUM NIT.	: A complimentary of Gelsemium specially, when diarrhea accompanies and there is a weak memory.
COCCULUS IND.	: Trembling of hands while eating. Legs tremble on walking, with a tendency to fall on the side.
GELSEMIUM	: Trembling on account of weakness of muscles and nervous system or impending paralysis. Gout causes staggering. For such conditions, it is an important remedy. Lack of muscular coordination. It reactivates and enlivens the dead cells.
KALIUM PHOS.	: Tremors due to nerve weakness.
LACHESIS	: Use it for trembling of the tongue.
LATHYRUS SAT.	: Trembling on account of slow nerve power and paralytic affec-

tions of the lower extremities. Reflexes are always increased and the movements of the fingers and toes are slow.

MAGNESIUM PHOS. 1000 :	Trembling of hands due to any cause and for general trembling. One dose a week.
MERCURIUS SOL. :	Trembling extremities, especially hands; paralysis agitans.
PHOSPHORUS :	Weakness and trembling from every exertion.
PLUMBUM MET. :	Trembling extremities, especially upper, cannot raise or lift anything with the hand.

TUBERCULOSIS

Tuberculosis is spread from person to person by coughing, sneezing, etc. Coughing not associated with large quantities of sputum but often streaked with blood is the first common symptom. Fever, loss of weight and profuse sweat specially at night, may follow. Under such circumstances, an X-ray of lungs will reveal the original defect.

Many think of TB as of lungs only, but a person can have TB of abdominal, urinary, reproductive systems, bones and joints including the spine. Homoeopathy offers a very successful treatment, in this respect. In advanced cases, bed rest with an adequate well balanced vegetarian diet and relief from emotional tension, is required.

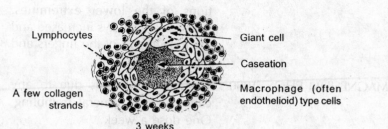

Lymphocytes

Giant cell

Caseation

A few collagen strands

Macrophage (often endothelioid) type cells

3 weeks

The tubercle at this state is just visible to the naked eye.

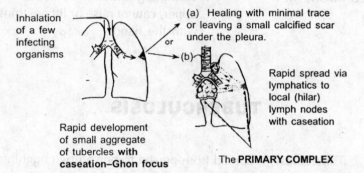

Inhalation of a few infecting organisms

(a) Healing with minimal trace or leaving a small calcified scar under the pleura.

or

(b)

Rapid spread via lymphatics to local (hilar) lymph nodes with caseation

Rapid development of small aggregate of tubercles with **caseation–Ghon focus**

The **PRIMARY COMPLEX**

General spread

Spread to individual organs

e.g. Tuberculous meningitis

TB of bone and adjacent joint

Bone

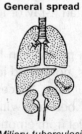

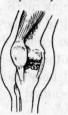

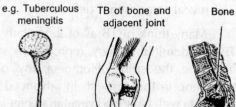

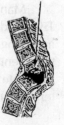

Miliary tuberculosis

Scattering of small pale tubercles throughout the body

ACALYPHA IND. Q	: Spitting of blood.
ALLIUM SATIVUM	: Four to six grams of raw garlic boiled in a little milk and given in divided doses, 3-4 times a day dries up the excessive phlegm in the patients of tuberculosis.
ARSENICUM IOD. 3X	: Phthisis with hoarse, racking cough and profuse expectoration of purulent nature. Cardiac weakness. Emaciation and debility. Chronic watery diarrhea. Appetite good. Anemia and dyspnea. Night sweats.
AVIAIRE 1000 (TUBERCULIN-FROM BIRDS)	: Has proved to be an effective remedy in tuberculosis, when there are symptoms of influenza and bronchitis. Relieves debility. Diminishes the cough. Improves the appitite and breaks up the disease. This should not be repeated before six months.
CALCAREA PHOS. 6X	: Weakness due to the disease. Consumption develops very rapidly.
CARBO ANIMALIS	: Ulceration of the lungs with a feeling of coldness in the chest. Cough with discharge of greenish pus.
CHININUM SULPH.	: Subnormal temperature. Chronic cough. Gradual loss of weight.
COCCULUS IND.	: Sensation of emptiness and cramps in the chest. Dyspnea. Constriction of the chest. Oppressed breathing, producing cough.
DIGITALIS	: Reduces the fever of the disease. Tuberculosis with heart disease.

DROSERA	:	Laryngeal phthisis with rapid emaciation. Hoarseness. Constriction of the throat at every word uttered.
GUAIACUM OFF.	:	Tuberculosis in rheumatic subjects. Suffocations. Dry, tingling cough. Stitches in the ribs and chest. Shortness of breath with expectoration.
HELIX TOSTA CM	:	Hemoptysis of consumption.
HYDRASTIS CAN.	:	To fatten patients after tuberculosis.
MILLEFOLIUM Q	:	Hemoptysis in incipient phthisis. Cough with bloody expectoration.
PHOSPHORUS	:	Tuberculosis in tall, rapidly growing young people. Do not give less than 30 potency and that also not too frequently. If given often, it may hasten the destructive degeneration of the tuberculoid masses. Repeated hemoptysis. Hard, dry cough with congestion of the lungs. Burning pains, heat and oppression of the chest. Tuberculosis of intestines.
SABAL SER.	:	Tuberculosis of larynx.
SACCHARINUM	:	For diarrhea in the disease.
SENECIO AUR.	:	Acute inflammatory conditions of upper respiratory tract. Hoarseness Chest sore and raw. Dyspnea on ascending. Dry, teasing cough with chest pain.
SILICEA	:	Large cavities in the lungs. Fever. Night sweats.
STANNUM MET. 3X	:	Phthisis of pulmonary mucous membranes. Violent, dry cough in

the evening and at night with copious green, sweetish mucus. Respiration short and oppressive. Fever. Hoarseness.

STREPTOCOCCINUM 200 : Reduces fever. Rapid action on temperature.

THUJA OCC.   : Tuberculosis of larynx.

TUMORS

ALUMEN 200   : Tumor of ovaries, with chronic constipation.

ARSENICUM ALB.   : For malignant tumors originating in the epidermis of skin, a carcinoma.

ASTERIAS RUB.   : Tumors of the breast. Acts on both the breasts but better on left.

AURUM MET.   : Useful in tumor of bones, when there are nocturnal bone pains.

AURUM MUR. NAT. 3X   : A very good remedy for uterine tumors.

AURUM ARS.   : Uterine cancer. Sexual desire increased. Inflammation of ovaries. Menses too copious, too frequent or absent.

BELLADONNA   : Painful tumors of the breasts.

BUFO RANA   : It is a palliative in cancer of breasts.

CALCAREA CARB. 200   : Brain tumor. Headache and vertigo on turning the head. Icy coldness of the head. May be used in fat patients. Pedunculated fibroid tumors with roots.

CALCAREA·FLUOR. 200 : Hard tumor of abdomen, scalp and left breast.

CALCAREA IOD. : Uterine fibroids.

CALCAREA PHOS. 200 : May be used in thin people. Brain tumor. Fibroid tumors without roots.

CHIMAPHILA Q : Woman with very large breasts and painful tumors of mammae, not ulcerated and with abundant milk.

COLOCYNTHIS : Cystic tumors of the ovary.

CONDURANGO Q : Hard tumor of the left breast.

CONIUM MAC. : Painful, hard tumor or cancer of either breast or both and that of the uterus and stomach, specially, if the trouble started after an injury to these parts.

CONIUM MAC., KALIUM CARB. : Tumors. Select the remedy according to the symptoms of the medicines.

EUCALYPTUS : Use externally and internally in vascular tumors of female urethra.

FRAXINUS A. Q : Fibroid tumors of the uterus with bearing down sensations. Dysmenorrhea.

HECLA LAVA : A general remedy for tumors anywhere.

HYDRASTIS CAN. : Tumors of breast, hard and painful. Nipple retracted. Menorrhagia.

HYPERICUM PERF. : Slow developing tumors specially on the passage of nerves.

KALIUM CARB. : Cancer of the womb with severe itching and cutting pains from hip to knee.

KALIUM IOD. CM   : Womb packed with tumors. Patient is tired with a sensation as if the legs were sleeping. It causes disappearance of long standing tumors and nodules.

KALIUM PHOS.   : Remember it in the treatment of suspected malignant tumors.

KREOSOTUM   : Cancer of the uterus with oozing of very fetid blood.

LACHESIS 200   : Tumor or cancer of the left ovary or both ovaries. Pain in the uterine region increases before menses and is relieved during menses.

LAPIS ALBUS   : Fibroid tumor or cancer of uterus with burning pain and debilitating bleeding.

MERCURIUS IOD. FLAV. : Mammary tumors with warm perspiration.

NITRICUM ACIDUM 200 : Cystic tumor in the region of the ear lobes.

PALLADIUM MET.   : Tumor of ovaries.

PHYTOLACCA DEC.   : Mammary tumors with enlarged axillary glands.

PULSATILLA NIG. 1M   : A dependable remedy for uterine fibroids, tumors situated near the fundus. A dose fortnightly.

SELENIUM MET.   : Tumor of right breast.

SOLIDAGO VIRGA. Q   : Uterine fibroids, tumors pressing down on the bladder causing difficulties in passing urine.

STAPHYSAGRIA,   : Sebaceous tumors of the eyes.
CALCAREA CARB. 200   Tumor of the eyes containing an oily, fatty matter.

TEUCRIUM MAR. CM	: Polyp in vagina.
THIOSINAMINUM 2X	: It is a great remedy for dissolving tumors. Use with indicated remedy.
THLASPI BURSA Q	: Cancer or fibroid of uterus accompanied with hemorrhage, cramps, clots and aching in the back.
THUJA OCC. 200	: Brain tumors with migraine, headache. Flatulence. Constipation. The patient is emotional and sentimental. Spongy tumors of the abdomen. Tumors of eyelids. Polypus of cervix. Lrregular menses.
THYROIDINUM 2X	: Fibroid tumor of breasts and uterus.
TRILLIUM PEND.	: Very useful for hemorrhage from fibroids.
TUBERCULINUM 200	: A dose of this remedy should be given at the commencement of all sorts of tumors. Specially, for benign mammary tumors.

TYPHOID FEVERS
(SEE FEVERS)

ULCERS

A lesion on the surface of the skin or on a mucous surface, caused by superficial loss of tissue, usually with inflammation.

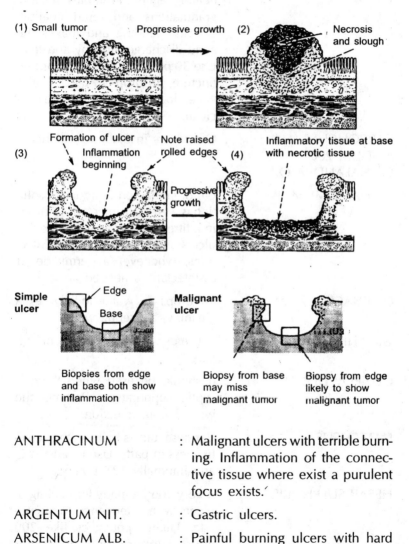

(1) Small tumor   Progressive growth   (2)   Necrosis and slough

Formation of ulcer   Note raised   Inflammatory tissue at base
(3)   Inflammation   rolled edges   (4)   with necrotic tissue
            beginning

Progressive growth

Simple ulcer   Edge   Base

Biopsies from edge and base both show inflammation

Malignant ulcer

Biopsy from base may miss malignant tumor

Biopsy from edge likely to show malignant tumor

ANTHRACINUM : Malignant ulcers with terrible burning. Inflammation of the connective tissue where exist a purulent focus exists.

ARGENTUM NIT. : Gastric ulcers.

ARSENICUM ALB. : Painful burning ulcers with hard margins. Ulceration of the heels.

ASTERIAS RUB. : Chronic ulcers,ulcers with sensitive edges and fetid discharges.

CALENDULA OFF. : Use locally for all kinds of ulcers and wounds. A most remarkable healing agent. Promotes healthy granulations and rapid healing. Checks bleeding and makes the acrid discharge, healthy and free. Use 30 potency orally and mother tincture, 50 drops to an ounce of water, locally. Ulcers must be kept clean.

CARBOLICUM ACIDUM 200, CEPHALANDRA Q. : Old ulcers in diabetic patients.

CINNAMOMUM : Oil of cinnamon in aqueous solution is a great disinfectant - 5 drops in a litre of water as a douche for ulcers of the vagina or other infections, whenever a germicide or disinfectant is needed.

ECHINACEA Q : 10 drops in water locally, as a cleaning, antiseptic wash.

GRAPHITES : A useful remedy for duodenal ulcers.

GUNPOWDER 3X : It should be used when there is septic suppuration. Protects the wound from infection.

HAMAMELIS : Varicose ulcers with great sensitiveness of parts. Use locally in Q and internally 12X potency.

HEPAR SULPHURIS : A very good remedy for healing of ulcers with a tendency to suppurate. Higher potencies like 200 abort suppuration and lower potencies 1X-3X promote it.

HYDROCOTYLE A.	: Ulcers of the womb.
KALIUM BICH.	: Round ulcer of the stomach. Dislikes water.
MERCURIUS SOL.	: Ulcers with thin purulent discharge, which is fetid.
MEZEREUM	: Sensitive and easily bleeding ulcers. Pain at night. Tendency to pus formation or pus already formed under the scab.
NITRICUM ACIDUM	: Ulcers that bleed when touched. Stinging pains. Sensation of a splinter; hard elevated irregular edges and growth of fungus on the ulcers. Syphilitic ulcers.
PAEONIA OFF.	: Ulcers caused by wearing shoes of a smaller size or misfitted shoes.
PHOSPHORUS	: Punched out ulcers. Ulcers that bleed easily. Ulcers surrounded by smaller ulcers. Healed ulcers break up again and again and show no tendency to heal.
SANICULA AQUA	: Ulcers between the toes.
SILICEA	: Simple ulceration and perforating ulcers which do not heal properly and quickly, and where granulations are taking time. Useful in ulcers of lungs and breasts.
STANNUM MET.	: Ulceration of ring hole in the lobe of ear.
SULPHUR	: Ulcers that itch a lot and where scratching causes burning.
SYMPHYTUM OFF. 1M	: For gastric and duodenal ulcers. It stimulates the growth of epithelium on the ulcerated surfaces.

URETHRA

It is a canal leading from the bladder, discharging the urine externally.

AMBRA GRISEA	: Itching in the urethra with burning micturition.
BERBERIS VULG. Q	: Burning between acts of urination.
CALCAREA CARB.	: Stone in urethra. Give every hour for it's expulsion.
CLEMATIS ERECTA	: Biting pain or tickling in the orifice of urethra, before urination. Burning, itching and stinging in the urethra after urination. Urine is emitted drop by drop. Interrupted flow, frequent and scanty.
EUCALYPTUS Q	: Use internally and externally in vascular tumors of the female urethra and also in carbuncles of the urethra.
FICUS IND. Q	: Bleeding from the urethra.
PAREIRA BRAVA	: Itching along urethra. Inflammation of urethra.
PETROSELINUM	: Intense itching, deep in the urethra. Constant dribbling of urine in open air. Has to get up several times during the night to void urine.
PHOSPHORUS	: Bleeding from the urethra after passing a catheter in it.
STAPHYSAGRIA	: When a stone has been removed surgically from the urethra; much pain and cold perspiration remains after removal or any other

difficulty after an opertion of the urethra.

THUJA OCC. : Burning in the urethra. Discharge thick. Urine stream splits.

URINE

ACIDUM PHOS., CINA : Urine becomes milky on standing, in children.

ACIDUM PHOS. 1C : Frequent, profuse and watery or milky urine. Frequent urination at night.

ACONITUM NAP. : Urine retained in infants. Hardly any other remedy will be needed.

ALOE SOC. : Cannot pass urine without passing stool.

ALUMINA, BARYTA CARB. : At night, frequent desire to pass urine in old people.

AMBRA GRISEA : Urine smells sour.

APIS MEL. : Desire frequent but passes in drops.

APIS MEL., SABAL SER. : Difficult urination due to affections of the prostrate gland.

ARGENTUM NIT. : Urine passes unconsciously day and night. Emission of a few drops after having finished urinating. Reduction of weight and loss of sleep. Large quantity of urine with or without diabetes.

ARNICA MONT. : Dribbling after labor.

ARSENICUM ALB. : Epithelial cells in the urine.

ARUM TRIPH.	: Starts the flow of suppressed urine within a short time, when it is suppressed for a day. There could be frequent, abundant, pale urine, alternately.
BARYTA MUR.	: Great increase in uric acid.
BELLADONNA 200	: Retention of urine in a otherwise healthy person, due to a kidney problem. Urine is dark and turbid. Involuntary passage of urine during sleep, at night.
BENZOICUM ACIDUM	: Dribbling of urine in old people with an enlarged prostrate. Urine has the smell of bitter almonds; the smell fills the whole room.
BERBERIS VULG.	: Sensation as if some urine remained after urinating.
BORAX	: Painful urination in children. Child is afraid to urinate and cries.
BRYONIA ALBA	: Urine brown like, beer.
CANNABIS IND.	: Urine is retained due to kidney or bladder inflammation.
CANTHARIS	: Burning urination. Voided drop by drop. Suppression with restlessness.
CAUSTICUM	: Urine retained after surgery or voided very slowly or retained after labor, which was strenous. Frequent desire at night in old people for passing urine. Loss of sensability in passing urine.
CHELIDONIUM, CHENOPODIUM AN.	: Urine profuse and foamy yellow, like beer. Dark and turbid, not clear.

CONIUM MAC.	: Frequent urination in old people at night, sometimes the urine cannot be retained and passes involuntarily. Dribbling in old people. Much difficulty in voiding. It flows and stops again.
COPAIVA OFF.	: Voided in drops with pain. Before micturition, burning pressure. Urine retained, with pain in the anus and rectum. Fetid smell, turbid and is green, in color.
CUPRUM ARS.	: Urine dark and scanty, specially in diabetic patients. Urine suppressed.
DULCAMARA	: Must urinate when getting chilled.
EEL SERUM	: In kidney affections from cold or intoxication, when there is diminished amount of urine or complete suppression of it, due to renal failure. The use of this remedy produces large quantities of urine and removes the infection. It also cleans the urine from albuminuria.
EQUISTEUM	: Painful urination with burning. Severe pain after urination. Urine is voided drop by drop.
FERRUM ACET., KALIUM ACET.	: Urine, alkaline.
FORMICA RUFA	: A useful remedy for Bacillus coli infection of urine. Large quantities of turbid and fetid urine is passed at night.
HAMAMELIS, ERIGERÓN	: Urine bloody with a stone in the bladder.
HELLEBORUS NIG.	: Urine suppressed. Unconsciousness. Convulsions. Body smells like urine.

HEPAR SULPHURIS	: Patient has to wait for sometime before he can pass urine. Takes a very long time to finish urination. Patient never finishes urinating. It seems as if some urine always remains behind.
KALIUM SULPH.	: A very useful remedy when there is excessive calcium oxalate and other oxalates in the urine.
LITHIUM CARB.	: Heavy deposits of mucus, uric acid or pus in the urine.
LYCOPERSICUM ESCU.	: Dribbling of urine in open air.
LYCOPODIUM, OCIMUM CAN.	: Head remedy for red sand in urine.
MAGESIUM MUR., CANNABIS IND.	: Must wait a long time before he can urinate.
MERCURIUS SOL.	: Frequent desire. Burning in urethra on beginning to urinate. It also cures urination on account of nervousness.
NATRIUM MUR., PULSATILLA NIG., CAUSTICUM, ZINCUM MET., KALIUM CARB.	: Urine escapes involuntary while coughing, sneezing, etc.
NATRIUM MUR., OXALICUM ACIDUM	: Oxaluria.
NITRICUM ACIDUM	: Urine is scanty and smells like horse's urine.
NUX VOM.	: Frequent urination due to digestive problems. Urine dribbles or is passed with great difficulty. Urethra and vulva feel itchy.
OCIMUM CAN.	: Red sand in urine. It is the most important characteristic of this

	remedy. Urine smells like musk. Uric acid diathesis.
OPIUM 200	: Retention or involuntry urination after fright.
PAREIRA BRAVA	: Dribbling after micturition. Constant desire. Flow starts after great straining.
PETROSELINUM	: Urine escapes, if not attended quickly. Intense biting, itching, deep in the urethra.
PLUMBUM MET.1M	: Urine extremely fetid. Urine suppressed. Frequent, ineffectual urge for urination. Tenesmus of bladder.
POPULUS T. Q	: Irritation of bladder. Urine contains mucus and pus. Urination painful and scalding.
PULSATILLA NIG.	: Frequent urination due to weakened pelvic muscles. Burning during urination.
RUMEX CRIS.	: Involuntary spurting of urine on coughing or sneezing.
SARSAPARILLA	: Dribbling while sitting.
SENEGA	: Involuntary passage of urine in sleep, during the day.
SEPIA	: Urine offensive. Slow micturition
SOLANUM XANTH. Q	: Give 5 drops every hour for retention of urine.
STAPHYSAGRIA	: Great and frequent urging to urinate after intercourse in young or newly married women.
SULPHUR, PSORINUM, CARBO VEG.	: These are other remedies for the infection of uninary tract.

SULPHUR	: Polyuria, specially at night. Burning in the urine lasts long after micturition. Must hurry. Sudden call for urination. Great quantities of colorless urine.
TEREBINTHINIAE	: Suppression of urine. Violent convulsions, all due to kidney trouble.
THUJA OCC. 1M	: A very good and curative remedy for Bacillus coli infection of urine. A dose every week.
URTICA URENS Q	: Give 5 drops dose in warm water in case of suppression of urine.
VERATRUM ALB.	: For suppressed urine in cholera.
VERBASCUM THAPS. Q	: Constant dribbling of urine and enuresis of long standing. 2 drops a dose, morning and evening.
VESICARIA COM. Q	: Cures polyuria, pyuria, albuminuria and hematuria.
VIOLA TR.	: Urine is copious and has a disagreeable smell like the smell of a cat's urine.

URTICARIA
(NETTLE RASH)

ANTIMONIUM CRUD.	: Urticaria on account of indigestion. Thickly coated, white tongue is a sure indication for its use.
APIS MEL.	: Sudden puffing up of the whole body, swelling like bites of honey

bee. Stinging and burning pains. Give it at the start of the disease.

ARSENICUM ALB. : Unquenchable thirst for small quantities of cold water. Restlessness. Burning, relieved by warmth. Intense itching.

ASTACUS FL. : Irritation is more at night in the warmth of the bed. Chronic urti-, caria. Liver diseases are generally present.

BOVISTA : Urticaria on excitement of any kind. Itching on getting warm. Urticaria on waking in the morning,worse bathing ; chronic urticaria.

CHLORALOSUM 1X : If Apis does not relieve, give four doses of this remedy in a day. It is a very successful remedy. It has red eruptions like measles with intense itching and sleeplessness.

DULCAMARA : Rashes all over the body due to chill and wet weather are characteristic.

FERRUM PHOS. 6X, KALIUM MUR. 6X : Three grains of each mixed together can be given in routine thrice daily. In most of the cases, when no other remedy is indicated, it suffices. It can be given in alteration with Thyroidinum which will clear the case.

HEPAR SULPHURIS : It is very useful in chronic and recurring urticaria.

HYDRASTIS CAN. 3X : Hives, rashes of various kinds accompanied by constipation.

NATRIUM MUR. 200	: If there is constipation alongwith the disease and the patient is emaciated with an earthy complexion. Two doses a day. Urticaria after taking quinine or after suppression of malaria.
PSORINUM	: Urticaria after exertion.
PULSATILLA NIG.	: Dyspeptic urticaria with vomiting and diarrhea.
RHUS TOX.	: Urticaria with restlessness and burning. Itching is better by the warmth of the bed. Uncovering aggravates.
SEPIA	: Urticaria worse in the open air and better in a warm room, after taking milk.
SKOOKUM CHUCK 3X	: When urticaria resists other treatment.
SULPHURICUM ACIDUM	: It relieves the troublesome itching and gives relief to the patient. Give 4 doses a day in between the treatment when the patient cannot tolerate itching. Chronic urticaria.
SULPHUR	: When there is aggravation at night and the rash is becoming chronic, Sulphur can be used as an intercurrent remedy.
THYROIDINUM 3X	: It is almost specific for the cure of this disease. More the swelling, more the area of infection, more the indication of this remedy.
URTICA URENS 1X	: Intense and intolerable itching of the skin. Face is swollen with the rash. Irresistible scratching. This can be applied externally.

UTERUS
(WOMB)

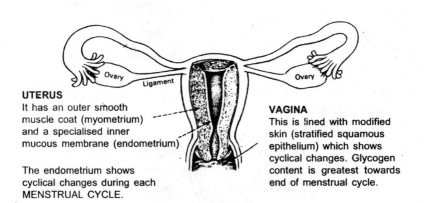

UTERUS
It has an outer smooth
muscle coat (myometrium)
and a specialised inner
mucous membrane (endometrium)

The endometrium shows
cyclical changes during each
MENSTRUAL CYCLE.

VAGINA
This is lined with modified
skin (stratified squamous
epithelium) which shows
cyclical changes. Glycogen
content is greatest towards
end of menstrual cycle.

Menstruation

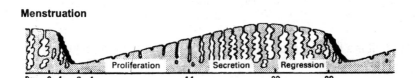

Proliferation   Secretion   Regression

Day 0 1   3 4   14   23   28

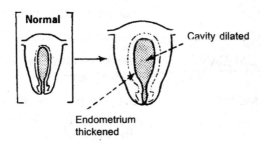

Normal

Cavity dilated

Endometrium
thickened

Tumors beneath the en-
dometrium tend to bulge into
the cavity and may eventually
develop to form a fibroid polyp.

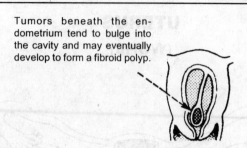

Endometriosis

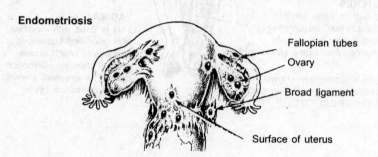

Fallopian tubes

Ovary

Broad ligament

Surface of uterus

It is a hollow muscular organ in which the impregnated ovum is developed into the child.

AGARICUS MUS. : Violent bearing down pains accompanied by sensation of coldness, numbness and tingling. Specially, after menopause.

AGNUS CASTUS : Hemorrhage. Vagina is relaxed.

APOCYNUM CAN. : Menses scanty. Yellow leucorrhea with dropsy.

ARNICA MONT. : Bruised pain in the uterus after scrapping the vagina and dilatation of the uterus, to cause surgical abortion or to remove unnecessary growths.

ARSENICUM ALB.	: Inflammation of the uterus due to excessive loss of blood from the uterus. Restlessness and weakness.
AURUM IOD.	: Inoperable fibroma or myoma of the uterus with very offensive hemorrhage. For ovarian cysts and pathological lesions.
AURUM MUR. NIT. 3X, FRAXINUS A. Q, CALCAREA IOD. 3X	: All the three medicines are to be given in one day after a gap of four hours. Aur-m-n. in the morning, Calc-i. 3X at noon and Fraxinus Q 10 to15 drops at bed time for the cure of uterine fibroma.
AURUM ARS.	: Cancer with increased sexual desire.
BELLADONNA	: Inflammation of the uterus after abortion. Face red. Sensitive to motion.
BROMIUM	: Loud emission of flatus from the uterus and vagina.
CADMIUM SULPH. CM	: After radium and other treatments for cancer, if the disease still persists, give this remedy. There may be persistent vomiting.
CALCAREA ARS.	: Cancer of the uterus.
CALCAREA PHOS.	: Polypus of the uterus.
CANTHARIS	: Inflammation of the uterus with cystitis. Burning pain and swelling.
CIMICIFUGA	: Pain travels from side to side.
COLOCYNTHIS 200	: Pain is severe. The patient doubles up by drawing limbs to the chest. Warmth and pressure relieves.

CONIUM MAC. 200	: Firm and hard fibroma in old maids or women who have been deprived of sexual pleasure.
EUPIONUM 3	: Hemorrhage from the uterus. Blood is thin. Gushing leucorrhea. Uterus is tilted.
FICUS REL. Q	: Hemorrhage from the uterus due to any cause, even cancer
HEPAR SULPHURIS	: Inflammation of the uterus with throbbing pain, worse by pressure, and cold.
HYDROCOTYLE A. Q	: Pain due to cervical cancer and ulceration of the womb.
KALIUM CARB.	: Cancer with severe pain in the legs and from hips to knees in cervical cancer.
KREOSOTUM	: Fibroids, cancerous tumors in the uterus specially of cervix with fetid discharge. Ulcer on the neck of the uterus or bleeding after sexual intercourse.
LACHESIS	: Pain on account of uterine displacement. Pain is more before menses but decreases after the flow.
LAPIS ALBUS	: Hemorrhage from cancer of the uterus. Patient is debilitated. Cancer with severe burning pain.
PHOSPHORUS 200	: Hemorrhage from the uterus. Blood is bright red. The patient is anemic.
PULSATILLA NIG.	: Fibroid tumor near the fundus.
PYROGENIUM 200	: Septic hemorrhage of the uterus after child birth.

RHUS TOX.	: Prolapse after child birth or straining.
SABINA	: Pain from sacrum to pubes, travelling upwards to the vagina after abortion. Inflammation.
SEMPERVIVUM TECT. 2X	: Cancerous tumor of the uterus. The vagina becomes very irritable and dry with tender ovaries.
SEPIA 1000	: Ulceration of the uterus with prolapse.
SILICEA 200	: Cysts in the uterus and vagina.
THLASPI BURSA Q	: Hemorrhage with violent uterine colic. Leucorrhea before and after menses. Recovers from one period when the other starts. Cancer or fibroma, hemorrhage with cramps and clots. Severe pain in the womb on rising.
TILIA EUR.	: Inflammation of the uterus after childbirth. Intense feeling about the uterus with bearing down sensation.
TRILLIUM PEND. Q	: Hemorrhage on account of fibroids.
VIBERNUM PRUN. Q, KALIUM PHOS. 6X, CALCARA FLUOR. 6X	: Uterine tonic and for displacement of the uterus.
VIOLA ODORATA Q	: Headache due to uterine fibroids.

UVULA
(AN APPENDANT FLESHY MASS)

ACONITUM NAP.   : For a constricted feeling of the uvula.

AMMONIUM CAUST.   : Deposition of a white, tenacious mucus on the uvula.

APIS MEL.   : It is a very good remedy for the elongation of uvula, when there is a feeling of burning and scraping in the throat.

CARBOLICUM ACIDUM   : Uvula withered and shrivelled.

IRIS VERS.   : Uvula enlarged like a cone with a thin tip.

KALIUM BICH.   : Ulceration of the uvula.

MERCURIUS BIN IOD. 3X : Elongated uvula, causing cough.

MERCURIUS COR. 3X   : When an elongated uvula is causing trouble, apply a little of this remedy on the uvula. It will relieve immediately and permanently.

TRIFOLIUM PRAT.   : Pain in the uvula.

VACCINATION
(ADMINISTERING A VACCINE)

ARNICA MONT.   : Relieves pain and discomfort of the needle without antidoting the effects of vaccination.

MALANDRINUM   : Acute ill effects of vaccination and eczema following vaccination.

Efficacious in clearing the remains of vaccination.

SILICEA : Ill effects of vaccination, checks the suppurative process.

THUJA OCC. 200 : Chronic ill effects of vaccination. Asthma alternating with eczema after more than one vaccination. The patient has never been well after vaccination. It also cures, fever after vaccination.

VAGINA
(GENERAL CANAL IN THE FEMALE)

AGNUS CASTUS : Inflammation of the vagina. Relaxation and prolapse with copious white discharge.

ALLIUM SATIVUM Q : Eruptions in the vagina and vulva during menses.

ALUMEN 200 : The vaginal canal is very narrow, causing pain and difficulty in penetration of penis. Chronic, yellow vaginal discharge. Apthhous patches in the vagina.

AMBRA GRISEA : Discharge of blood from the vagina while straining at stool. Inflammation of the vagina.

BROMIUM : Loud emission of flatus from the vagina.

CALCAREA CARB. : Fungal infection of the vagina with itching and a milky discharge, worse before menses.

CIMEX LECT.	: Shooting pain from vagina, up towards the left ovary.
FERRUM MET.	: Soreness and cutting in vagina during coition.
HYDROCOTYLE A. 3X	: For heat in the vagina. Pruritis of vagina. Granular ulceration of the vagina.
KREOSOTUM	: Chronic itching within the vulva, burning and swelling of labia, violent itching inside the vagina during menses. Bleeding from the vagina on the day after coitus.
LAC CAN.	: Physometra.
LYCOPODIUM	: Dryness of the vagina with burning pains during and after coition. Physometra during intercourse.
NATRIUM MUR. 200	: Dryness of the vagina and aversion to coition.
PHOSPHORUS	: Absence of sensation in the vagina during coition.
SEPIA	: Vagina painful during coition. Bearing down sensation as if every thing would escape through the vulva. Prolapse of vagina and uterus. Fungal infection with a very offensive discharge, worse on coition.
SILICEA	: Bleeding from the vagina after suckling the child. Patient is chilly. Vaginal cysts.

VARICOSE VEINS

Dialated veins at lower end of oesophagus

Dilated vessels around umbilicus (caput medusae)

Dilated hemorrhoids

ALLIUM CEPA	: Varicose veins after Cesarean section.
AMBRA GRISEA	: Varicose veins of the left leg, very painful.
CALCAREA FLUOR. 6X	: Varicose veins are knitted in hard lumps, in chronic cases.
FLUORICUM ACIDUM	: In all cases of varicose veins of the legs, specially old standing cases. Veins in the legs tending to ulceration. Burning.
FORMICA RUFA 3X	: If there is debility on account of varicose veins.
HAMAMELIS 1X	: Excess of pain; when applied externally causes the vessels to shrink. Use externally for varicose ulcers. It is almost specific in all cases.
HIPPOZAENNUM	: Scrofulous swelling of the veins with formation of pus.
PULSATILLA NIG.	: In cases of varicocele and varicose veins, when constitution and symp-

toms of this remedy are present. Varicose veins during pregnancy.

PYROGENIUM 200 : Ulceration of varicose veins with fetid discharge and pain.

VIPERA : The patient has to keep the legs elevated due to the bursting sensation in the veins while hanging the legs.

VERTIGO

ACIDUM PHOS. 1X : Vertigo in the evening while walking or standing. Stumbles easily and makes mis-steps.

ACONITUM NAP. : Vertigo on rising.

AGARICUS MUS. : Vertigo from sunlight and looking at passing cars and other vehicles. Feeling of coldness in the head with a desire to cover it warmly.

AMBRA GRISEA : Vertigo of old people, due to any cause. Has to lie down, to avoid vertigo.

ARNICA MONT. : Long standing vertigo is cured by the use of this remedy, specially when the objects whirl about while walking.

BELLADONNA : Vertigo on stooping or when rising from a seat.

BORAX : Vertigo while descending.

BRYONIA ALBA : Vertigo on moving the head or when rising from a seat.

CALCAREA CARB. : Vertigo from ascending.

COCCULUS IND.	: Vertigo on watching a hockey match or from loss of sleep.
CONIUM MAC.	: Vertigo on turning the head sidewise, turning in bed, looking around sidewise or while lying down.
DIGITALIS	: It is very efficacious in severe cases of vertigo. It is specially indicated when the pulse is very slow.
FERRUM PHOS.	: Vertigo due to anemia or loss of blood.
GRATIOLA OFF.	: Vertigo during and after meals.
LACHESIS	: Vertigo on rising from the bed in the morning and after sleep.
NATRIUM MUR.	: Vertigo on studying.
NUX VOM.	: Vertigo from stooping, after eating, from odor of flowers, from loss of sleep or from walking.
PHOSPHORUS	: It displays great curative powers in every imaginable case of vertigo. Vertigo on looking down and from odor of flowers.
PULSATILLA NIG.	: Vertigo on looking up or from suppressed menses.
SEPIA	: Vertigo from suppressed menses.
THERIDION	: Vertigo on least noise and on closing the eyes.

VISION

In all cases of eye troubles, it is advisable to get the eyes examined, by an efficient eye specialist. When ocular symptoms exist but no organic defect is found in the eyes, one or more of the following remedies may be tried, according to the symptoms.

ACONITUM NAP., BELLADONNA	: Patient becomes almost blind at night but is okay during the day.
AURUM MET.	: Lower or upper half of vision is invisible.
BELLADONNA	: Flashes before the eyes.
CALCAREA CARB.	: Left or right half not visible.
CARBONEUM SULPH.	: Sensation of a cobweb before the eyes.
FERRUM MET.	: The patient can see equally during day and night.
HYOSCYAMUS NIG.	: Red spots before the eyes.
LITHIUM CARB.	: Right half of an image is invisible.
LYCOPODIUM	: Night blindness with black spots before the eyes.
PHOSPHORUS 200	: Blindness on account of lightening. Give four doses in a month after a gap of a week between each. If there is no improvement at all, consult an eye specialist. It is also used for color blindness.
PILOCARPUS M.	: It improves far sightedness, specially when there appears to be a mist before the eyes.
RUTA G.	: Eyes are fatigued easily on reading or watching TV.

SEPIA	: Dimness of vision after coition.
SULPHUR	: Black spots before the eyes. Patient's eyes resemble the eyes of an owl,who can see during the night but not during the day. Mist before the eyes.

VITAL FORCE

ARMORACIA SAT.	: Use thrice daily to raise vital force, for quite sometime.
CARBO VEG.	: An acute disease has greatly depleted the patient. Patient is incapable of any movement and his fingers become blue. Cold, copious sweat, cold breath, cold tongue and cold body as if, there is no life in it. Loss of voice. Carb-v. saves the life where vital force is nearly exhausted.
COCA Q	: Exhausted nervous system. Loss of voice. 5-6 drops thrice daily.
LOBELIA PURP.	: All the vital forces are weak. Nervous prostration. Intense feeling of chill without shivering. Tongue, heart and lungs feel paralysed. Use it in lower potencies.
PICRICUM ACIDUM	: Vital force is weakened. There is excessive and persistent tired feeling all over the body. Want of will power. Weakness of mind.
SILICEA 6X	: It strengthens the vital force and cures very deep seated diseases.

Here also the patient feels cold
and likes to keep his head covered
always.

VOICE - LOSS

ANTIMONIUM CRUD.   : Loss of voice on account of exces-
                      sive heating of the body.

ARGENTUM NIT.   : Loss of voice from too much sing-
                      ing or shouting. Voice breaks dur-
                      ing singing. Hoarseness may re-
                      sults from much singing or shout-
                      ing.

AURUM MET. 1M   : Sudden loss of voice in singers or
                      public speakers after lengthy speak-
                      ing. It also cures hoarseness in
                      such cases.

BORAX 1X   : A piece of Borax 1X (sodium
                      borate) of the size of a pea, dis-
                      solved slowly in the mouth, acts
                      magically in restoring the voice in
                      case of sudden hoarseness brought
                      on by cold. For an hour or so, it
                      renders the voice clear and silvery.

CARBO VEG.   : Loss of voice with hoarseness after
                      a debilitating disease.

CAUSTICUM   : It is worth trying for loss of voice
                      whether from psychological or
                      inflammatory causes, when there
                      are no other symptoms for accu-
                      rate prescription.

COCA Q   : When a singer or a public speaker
                      experiences loss of voice during

singing or speaking, give5-6 drops every half an hour, about two hours before the expected demand on the voice.

CROTON TIG. : There is complete loss of voice from drinking cold water or cold beverges, when overheated.

FERRUM PIC. : Voice fails after public speaking. or during speaking or singing.

PHOSPHORUS : Loss of voice with laryngitis and constant hawking.

POPULUS CAN. Q : It is a remarkable voice producer and restores the voice, instantly. It removes hoarseness and dryness of the larynx and pharynx, rawness and soreness of the throat and tones up the voice.

VOMITING

AETHUSA CYN. : Vomiting after drinking milk.

AMYGDALUS PER. Q : Very useful in all kinds of nausea and vomiting, morning sickness or vomiting in pregnancy. Children do not digest any kind of food, which is vomited out.

ANTIMONIUM CRUD. : Vomiting after eating or drinking due to indigestion.

APOCYNUM CAN. Q : Excessive vomiting. Nausea with drowsiness. Food and water are immediately ejected. Dull and sinking sensation in the stomach.

Oppression in the epigastrium and chest with difficulty in breathing.

APOMORPHINUM H. Q : The chief power of this remedy is that it produces vomiting. 25 drops in a little water will cause full vomiting in 5-15 minutes. It is used when some poison has been swallowed.

AQUILEGIA VUL. : Vomiting after menopause or hysterical vomiting.

ARSENICUM ALB. : Vomiting of all kinds of foods and drinks due to acidity, specially after eating and drinking.

BELLADONNA : Incessant, uncontrollable vomiting.

CARBOLICUM ACIDUM : Vomiting due to cancer of the oesophagus or stomach.

CINA : Vomiting with worm symptoms.

COCCULUS IND. : Vomiting while travelling by bus or car.

CROTALUS H. : Vomiting after menstruation.

EUPHRASIA, BRYONIA ALBA : Clearing throat of mucus in the morning causes vomiting.

FERRUM MET. : Vomiting immediately after eating.

IPECACUANHA : Good for all kinds of vomiting.

IRIS VERS. : It is a good remedy for habitual vomiting of babies.

KALIUM BICH. : Vomiting after drinking beer.

LYSSINUM : Vomiting at the sight of running water.

NUX VOM. : Vomiting in the morning after drinking whisky at night.

PHOSPHORUS	: Vomiting after an operation.
PLUMBUM¯MET.	: Continued and violent vomiting of food or of greenish, yellowish or blackish matter with violent pain in the stomach and abdomen. Vomiting of bile or blood. Vomiting of fecal matter. Colic with constipation.
PYROGENIUM	: Coffee ground color of vomiting.
SYMPHORICARPUS 200	: This is a routine remedy for the cure of persistant vomiting of pregnancy and nausea during menstruation. Nausea is worse by motion.
SEPIA, COLCHICUM AUTUM., STANNUM MET.	: Vomiting during pregnancy. : Smell of cooking food causes vomiting. Sensation of emptiness in the stomach.
STAPHYSAGRIA	: Vomiting due to insults inflicted upon her.
THYROIDINUM 3X	: Vomiting of pregnancy. Give a dose early in the morning before the patient gets up.
VALERIANA	: Vomiting due to anger in a nursing woman. Child vomits curdled milk after nursing.
VERATRUM ALB.	: Thirst for cold water which is vomited out, as soon as, swallowed.

VULVA

BROMIUM, LAC CAN., LYCOPODIUM	: Emission of flatus from the vulva.
COPAIVA OFF.	: Inflammation of the vulva with itching.
EUPIONUM	: Sore pain between labia during urination. Swelling of labia. Pruritis vulva.
KALIUM IOD., SANGUINARIA CAN.	: Burning of vulva.
PLUMBUM MET.	: Eczema on the vulva.

WALKING

ACIDUM PHOS., GELSEMIUM	: Walks slowly without a reason and easily makes mis-steps and stumbles.
ARGENTUM NIT.	: Gait unsteady and staggering when not noticed.
BARYTA CARB., CALCAREA CARB., CALCAREA PHOS.	: Child is slow to learn walking.
CAUSTICUM	: Patient is slow in learning to walk. Unsteady gait, falls easily.
COFFEA CRUDA, SEPIA	: Walks fast and quickly without any reason.
CONIUM MAC.	: Sudden loss of strength while walking.
CROTALUS H.	: Walks on the toes.

HELODERMA	: When walking, lifts feet higher than usual and brings them down with a thud.
KALIUM PHOS., SILICEA	: Walks half-consciously in sleep.
LACTICUM ACIDUM	: While walking, trembles all over.
LAC CAN.	: When walking, seems to be walking in air.
LACHESIS 200	: Knees knock against each other while walking.
LATHYRUS SAT.	: When walks, heels do not touch the ground.
LATHYRUS SAT., MEZEREUM	: Must stoop when walking.
MAGNESIUM CARB.	: Suddenly falls to the ground while walking.
MANGANUM ACET.	: Cannot walk backwards without falling forward. Walks stooping forward. Peculiar slapping gait. Walks on metacarpophalangeal joints. Walks on the toes.
MEDORRHINUM	: While walking, legs feel heavy as lead. Cannot walk on soles. Walks on the heels.
NUX VOM.	: Drags feet, while walking.
OXYTROPIS L.	: Staggering gait. Walks backwards.
SILICEA	: Scrofulous, rachitic children with large abdomen. Slow in walking, night walking,gets up while asleep.
THUJA OCC.	: Legs feel heavy as if made of wood or glass.

WARS

ACONITUM NAP.

: A soldier becomes nervous on taking part in a war for fear of death or other horrors of war and is reluctant to fight,a dose of this remedy will remove his fears and nervousness.

ARGENTUM NIT.

: By the use of this remedy, anxiety on account of air raids is diminished.

ARNICA MONT.

: Any person who has been too close to the site of a bomb explosion and is not hurt, but feels fear and anxiety, will be comforted by a dose of this remedy.

ARSENICUM ALB.

: Sleeplessness due to fear of air raids is cured by this remedy.

BORAX 3X

: Violent fright from the sound of a firing gun even at a distance.

CONVALLARIA MAJ. Q

: Palpitations and impending heart failure of the aged from a sudden explosion of a bomb. Extremely rapid and irregular pulse.

HYPERICUM PERF. Q

: For healing the wounds produced by gun shots and after the lead has been take out surgically, apply externally and take orally for injury of the nerves.

IGNATIA AMARA

: Fear and anxiety of air raids is removed by the use of this remedy.

KALIUM IOD. 1X

: It protects the thyroid gland in case of an accidental release of radioactivity from the nuclear stations. People living near, in about a 10 kilometer radius of nuclear generating plants, should keep such tablets handy in their houses and take them as soon as possible, after the radiation leak, in order to avoid permanent damage to their thyroid gland and should move to a far off place quickly.

PHOSPHORUS, STRONTIUM CARB. : Removes bad effects of the radiations on account of an atom bomb explosion.

SYMPHYTUM OFF. Q, TRILLIUM PEND. Q : When the bones have been pierced by gun shots which have been removed surgically, take Symphytum Q internally and apply Trillium Q externally to arrest bleeding.

THALLIUM : Loss of hair due to an atom bomb explosion.

WARTS

(PAPILLOMA)

ACIDUM PHOS., SABINA : Black warts.

ANACARDIUM ORI., DULCAMARA, NATRIUM MUR. : Warts on the palms of hand.

ANAGALLIS 1X : It possess the power to soften flesh and destroy warts.

ANTIMONIUM CRUD.	: Warts on the soles ,palms and neck.
ARSENICUM ALB., NATRIUM CARB.	: Warts on the back of the hand.
ARSENICUM ALB.	: Warts on the right hand.
AURUM MUR.	: Warts on the tongue and genitals.
CALCAREA CARB.	: Red warts on the fingers. Warts on the face and hands.
CALCAREA CALCIN. 3X	: It is a remedy for all kinds of warts.
CANNABIS IND., ACIDUM PHOS.	: Warts situated on the prepuce.
CARBO ANIMALIS	: Warts on hands and face of old people.
CASTOR EQUI	: Warts on the breasts.
CASTOREUM CAN.	: Warts on the forehead.
CAUSTICUM	: Warts on finger tips and right index finger, on the face, eye lids and nose. Burning and bleeding easily. May be situated all over the body.
DULCAMARA	: Warts on the lower eye lid of the eyes.
FERRUM MET., PSORINUM	: Warts on the left hand.
FICUS CARICA (FIG)	: The fresh milky juice obtained by breaking the stalk, when applied externally on warts causes their disappearance.
KALIUM CARB.	: Warts on the fingers.
NATRIUM CARB.	: Warts on the forearms.
NATRIUM MUR.	: Warts on the palms or hands.

NATRIUM SULPH.	: Red warts all over the body.
NITRICUM ACIDUM	: Cauliflower like warts on lips or anywhere hard, with cracks, sometimes emitting fetid a fluid. Warts on genitals. Warts bleed on washing.
SARSAPARILLA	: Warts around the joints of fingers.
SEPIA	: Warts situated all over the body.
THUJA OCC. 1M	: Warts on the anus, thumb, sides of the fingers and left index finger. Warts in crops, sometimes oozing moisture or blood. Warts on the genitals and anal surface.

WATER

AMMONIUM CARB.	: Great aversion to water. Cannot bear to touch it.
CALCAREA CARB.	: Aversion to water and washing as it aggravates the ailments.
FERRUM MET.	: Sight of flowing water causes vertigo.
HYDROPHOBINUM	: Dread of flowing water.
HYOSCYAMUS NIG.	: Dislikes water as he cannot swallow liquids.
SEPIA	: It is called a washer woman's remedy,because the ailments worsen due to laundry work.
SULPHUR	: Dislikes water. Aversion to being washed.

WEAKNESS (DEBILITY)

ACETICUM ACIDUM : Prostration after surgery and due to use of anesthesia.

ACIDUM MUR. 3X : Debility during low and septic fevers. Involuntary stools while passing urine.

ACIDUM PHOS. Q : 5 drops of it in a tumbler full of water as a beverage alongwith meals for debility by loss of vital fluids, sexual excesses and disappointed love. Debility, both sexual and physical.

ALETRIS FAR. : Debility due to prolapse of the uterus.

ARGENTUM NIT. : Debility of the calves. Walks and stands, unsteadily.

ARNICA MONT. : Muscular fatigue due to over exertion or due to injuries.

ARSENICUM IOD. 3X : General weakness. Tendency to faint. Loss of appetite. Thrice daily after food, with an interval of a day or two after a week of its use.

ARSENICUM ALB. : Debility resulting from overtaxing the muscular system by exercise, etc.

AVENA SAT. Q : Debility after exhausting diseases.

CADMIUM SULPH. : Exhaustion of mind and body. Declining to work after chronic post influenzal states. Extreme prostration in low forms of the disease.

CALCAREA CARB. : Debility in fat children.

CALCAREA PHOS. 6X : Debility after acute diseases, overwork and worry.

CARBO VEG.	: Debility without fever, with blueness and coldness. A lowered vital force from loss of fluids or after drugging. Debility in people due to disintegration and imperfect oxidation.
CHINA OFF. 1M	: After profuse bleeding in delivery, a dose of it will recover the strength of the patient.
CHINA OFF. 1X, CURARE	: From loss of blood and other animal fluids like semen or leucorrhea.
COLCHICUM AUTUM.	: Prostration and feeling of internal coldness as an effect of hard study or night watching. A peculiar symptom of this remedy is that the patient complains of prostration and weakness, though apparently, he looks well.
CONIUM MAC., LYCOPODIUM, BARYTA MUR.	: Great debility in the morning, in the bed.
CONIUM MAC.	: General debility of the body and mind, greatly felt in the morning while in bed. Feeling as if bruised by blows. Difficult gout,trembling and sudden loss of strength while walking.
CURARE, AMBRA GRISEA, BARYTA MUR.	: Debility in aged people.
FERRUM PHOS. 6X	: Debility due to anemia. Tired feeling in the brain. Depression.
GINSENG	: Removes weakness and produces a sense of general well being.

HELONIAS	:	Debility and dragging in the sacrum and pelvis.
IODIUM	:	Great unaccountable sense of debility. Least effort induces perspiration. Loss of breath on going upstairs. Feels better,for the time being, while eating.
KALIUM CARB.	:	Muscular debility combined with a weakened condition of the nerves. This makes him very sensitive. He is easily frightened, shrieks about imaginary appearances, cannot bear to be touched and startles when touched.
KALIUM PHOS. 6X	:	Debility from mental strain.
LATHYRUS SAT.	:	Debility after influenza and other diseases.
LECITHINUM 3X	:	Acts as tonic during convalescence and in anemia.
NATRIUM CARB.	:	Debility due to summer heat.
NATRIUM MUR. 200	:	Weakness of the spine. Mental and physical debility. Weakness of the limbs like half paralysed extremities. Physical and mental labour is prostrating.
NATRIUM SAL.	:	One of the best remedies for the prostrating after effects of influenza.
PSORINUM	:	Debility after acute diseases such as typhoid, chilliness. Desire to lie down.
SELENIUM MET.	:	Mental and physical weakness in old age. Debility due to summer heat and after exhausting diseases.

Weakness, after exercise and in the hot weather. Strength rises as the sun sinks.

SILICEA : Prostration of mind and body. Want of grit or grit all gone. It builds up such people, raises spirits, revives hopes and weakness, and depression gives way to the feeling of returning strength and health. Debility of thin, rickety children.

STROPHANTHUS HISP. : Severe prostration from hemorrhage after surgery and acute diseases.

SYPHILINUM 1M : Weakness and all other symptoms like pain, etc. are worse from darkness to daylight, sunset to sunrise, they decrease and increase gradually. Utter prostration and debility in the morning.

THYROIDINUM 2X : Weakness, sensation of faintness and nausea. Sensitive to cold. Weakness after an acute disease. Easily fatigued, weak pulse, palpitations, cold hands and feet, chilliness and low blood pressure. Specially indicated in patients with thyroid dysfunction.

VERATRUM ALB. : Cardiac and general muscular depression and weakness. A good heart tonic.

WEATHER

COLD WEATHER

ANTIMONIUM SULPH.	: Winter cough, with soreness all over the body.
ARGENTUM NIT.	: Cannot withstand hot and very cold weather.
ARSENICUM ALB.	: Skin diseases become worse during winter.
AURUM MET.	: All complaints are worse in cold weather and when getting cold. Many complaints come only in winter.
CUPRUM MET.	: Asthma, worse cold weather, cold wind and dampness.
DULCAMARA	: Complaints, worse during rains in winter.
MERCURIUS SOL.	: All complaints are worse during winter rains and dampness.
PETROLEUM	: Diseases are worse in cold weather.
SILICEA, PETROLEUM	: All symptoms are worse in the cold weather.
TEREBINTHINIAE 1X	: Winter cough, bronchitis and sub-acute inflammation of the respiratory tract. Makes expectoration easy.

CHANGE OF WEATHER

CALCAREA CARB.	: Takes cold at every change of weather, specially fat persons.
CALCAREA PHOS.	: Diseases are worse, during change of weather.

CHELIDONIUM	: Ailments brought on or renewed by change of weather.
COLOCYNTHIS	: It is often indicated in the transitional season, when the air is cold, but the sun is still powerful enough to heat the blood.
PSORINUM	: Diseases are worse during change of weather.
RHUS TOX.	: Rheumatism is worse during storm, spring and changing weather.

HOT WEATHER

ACONITUM NAP.	: Complaints of very hot weather specially diseases relating to digestion.
AETHUSA CYN., CHINA OFF.	: Diarrhea and indigestion during summer, specially of children.
ANTIMONIUM CRUD.	: The patient feels exhausted during warm weather and his gastric problems increase in the hot season.
ARGENTUM NIT.	: Cannot withstand hot and very cold weather.
BRYONIA ALBA., NUX VOM., PULSATILLA NIG.	: Diarrhea in summers after over eating. Nux - diarrhea is worse in the morning and Puls.-diarrhea is worse at night.
NATRIUM CARB., SELENIUM MET.	: Debility due to summer heat.
PICRICUM ACIDUM	: It is a hot weather or summer remedy. Prostration and tired feeling. Aversion to food. Feet cold, cannot get warm enough.

PODOPHYLLUM : Diarrhea of children during summer and after eating acidic fruits.

RHODODENDRON CH. : Rheumatism and gouty symptoms, worse in hot weather and before a storm.

SPRING WEATHER

NATRIUM SULPH. : Skin troubles return every spring.

RAINY WEATHER

BLATTA ORIENT. : Asthma is worse in the rainy weather.

DULCAMARA : Aggravation of skin problems during rains and damp climate.

HEPAR SULPHURIS : Strong amelioration of respiratory diseases in damp weather.

MERCURIUS SOL. : All complaints worse from damp, cold and rainy weather.

NATRIUM SULPH. : Aggravation of asthma and other respiratory troubles in rains and dampness. Every change of dry to wet has an effect. All troubles are worse during rains.

RHODODENDRON CH., RHUS TOX. : Pain and all the other symptoms are worse during winter rains and dampness.

WEEPING

MANGANUM ACET. : Involuntary laughter and involuntary weeping. Makes fun of other's gait.

MEDORRHINUM	: The patient cannot speak without weeping and speaks hurriedly. The patient loses thread of conversation.
NATRIUM MUR. 200	: The patient is secretive, holds her secrets, wants to be alone and weep. She has tears even with laughter.
PULSATILLA NIG. 200	: A mild, timid, reserved and yeilding patient, weeps while talking.
SEPIA 200	: The patient dreads to be alone and is easily offended. Weeps while telling symptoms.

WEIGHT

ALFALFA Q	: 10 drops taken thrice daily produces more fats and subsequent gain in weight.
ARSENICUM ALB.	: Gradual loss of weight due to impaired nutrition.
IODIUM	: In high potencies 200 and 1000, increase weight, while in low potencies i. e. 2x and 3x, it reduces weight, flesh and obesity. Patient eats well but loses weight and flesh.
KALIUM HYDRIOD.	: Gradual loss of weight is stopped by the use of this remedy.
LECITHINUM 3X	: Improves nutrition and increases flesh and weight.

NATRIUM MUR. 30-10M : Losing weight gradually due to overwork, disappointment and suppressed menses.

TUBERCULINUM : Loss of weight due to respiratory diseases and enlarged tonsils.

WENS
(SEBACEOUS CYSTS)

A cyst resulting from the retention of sebaceous gland secretion. It is round in shape, varying in size from the size of a pea to the size of a walnut. May appear anywhere on the scalp, face, back, etc. It is soft and painless.

BARYTA CARB. : For recurring cysts around the eyes.

BENZOICUM ACIDUM : In gouty subjects with strong smelling urine.

CALCAREA FLUOR., : Cysts on the eye lids.
NITRICUM ACIDUM

CONIUM MAC. 200 : Cysts in breasts.

GRAPHITES 200 : It is one of the best remedies for people prone to eczema and other skin troubles.

HEPAR SULPHURIS : Suppurating wens.

PHYTOLACCA DEC. : Glandular swelling with heat and inflammation.

THUJA OCC. 200 : Soft fleshy excrescences and spongy wens. Cysts on the covered parts only.

KALIUM IOD. : Wens in the scalp.

WHISKERS

(ALSO SEE THE HEADING BEARD AND BALDNESS)

ARSÉNICUM IOD. : Eczema of the bread and mous-
tache. Eczema itching, watery
oozing; worse washing.

BARYTA CARB., : For falling of hair from whiskers.
CALCAREA CARB.,
KALIUM CARB.,
SPHINGURUS MAR.

GRAPHITES : Ringworm of moustaches.

WHITLOW

(SUPPURATIVE INFLAMMATION AT THE END OF A FINGER OR TOE)

LEDUM PAL. 200 : Abscess on the finger tip caused by
a thorn, needle or sharp pointed
instruments. It not only cures but
acts as an anti-tetanus.

MYRISTICA SEB. : It acts more powerfully than Hepar
and Silicea. It has a specific action
on whitlow. It hastens suppuration
and shortens its duration and often
does away with the use of a knife.

SILICEA : If administered early, generally
prevents the development of whitlow.

WHOOPING COUGH
(SPASMODIC COUGH)

AMBRA GRISEA : Convulsive cough with flow of warm water from the mouth.

BELLADONNA 200 : In the first stage of cough. Dry cough with a red face. 3-4 fits at a time. If there is no improvement within 24 hours, do not repeat it. Choking. Sputum may be blood streaked. Vomiting may occur. Expectoration is scanty and tenacious.

COCCULUS IND., NATRIUM MUR. : Spells of vomiting and coughing with tears in the eyes.

CORALLIUM RUB. : Spasmodic whooping cough. Attacks follow and run into each other. Profuse secretion of mucus, mucus drops through the posterior nares. Feels as if cold air was passing through the head and air passages. Cough is worse in open air.

DROSERA 30 : It is a true remedy for whooping cough. Cough is barking and choking. Sputum may be blood streaked. Vomiting may occur. Give only one dose and await results for four days. Cough may not come all day long but commences as soon as the head touches the pillow, at night. Patient cannot speak due to asthma.

IPECACUANHA : Whooping cough with wheezing, nausea and vomiting.

KALIUM CARB.	: Dry, hoarse cough worse about 3 A.M. with stitching pain in the chest and dryness of the throat, worse in cold and better in warm climate. Expectoration is scanty and tenacious.
MAGNESIUM PHOS.	: Voice hoarse. Cannot lie down, suffocating cough.
NAPHTHALINUM	: Long lasting, choking cough with sneezing. Throat appears constricted.
PERTUSSINUM	: It is a nosode of whooping cough and if given in the beginning of the disease, cut shorts its duration.
THYMUS SERP. Q	: Whooping cough of children. Sore throat and burning in the pharynx. Severe spasms, but only a little sputum is expectorated.

WORMS

CARBONEUM TETRAMUR. Q	: It has given wonderful clinical re sults in the treatment of hookworm infestation.
CHELONE Q	: It is an enemy to every kind of worm, infesting the human body including round worms and thread worms.
CINA 200	: It is a remedy for round, thread and tape worms. The patient usually rubs the nose and is restless. Grinding of teeth during sleep is a

guiding symptom, for it's use. One dose daily.

CUCURBITA PEPO Q : One of the most efficient and least harmful remedies for expulsion of tape worms.

CUPRUM OXYDATUM NIG. 1X : It expels all kinds of worms including tape worms and trichinella (a hair like worm). One gram a dose, thrice daily.

HELMINTHOCHORTOS : It acts very powerfully on the intestinal worms specially round worms, and earth worms (Lumbricoids).

HYDROCOTYLE A. 6X : It is a very near specific, in treatment of expulsion of filaria and thread worms from the intestines.

TEUCRIUM MAR. : It is a very near specific, for the treatment of ascarides, pin worms and round worms in the intestines. Tingling and tickling in the nose is an important symptom in children.

THYMOLUM 6 : It is specific for hookworm infestation. A single dose of 3 ml removes 95% of the hookworms in adults.

SANTONINUM 3X : It is of unquestioned value in the treatment of worms. Itching in the nose, restless sleep and twitching of muscles indicate this remedy in the treatment of thread worms and round worms. It has no effect on tape worms.

NOTE: All worms infesting the human body are parasites and they consume the patient's nutrients. Hundreds of human parasites are known. Conventional anti-parasitic drugs cure only a few types and tend to cause side effects. General symptoms are constipation or diarrhea, gas and bloating, anemia, grinding teeth, chronic fatigue and other immunity problems. Anti-parasitic foods include garlic, onions, raw pumpkin seeds, raw beets, carrots, figs, papaya seeds and pomergranate.

WORRY

BUTYRICUM ACIDUM : Worries over little trifles. Impulsive thoughts of suicide. Constant state of fear and nervousness. Headache on account of worries over trifles.

IGNATIA AMARA : Sighing and sobbing on account of worries.

KALIUM PHOS. 6X : Ill effects of worries like mental and physical depression are wonderfully relieved by the use of this remedy.

WOUNDS

CALENDULA OFF. Q : It is a very good remedy for wounds. When applied locally, open wounds and ulcers heal quickly as it promotes healthy granulation. Use 20 drops of Calendula Q in an ounce of water for cleaning the wound and for dressing, use Calendula Q.

HYPERICUM PERF. Q   : Use externally as well as internally for lacerated wounds, injured nerves and also punctured wounds.

IODIUM Q   : It is a very good remedy for keeping wounds clean and disinfected. Use it in gunshot wounds after removing the pellets, and in bites of insects and reptiles.

LEDUM PAL.   : Use externally and internally for punctured wounds. In 200 potency, give a dose daily for three days, it acts as an anti-tetanus.

OLEUM JEC.,
CINNAMOMUM   : 10 drops of cinnamonum oil in a litre of water acts as a germicide and disinfectant. It can be used as a vaginal douche and if used after intercourse, it sometimes proves to be as an effective contraceptive. It can be used for washing the wounds.

STAPHYSGARIA   : Incised wounds. Clear cut wounds. Cut with a knife, sharp instruments or weapons like sword..

WIESBADEN   : Gunshot wounds which are slow to heal, are benefited by this remedy.

NOTE: For healing a wound, three factors are necessary :

1.   CLEANLINESS : For this purpose, the dirt, sand, splinters, small pieces of glass, etc. should be removed and the wound should be washed with cold water to which a few drops of Calendula Q have been added.

2.   DRESSING OF THE WOUND: It is important to bring the sides of the wound together and to exclude the air. It can be done by stitching if the wound is large or by applying pressure with fingers. Thereafter, a lint dipped

in Calendula Q should be placed over it with a little cotton. Thereafter, bandage it tightly to keep the ends of the wound together.

3. BLEEDING: If the wound is bleeding profusely, the bleeding should be stopped before step no. 2. A bandage should be tied above the wound, towards the heart, tightly. It will stop the bleeding. Thereafter, a lint piece dipped in Trillium pendulum Q should be applied over it, as in step no. 2. In deep and dangerous wounds, help of a surgeon may be obtained. The above mentioned medicines should be used internally as indicated.

WRINKLES

ABROTANUM	: Wrinkles on the face.
AURUM MUR.	: Wrinkles on the face, in a syphilitic patient.
CALCAREA CARB.	: These are formed due to relaxation of abdominal muscles in a woman, who has given birth to several children. There are folds of skin on the abdomen, which are loose and hanging. These may be formed in case of a fat man who exercised to reduce fat and girth of the abdomen and then suddenly left exercising.
CALCAREA PHOS.	: The entire skin of the body is wrinkled, giving a withered look. It is a good remedy for these conditions, specially when the person is thin.
NATRIUM MUR.	: Wrinkles on the neck.

LYCOPODIUM : Wrinkles on the forehead.

SILICEA 6X : Wrinkles on the face of a child like that of a monkey. Weak child having a big abdomen.

NOTE: My own experience shows that wrinkles can be prevented to a great extent by using the following tips:

1. Massaging the face with an upward motion from the cheeks to the forehead.

2. Vitamin E mixed with any oil should be used for the massage.

3. Onion juice mixed with honey is an excellent anti-wrinkle paste. Before application, the face should be washed with soap and water, and dried

4. Plenty of rest and sleep helps to keep the looks young and fresh.

5. Scientists have long known that sunlight can cause the skin to wrinkle and turn leathery. Skin damage is caused by ultra violet solar rays which are absorbed by urocanic acid,a natural molecule, made by the outer most skin cells. Sun rays chemically change this molecule making it free of oxygen thus degrading, collagen and elastin, which are the major molecules that make the skin. Elasticity of the skin is reduced making a person looks older than he is.

WRISTS

WRIST CURLS

A.) Hold a tin can (i.e. beans).
Place forearm on table with
wrist free over the edge. Do 15
wrist curls with palm facing up,
15 with palm facing down.
Repeat 3 times. Doing this
exercise with a shopping bag will
alow weight to be added as your
strength improves.

B.) Squeezing a rubber ball
will also strengthen the
injured area. Carry one
with you and squeeze it
as often as you can.

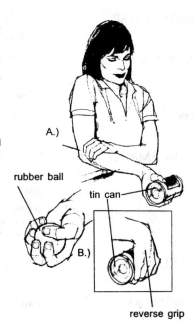

reverse grip

ACTAEA SPIC. 3X	:	Rheumatism of the wrist joint.
CAULOPHYLLUM 3X	:	Aching in the wrists.
EUPATORIUM PERF.	:	Aching in the arms and wrists.
KALIUM CARB.	:	Lacerating pain in the wrist joint. Better by moving the wrist and warmth.
MAGNESIUM PHOS. 3X	:	Pain in one or both wrists with tension in nerves. Give 3 tablets every two hours.
NATRIUM PHOS.	:	Aching in the wrist joint.
TRIMETHYLAMINUM Q	:	Rheumatic pain in the wrist. 10-15 drops in a glass full of water, a teaspoonful every 2 hours.

YAWNING

ACONITUM NAP.	: Frequent yawning in the evening without feeling sleepy.
CHELIDONIUM	: Frequent yawning with stretching and sleepiness, as if remained awake, the whole night.
EUPHRASIA	: Yawning while walking in open air.
IGNATIA AMARA	: Yawning after a sleep, with flow of tears. Excessive yawning as if the jaw would be dislocated. Yawning while eating. Yawning interrupted by spasmodic rigidity of the chest walls.
LATHYRUS SAT.	: Constant yawning and feeling sleepy.
LYCOPODIUM	: Yawning after dinner and supper.
NATRIUM MUR.	: Yawning with internal chilliness.
NUX VOM.	: Yawning for hours after eating and immediately after waking.
RHUS TOX.	: Yawning with crackling of jaw bones as if the jaw bones will dislocate.
SULPHUR	: Frequent yawning with eructations during the day.

YOUTHFUL LOOKS

(SEE REJUVENATION ALSO)

BREWER'S YEAST 1X : Two tables (2 grains) of brewer's yeast taken with meals twice daily brings back youthful look. This yeast is obtained during the brewing of beer. In the dried form, it is a very good source of vitamin B. In the raw form, it is bitter in taste.

GINKGO BILOBA Q : Its use slows down the aging process, increases the vitality, improves the memory, removes physical fatigue and tones up the immune system of the body. It is credited with a beneficial effect on blood circulation and it strengthens the capillaries.

THIOSINAMINUM 2X : It is said to be useful for retarding old age and maintaining youthful looks.

NOTE: Here are some tips, as how to feel mentally young and psychologically fit, in senior years:

1. Maintain regularity in life by getting up early in the morning, taking a bath regularly and eating at regular intervals. Break the boredom by eating out at a reputed restaurant, once in a while.

2. Exercise the brain by reading or listening to books on subjects which were liked in the younger years. Keep busy.

3. Keep company of stimulating and agreeing younger companions. This can have a positive effect on mental sharpness and happiness.

4. Do not feel lonely,bored or unhappy. These feeling make one sick. If weather permits, go out for a short walk or watch a movie, it breaks such feelings.

5. Cosmetic laser surgery can also bring back youthful looks by removing bags and lines from eyelids, wrinkles and sun damaged skin of the face, removal of unwanted hair, reshaping of lips, nose, breasts, buttocks, etc.

6. Body has an enzyme called Telomerase. It is also called "immortality enzyme" in layman's language. It encourages cells to keep on dividing indefinately instead of dying with age. It is said that it does not turn healthy cells into malignant or cancer cells. In course of time, homoeopathic researchers may develop potenctized Telomerase which may prove to be an anti - aging drug.

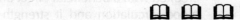